Human Services and the Afrocentric Paradigm

Human Services and the Afrocentric Paradigm

Jerome H. Schiele, DSW

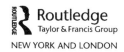

Routledge
Taylor & Francis Group

NEW YORK AND LONDON

First Published by

The Haworth Press, Inc., 10 Alice Street, Binghamton, NY 13904-1580

Transferred to Digital Printing 2010 by Routledge
270 Madison Ave, New York NY 10016
2 Park Square, Milton Park, Abingdon, Oxon, OX14 4RN

Cover design by Jennifer M. Gaska.

Library of Congress Cataloging-in-Publication Data

Schiele, Jerome H.
  Human services and the Afrocentric paradigm / Jerome H. Schiele.
      p.   cm.
  Includes bibliographical references and index.
  ISBN: 0-7890-0565-4 (hard)—ISBN0-7890-0566-2 (pbk)
  1. Social work with Afro-Americans. 2. Social service and race relations—United States.
3. Human services—United States—Philosophy. 4. Afrocentrism—United States. I. Title.

HV3181 .S35 2000
362.84′96073—dc21   99-055441

To the Spirit of those upon whose shoulders I stand

ABOUT THE AUTHOR

Jerome H. Schiele, DSW, is Associate Professor and Director of the PhD program at Clark Atlanta University School of Social Work in Atlanta, Georgia, and Research Associate-at-Large for the Institute of Africana Social Work at Temple University's School of Social Administration in Philadelphia, Pennsylvania. Dr. Schiele was previously Assistant Professor of Social Welfare at the State University of New York at Stony Brook.

A nationally and internationally known scholar in the field of Afrocentric human services and social theory, Dr. Schiele has written numerous articles and book chapters and has conducted manifold workshops on the Afrocentric paradigm. He also serves on the editorial board of the *Journal of Black Studies* and on the Editorial Review Board for the National Association of Social Workers' *Social Work Dictionary* (Fourth Edition). In addition, he is a member of the Advisory Council for the National Academy for African-Centered Social Work for the National Association of Black Social Workers. Dr. Schiele's primary teaching areas are social welfare history and policy, social research, and human behavior theory.

CONTENTS

Foreword

The Afrocentric paradigm, in its currently articulated form, is a development from the last quarter of the twentieth century. It has emerged as a consequence of the reconstructive efforts of African-American and African-diasporic scholars seeking to relocate a perspective for understanding the African experience in the world. Certainly the need for such a paradigm was not new to this period in time, nor did its details emerge exclusively from this recent era. The recognition that African people had been systematically omitted or distorted by the world's scholarship is a fact firmly articulated by African scholars for as long as there have been written records available regarding the African encounter with European invaders. Certainly, during the entirety of the twentieth century as African people began to reclaim their ability and right to describe their own circumstances, more and more scholars protested the obvious distortion of the African experience in the world, particularly as revealed in European scholarship.

This outcry, heard as early as the "Appeals" of David Walker and the writings of Frederick Douglass in the nineteenth century, was the harbinger of a much more concerted intellectual reckoning to come as the literacy-deprived former slaves began to reclaim their self-defined reality in the twentieth century. The West Indian-born theologian, Edward Blyden, continued this thrust with his writings as he increasingly looked to Africa as the prototype for the cultural ethos of African people. The highly popular movement of the Honorable Marcus Moziah Garvey during the 1920s inspired a growing identification of African-Americans with the African continent. Of course, W. E. B. Du Bois and Carter G. Woodson became the real patriarchs for this deconstructive scholarship that gradually dawned into the reconstructive paradigms which increasingly pointed back to Africa as the norm and model for African thought and scholarship.

The early recovery from the literacy deprivation, which had characterized most Africans since their enslavement by Europeans in the sixteenth century until the very end of the nineteenth century, initially required demonstration of basic levels of competence at utilizing European academic tools. Therefore, the first several generations of literate Africans spent considerable effort demonstrating to their former masters their ability to conduct the rudiments of European scholarship. Of course, the teachers, the content, and the methods for these skills were all managed, controlled, and defined by the former captors. Even the most well-meaning teacher could only teach from the perspective that he or she understood and this was the perspective that had engendered European effectiveness and progress. The African beneficiaries of these teachers and their scholarship could only imitate their mentors until their reservoir of understanding permitted them to critique the content of what they had been given. As we progress through the twentieth century, not only do we see the critique expanding in terms of protest and demands for social, legal, political, and educational reorganization, it also begins to challenge the basic epistemology or knowledge standards of the European-American-based academy. By the third quarter of the twentieth century, African-American scholars had well demonstrated their recovery from the shackles of enforced illiteracy and had achieved prominence in every area of European-American thought and scholarship.

This phenomenal achievement, accomplished in less than a century after the Emancipation (which only removed formal and legal slavery from the American scene) did not develop without critical observation. As had been the case from the earliest demonstrated masters of European scholarship such as Du Bois and Woodson, African Americans increasingly began to raise very fundamental questions about the presentation or lack of presentation of Africans and African reality in European scholarship. The question of the omission and distortion of African presence in world reality increasingly raised fundamental questions about the validity of social, historical, legal, and even scientific conclusions that had been reached without the inclusion of African-American scrutiny, input, or even consideration. This led to an explosion of the deconstructive scholarship initially coming from the arts and scholars of history. Such deconstruction challenged the "miseducation" as defined by Dr. Carter G. Woodson, which thwarted the social, political, economic, and personal development of African Americans who only mastered European-centered education.

By the time we reach the last quarter of the twentieth century, African-American scholars have evolved from a purely deconstructive response to European-American-centered scholarship to the formulation of a reconstructive approach to African-American scholarship. The development of this approach, which is thoroughly reviewed in this volume, came to be designated as an African-centered approach. In its earliest articulation, emerging from the work of several African-American psychologists and subsequently other social scientists, the argument was for a perspective that offered a constructive view of African-American behavior. The frustration of these scholars with the destructive, pathology-ridden, biased assumptions of black life from European-centered social science gave birth to a clamor for another perspective. The deconstructionist writings of so many African-American scholars had well documented the invalidity and limitations of the European-centered approach. The early Afrocentric scholars, as they came to be known, began to formulate a conception of African-American life that identified African people with their cultural origins as Africans rather than with their cultural origins as Europeans, which was the overriding assumption of Eurocentric scholarship.

This simple assumption had significant implications, not only for understanding but also for addressing the needs of African people. Perhaps the best example of the implications of the significance of this paradigm shift can be seen in the perception and conceptualization of the African-American family. Within the Eurocentric paradigm, the extended, matrifocal family of African Americans had been identified as a pathological and dysfunctional family structure because it failed to comply with the European assumptions of patriarchal nuclear family structures. Once the African-American family was conceptualized from the African framework as was done with the early work of the Afrocentric pioneer, Wade Nobles, the family structure became not only "normal" but also desirable and beneficial for African Americans. This had important service implications for how practitioners should approach problems of African-American family life.

In addition to the focus on African origins, the Afrocentric paradigm required the evaluation of models and methods on the basis of their effectiveness in alleviating the acquired suffering of oppressed people. Concepts were meaningful and valuable to the degree that they more effectively equipped social scientists to improve the life circumstances of African-American and other oppressed people. The model required an immediate and urgent relevance without the luxury of esoteric, abstract, and long-term probabilities.

Not unlike the budding phases of any new paradigm, much of the early work by Afrocentric scholars was conceptual. Much time and scholarship were devoted to formulating an epistemological framework that could serve as the parameter of this African paradigm. The formulators of the new paradigm continued to devote a great deal of energy to the deconstruction of the Eurocentric paradigm while identifying the basic concepts in the reconstruction of the new African-centered model of study.

This volume, under the careful construction of Dr. Jerome Schiele, is representative of the "Next Generation" of Afrocentric scholarship. It takes the paradigm formulation to its next logical level and opens the door for the real value of a new paradigm in any scientific endeavor, which is its greater utility in formulating the issues and offering solutions to the problems confronted by African people specifically but all people generally. As Dr. Schiele effectively documents in the introductory chapter of this volume, he builds his ideas on the conceptual basis that has been established by the first generation of Afrocentric scholarship. The "New Generation" work that he has already spearheaded in so many of his publications, and further augments with this volume, establishes him firmly as a key figure for the next phase of this scholarship.

There are two basic developments that should emerge from this new-generation phase of expansion of the Afrocentric paradigm. The first development has begun with the growing number of Afrocentric scholars who are already engaged in establishing research models and measurement scales to investigate the validity of the concepts articulated in the conceptualization of the paradigm. An example of the research on measurement is the development of the African self-consciousness personality scale by Kobi Kambon, his colleagues, and students. Researchers such as Darryl Rowe and Cheryl Grills are doing intense and creative investigations of African traditional healing and its usefulness in working with African-American people.

The research done by both of these groups has grown very directly from the foundations established in the laborious conceptualizations of the builders of the Afrocentric paradigm. Most important, these research developments have been creative in their commitment to offering meaningful advancement to the members of the African-American community and humanity as a whole. These researchers have followed the mandate of the builders of the Afrocentric paradigm. That mandate demanded that the work from the Afrocentric paradigm should always provide some immediate applicability to the resolution of problems of a community with urgent needs created by conditions of sustained oppression. The emphasis was that Afrocentric research should always have heuristic value greater than just documentation for the paradigm or the expansion of knowledge. This deliberately subjective motive represented a radical departure from the so-called "objective" demands of Eurocentric research.

The second major expansion from the early reconstructive formulations of the Afrocentric paradigm has been the institutionalization of structures to more appropriately serve African-American people and others whose needs had been violated by the preservation of an alien conceptual framework. Although Chapter 10 in this volume contributes substantially to the first aspect of the new generation's thrust, it is in this second expansion that Jerome Schiele's book provides a monumental contribution. His insightful and useful application of Afrocentric theory to the broad area of human services based on appropriate and relevant cultural understanding not only typifies the form of such applied scholarship, it provides critical elaboration of the paradigm itself. In his loyalty to the service and commitment of Afrocentric scholarship demonstrated in this volume, Schiele articulates specific discussions of relevant problems confronting the African-American—and the general human—community and examines the applicability of this conceptual framework to the treatment of these problems. He offers suggested approaches for the resolution of youth violence and substance abuse and the analysis of social welfare policy that could completely change the human services field.

This book is a compendium of some of the most significant thought of this century that has emerged from African-American scholarship. Its emergence from African-American thought makes it noteworthy because African-American scholars have been required to master the Eurocentric paradigm to legitimize their involvement in the dialogue regarding their survival and advancement as human beings. In mastering the Eurocentric concepts, they have evolved a critical perspective unavailable to those of European descent. So these scholars have come with the best of the European-American conceptualization of themselves, and also the unique perspective gained from being participant-observers of a system that has constrained their progress and simultaneously has benefited their oppressors. With the benefit of this painfully gained "double-consciousness," African-American scholars have a perspective unlike any other for assessing European-American thought and for compelling them to engage in their collective liberation.

Dr. Jerome Schiele has given us a gift at the beginning of this new century. This gift is a forerunner of the significant scholarship that the world can expect from the Afrocentric paradigm, which has been so brutally maligned, not unlike African-American people, from its early days at the end of the twentieth century. It comes as a triumphant declaration of the irrepressible nature of Truth as it applies to ultimate restoration of the unjustly disparaged. Jerome Schiele's keen insights, his thorough analysis of the work that has preceded him, and his passionate commitment to bring tools that will serve his community have forged this document as a wonderful light in the dark cave of human services doomed to failure because of their formulation in an alien framework. Professor Schiele typifies the "new generation." He comes with the full armaments of the perspectives of multiple worldviews and the capability to select those ingredients that are most appropriate for any given situation. He is the rightful heir of generations who were not permitted to know, who came to know despite protest, who deconstructed the flaws of the errant, and who reconstructed appropriate reality and ultimately ideas and strategies to restore health to all of the violated in the land. Welcome to the beginning of the new generation's legacy.

Na'im Akbar, PhD
Florida State University
Tallahassee, FL

Acknowledgments

Books, as with any written treatise, reflect the experiences and interpretations of the author. There are many who have helped to shape both my experiences and interpretations. Considerable credit should be given to my immediate and extended families. Using the African proverb "I am because we are and because we are therefore I am" as a backdrop, my immediate and extended families provided the foundation for the collective "we" in my life. Although my extended family complemented and reinforced the socialization I experienced in my immediate family, my parents deserve primary credit for influencing who and what I have become. In this regard, preeminent gratitude is extended to my father, Dr. William Bernard Schiele, and my mother, Mae Schiele. My parents were my first teachers, and they not only gave me life, but also the socioemotional and financial support necessary to advance in America.

Though my parents gave me life and established a home milieu supportive of positive growth and potential, it was my only sibling and elder brother, Dr. Adib Shakir, who was the main person who accelerated my exposure to, and insights about, the Afrocentric paradigm. His receipt of a student fellowship in college to travel to Africa in 1974, and his personal relationship with his then-Morehouse College psychology professor, Dr. Luther B. Weems (now known as Dr. Na'im Akbar, the eminent Afrocentric psychologist), afforded me an intimate window into the history, culture, and contributions of Africa that most teenagers in the 1970s probably did not have. In fact, after he returned from Africa, and via a community slide show presentation, Adib was the one who gave me my first formal Afrocentric lecture. Adib, thank you immensely for rescuing me from my miseducation!

I also would like to offer my appreciation to the academic institutions that trained me. My experiences and training at Hampton and Howard Universities, both historically black universities, helped me to master Eurocentric paradigms in sociology and social work and offered me opportunities to explore conceptual models established by prominent African-American scholars. Although Hampton furnished me with rudimentary social science and social work skills, my matriculation in Howard University's MSW and DSW programs provided the icing on the cake.

Partly because of my greater maturity, and because of the outstanding and supportive administration, faculty, and staff, my academic skills and enthusiasm blossomed at Howard. Howard afforded an open intellectual environment for me to explore all kinds of ideas while concomitantly helping me to focus my personal interest in Afrocentricity. As a demonstration of Howard's intellectual elasticity and motivating force in my academic life, my very first publication—which was on the Afrocentric paradigm—was developed from a paper I had written for a Communities and Organizations seminar in the doctoral program.

Although my academic training and experiences at Howard did much to nurture my ideas on Afrocentricity and its applicability to social work, my participation in, and exposure to, grassroots community-based organizations and advocates in the African-American communities of Washington, DC (and later on in New York) also helped to crystallize my thinking on the Afrocentric paradigm. Organizations such as the Association for the Study of Classical African Civilizations, black-owned bookstores such as Pyramid Books in DC and Pan African International in Hempstead, New York, events such as the weekly Afrocentric lectures at the Slave Theatre in Brooklyn, New York, and daily talk radio programs sponsored by WUDC and WPFW in Washington and WLIB in New York gave me a wealth of information and analysis on the Afrocentric paradigm. The experiences with these African-American community entities oftentimes provided me with a much more incisive, substantial, and emotional understanding of the Afrocentric paradigm than the confines of traditional Eurocentric academic training, even at historically black colleges and universities, could offer.

I also would like to thank all of my personal friends who have provided encouragement, constructive criticism, and much-needed fun along the way. Although all of my personal friends have been very special to me, a few have been enormously helpful in the process of either conceptualizing or writing this book. Special thanks to Ms. Valerie A. Crawford, Dr. A. Kareem Abdullah, Ms. Robin S. Brazley, Dr. Alfrieda A. Daly, Dr. Leslie Fenwick, Mr. Alphonso Murrill, and Dr. Ronnie Stewart.

Since one cannot write a book without sufficient time, I extend special thanks to Dr. Dorcas Bowles, Dean, and Dr. Richard Lyle, Associate Dean, of the Clark Atlanta University School of Social Work. Both Dean Bowles and previous acting Dean Richard Lyle granted me permission for a reduced teaching load so that I could complete this book. I also offer my sincere appreciation for the support received from the faculty, students, and staff in the School of Social Work at Clark Atlanta University.

Although Dean Bowles and Associate Dean Lyle gave me the time to write, it was Dr. Molefi Asante, the renowned Afrocentrist and former chairperson of Temple University's black studies department, who planted the idea of this book in my head, and, more important, my heart. In the Summer of 1994, Dr. Asante invited me to present at the Sixth Annual Chiekh Anta Diop Conference held in October of that year in Philadelphia, Pennsylvania. It was there that he suggested I write a book on Afrocentric social work. Asante Sana (thank you, thank you) Dr. Asante.

I would also like to offer my sincere appreciation to The Haworth Press, Inc., for publishing the ideas in this book. Although I am appreciative of all who had a hand in the book's production, special gratitude is offered to Mr. Bill Palmer, Vice President/Managing Editor, Book Division; Dr. Carlton Munson, Social Work Editor; Ms. Melissa Devendorf, Administrative Assistant; Ms. Marylouise Doyle, Cover Design Director; Ms. Dawn Krisko, Production Editor, Mr. Andy Roy, Production Editor; Ms. Patricia Brown, Editorial Production Manager; Ms. Nancy Foster, Typesetter; and Ms. Jennifer Gaska, Cover Designer.

Last, but certainly not least, I offer the greatest and most humble appreciation to the Creator or God. I sincerely believe the Creator has worked positively through the actions of others to help bring me to this point. Indeed, all praise is due to God.

Jerome H. Schiele
Atlanta, GA

Chapter 1

Introduction

WORLDVIEWS AND CULTURAL OPPRESSION

The struggle for liberation and advancement of an oppressed group is not limited to its goals of equal rights and economic empowerment. The struggle fundamentally is to affirm the traditions, history, and humanity of the oppressed by validating and promoting their cultural worldviews. The notion of worldview has received increasing attention in the social science literature (see, for example, Ani, 1994; Baldwin and Hopkins, 1990; Dixon, 1976; English, 1984, 1991; Myers, 1988; Schiele, 1994). A worldview can be defined succinctly as the overarching mode through which people interpret events and define reality. It is a racial or ethnic group's psychological orientation toward life (Kambon, 1992; Schiele, 1993). It provides a group with a structure for expressing its own cultural truths (Karenga, 1996), a way to organize its experiences and interpretations into a logical and fairly stable conceptual scheme.

This conceptual scheme, some believe, is the basis for knowledge development in a given culture or society. Though there may be common elements of knowledge development across various cultural groups, it is generally believed that these groups have their own unique cultural ethos (Chau, 1991; Hutnik, 1991). Under the unnatural conditions of cultural oppression, the worldviews of various cultural groups who occupy a common space and time are not equally validated. This is because in a society that practices cultural oppression, the dominant group uses its control to universalize its experiences, history, and interpretations, thereby establishing them as the norm (Blauner, 1972; Kambon, 1992; Young, 1990). The fallout of this is that a false sense of cultural superiority of the dominant group's ethos takes hold in the minds of not only the culturally dominant but also the culturally oppressed. More seductively, both the culturally dominant and the culturally oppressed are susceptible to the belief that the variance in human interpretations, experiences, and values is minimal and that these differences should be downplayed. Furthermore, the social construction of how others differ from the culturally dominant is often couched in language that vilifies and negates the humanity of these oppressed "others" (Rothenberg, 1990). The significance this has for the culturally oppressed is that they are at risk of viewing their own unique history and culture as nonexistent, illegitimate, or marginal to that of the history, experiences, and interpretations of the culturally dominant (Asante, 1988; Cabral, 1973; Schiele, 1993). From this, a sense of low cultural self-esteem can emerge that precludes the culturally oppressed from having the complete knowledge of themselves that is essential for a group to maximize its self-perceived humanity, its level of group self-determination, and its contributions to the advancement of the human family (Akbar, 1996; Karenga, 1993, 1996).

CULTURAL OPPRESSION AND SOCIAL SCIENCE

The dynamics of cultural oppression that are played out in the wider society are also manifested in the social sciences and professions, such as the human services, that apply social science theory and knowledge. Many American scholars of African descent, over the last twenty to thirty years, have suggested that the knowledge base of the social sciences is characterized by a European-American cultural hegemony that validates the paradigms and theories that have emerged from European-American and European intellectual history and thought (see Akbar, 1976, 1979, 1984, 1994; Ani, 1994; Asante, 1980, 1988, 1990; Baldwin, 1981, 1985; Baldwin and Hopkins, 1990; Boykin, 1983; Cook and Kono, 1977; Dixon, 1976; Hale-Benson, 1982; Hilliard, 1989; Kambon, 1992; Karenga, 1993; Khatib et al., 1979; Myers, 1988; Nobles, 1974, 1980; Semmes, 1981). These writers believe, as intimated by Billingsley (1970), that "American social scientists are much more American than social and much more social than scientific" (p. 127). Still others, such as Nobles (1978), contend that, similar to the political and economic institutions in society, Western social science is a tool to achieve the more efficient domination of people of color, generally, and people of African descent, specifically. Thus, increasingly, among many African-American social scientists, social science in the United States is conceived as a subjective and political enterprise that primarily, if not exclusively, reflects the ideas, interpretations, and racism that imbue European-American culture. For this book's purpose, European-American culture (also referred to in this book as "Eurocentric" culture) is defined as a collective hybrid of European traditions that have been maintained and modified by the unique history and experiences of the descendants of Europe who occupy the United States.

The Afrocentrists

Many of these African-American social scientists who have critiqued the hegemony of European-American cultural ideas in the social sciences have begun to refer to themselves as *Afrocentrists*. They are Afrocentrists in that they believe that social science should and does reflect the worldviews of a particular cultural group and that since they are social scientists of African descent, the worldview that should inform their research and scholarship is that which emerges from traditional West African societies and is assumed to have been preserved by the descendants of West Africa in the United States, known as African Americans. For Asante (1987, 1988), one of the leading proponents of Afrocentricity, who is often credited with coining the term, this emphasis on Africa as the basis from which African-American social scientists interpret social reality fosters the belief in the centrality of African culture and history as valid frames of reference. This, according to Asante (1987, 1988), can encourage a new conception of Africa and people of African descent as subjects and not just objects of Eurocentric interpretations. In this way, Asante maintains that an Afrocentric framework centers the scholar of African ancestry in his or her own history and culture and that this "centering" can help the scholar of African descent recapture and resurrect traditional African cultural values and worldviews, from which a more authentic narrative of African people can take form.

As implied by Asante's comments, Afrocentrists contend that although slavery and Eurocentric cultural oppression have caused considerable psychological, physical, and political harm to African Americans, the vilification of African culture inherent in both slavery and Eurocentric cultural oppression did not destroy all relics of traditional African culture for African Americans. Traditional African culture is defined here as those cultural beliefs and traditions which predate the effects that European colonization and enslavement have had on continental and diasporic Africans and which are assumed to continue today among the descendants of Africa, albeit to varying degrees. The assumption about the survival of traditional Africa among African Americans is best captured in Nobles' (1974) assertion that African Americans are of "African root and American fruit." This assumption implies that African Americans have retained some of their fundamental "Africanisms" and have adapted them to the unnatural conditions of Eurocentric cultural oppression that shapes the character of the American cultural landscape. In this vein, some Afrocentrists, such as Boykin (1983), posit a tripartite influence on African-American behavior and worldviews. The elements of this influence are (1) the survival of traditional African culture, (2) the experience of racial discrimination and injustice, and (3) the overlay of European-American culture.

The Dual Disservice of Cultural Oppression

For Afrocentrists, the imposition of paradigms and theories in the social sciences that emerge from European and European-American intellectual thought and history does a disservice to social scientists of African and European ancestry. For both groups, the imposition of Eurocentric paradigms and theories creates the illusion that social science ideas are culturally universal and applicable to all cultural groups in all time periods, or at least time periods with similar technological and economic circumstances. To this extent, an illusion that promotes the notion that the paradigms and theories of Eurocentric social science can be employed to explain events of the contemporary world and of history develops. Afrocentrists assert that the belief in Eurocentric or Western social science universalism among social scientists of European descent can engender a sense of sociocultural arrogance, the kind that implicitly reinforces the idea of the intellectual superiority of people of European ancestry. It also can effectuate sociocultural ignorance among this group's members in that their opportunities to gain insight into the worldview integrity of other cultures and to acknowledge the significant contributions to human history and thought made by these cultures are restricted, at best, and precluded, at worst.

For social scientists of African descent, Afrocentrists claim that Eurocentric social science universalism has created ignorance among this group and, more important, has restrained this group's ability to materially liberate itself from political and economic oppression. Because African-American social scientists, similar to European-American social scientists, are trained in paradigms and theories that advance ideas about human nature, morality, and behavior emanating from European-American culture, they are not exposed in their training to ideas about human nature, morality, and behavior stemming from traditional African culture (Hilliard, 1995; Woodson, 1933). This renders them incognizant of the traditions of their ancestors, and there are few incentives for them to construe these traditions as a foundation for establishing alternative social science paradigms and theories.

Second, the lack of exposure to the intellectual traditions of Africa in their training prevents African-American social scientists from tapping into an essential source of their liberation: a sense of pride in the intellectual contributions of Africa. This absence of pride in, and knowledge of, the intellectual contributions and traditions of Africa can influence African-American social scientists to become what Kambon (1992) calls psychologically or culturally misoriented. Psychological/cultural misorientation describes African-American social scientists, and other African Americans, who mentally affirm the traditions and worldview of European-American culture to the oblivion and self-degradation of their African/African-American cultural worldview and traditions. In essence, they run the mental risk of internalizing the demeaning values and images of Africa, and by extension people of African descent, as uncivilized, culturally impotent, and intellectually inferior. These images of Africa have been perpetuated historically by such works as Hegel's (1837/1956) *The Philosophy of History* and other social science theories that have portrayed people of African descent as mentally inferior, as having unstable and dysfunctional families, and as being inherently criminal. This unfavorable image of Africa continues to be promulgated through recent news stories underscoring African famine and political chaos without examining the lingering and pernicious effects of European colonialism on the continent's stability.

Afrocentrists believe that the pejorative internalization of Africa among African-American social scientists can restrict their capabilities in contributing to African/African-American liberation because they fail to acknowledge the importance of using traditional African philosophical concepts, (1) as a means to validate and codify the collective narratives and experiences of people of African descent as a basis for creating new paradigms and theories, and (2) as a method to organize these collective narratives and experiences as a foundation to advance new models of societal relationships that can help people of African descent to empower and liberate themselves economically. In short, Afrocentrists firmly believe that African-American social scientists should use their scholarship and knowledge to critique Eurocentric social science universalism and to liberate people of African ancestry from political and economic oppression.

TOWARD AN AFROCENTRIC HUMAN SERVICE PARADIGM

Since the knowledge base of those who work in the human services (e.g., social workers, case managers, human service administrators, psychologists) is heavily dependent upon social science theory and research, human service paradigms also suffer from the Eurocentric cultural universalism previously described. In the human services, this hegemony is best expressed through two modes: (1) the theories and models for explaining and solving social problems arise from a Eurocentric conception of human behavior and social problems, and (2) the cultural values of people of color, generally, and African Americans, specifically, have not been used sufficiently as a theoretical base to establish new human service practice paradigms and methods.

Attributes of Eurocentric Knowledge Base in the Human Services

As it concerns the first mode, the theoretical foundation of the human services' knowledge base is not only shaped immensely by European American intellectuals but also tends to have an individualistic, materialistic, mechanistic, and pessimistic character. The individualistic focus is manifested in human service paradigms that spend an inordinate amount of time delineating and explaining individual traits/attitudes, personality dispositions and disorders, ego functions or dysfunctions, or individual psychosocial crises. Indeed, personality characteristics such as independence, internal locus of control, and assertiveness are generally valued over attributes such as dependence, external locus of control, and submissiveness (Akbar, 1984; Baldwin and Hopkins, 1990; Cook and Kono, 1977). The fundamental problem is that although there are human service paradigms, such as the ecological and systems approaches, that contextualize the individual and his or her problems, there is still a penchant to view the individual as a sort of isolated, autonomous entity. The tendency is to impose dichotomous logic to separate or decontextualize the individual from his or her immediate and wider social milieu. This is best expressed in the social work profession's "person in situation" paradigm. Even though the situation or milieu is acknowledged, considerable emphasis in social work is placed on the "person" side of the equation (Rose, 1990). In addition, the concept of situation often is restricted to connote the immediate environment, such as the individual's family. Furthermore, the ecological and systems approaches have received wide exposure recently in the social work literature, but rarely—if ever—is there a connection made that demonstrates how the African and Eastern worldviews can complement these approaches. Because both worldviews are more holistic in their focus than is the fragmentary logical character of the Eurocentric worldview (Cook and Kono, 1977; Myers, 1988), the application of philosophical concepts inherent in each might better elicit the holistic conception of human beings and social problems that could facilitate smoother integration of the "person" with the "situation."

The dichotomy between the person and situation is also found in the bifurcation of practice methods within social work training. These methods are usually bifurcated along the dimensions of those who desire to specialize in the individual or person (direct practice) and those who desire to specialize in the situation (i.e., macro/policy practice and administration). Though appropriate within the context of the broader professional marketplace in which specialization is encouraged, the separation of the person and the situation limits the ability to integrate knowledge of the two in a way that prevents further understanding of human behavior and social problems. From an Afrocentric viewpoint, this excessive focus on fragmentation reflects the particular logical style of European-American culture, which, at least in the professional world, has been significantly influenced by Cartesian dualism (see Descartes, 1641/1986).

The second feature of the current knowledge base in the human services is that the models tend to be heavily materialistic. They are materialistic in that an intense, almost exclusive, focus is placed on sensory perception as a means of determining reality, and there is a proclivity to downplay or reject the legitimacy of the unseen. In this way, information on how the unseen or spiritual world affects human behavior and human values and how this world can be a means for positive human and societal transformation is usually suppressed. The materialist focus, which nurtures a conception of humans as primarily material and physical beings, can considerably confine human service practitioners' understanding of the extensive and latent capabilities of their consumers and themselves.

Except for those human service practitioners who rely on the existentialist, humanistic, and transpersonal schools of thought, including the works of Carl Jung, most human service paradigms have omitted content on spirituality and the soul (Myers, 1988; Schiele, 1996; Sermabeikian, 1994). Eurocentric human service and social science paradigms have traditionally viewed spirituality as too esoteric to examine and as fitting better within the domains of theology or philosophy (Akbar, 1984; Canda, 1988, 1998; Myers, 1988; Sermabeikian, 1994).

Eurocentric human service paradigms, with some exceptions, also tend to be mechanistic. This mechanistic flavor and feature is manifested poignantly in the predominance of stage theories and the reliance on unilinear causation. The reliance on stage theories is best discerned in the preeminence of the psychosocial model used to explain normal human growth and development. Based on the assumption that psychosocial development at a previous stage will have a significant impact on psychosocial development at a subsequent stage, human development and interpersonal problems are primarily conceived as sequential and additive, with limited focus on the human being's capacity for spontaneous change that nullifies the influence of previous psychosocial dysfunctions. The tendency exists, therefore, to conceive the individual as a machine or robot with a predetermined path or set of rules by which he or she must abide to become a fully functioning human being. Although some paradigms, such as the strengths perspective (see Saleebey, 1992, 1996), promote a more spontaneous concept of human change and development that is not bounded to the individual's past, they have not gained widespread popularity among human service practitioners.

The focus on unilinear causation, which is also found in the predominance of stage theories, is best expressed in the epistemological model used to explain human behavior and to evaluate human service interventions. Known as empiricism, positivism, or, more recently, postpositivism (see Fraser, 1993; Smith, 1993), the model assumes that cause and effect are invariably separate entities in human behavior, and thus, should be treated as such when attempting to explain behavior or to evaluate the effectiveness of interventions. The notion of a variable being independent of another that is assumed to be dependent on the one preceding it reinforces this fragmentary, unilinear model. Furthermore, the practice of attempting to isolate the effects of a human service intervention on some desired treatment outcome and referring to extraneous factors as "threats" to internal validity, without considering the value that those "threats" might have in human transformation, also demonstrates the allegiance to unilinear causation. Like stage theories, unilinear causation imposes a deterministic view of human behavior, one that not only deemphasizes the possibility of reciprocity and interchangeability between cause and effect but, because of the materialistic thrust, also rejects the interaction of the material with the spiritual.

Last, the Eurocentric hegemony in human service paradigms has been manifested in the ascendency and popularity of human behavior theories that are pessimistic about people's intentions. For example, in Freud's psychodynamic theory, humans are conceived as being motivated by sex and aggression, and civilization as an essential structure to monitor the drives of an uncontrollable id seeking immediate pleasure. In ego psychology, the ego is thought to experience perpetual conflict in not only adapting to the outside environment but also in regulating anxiety produced by unacceptable instinctual impulses and intrapsychic dissonance. In both classical and operant behavioral conditioning, the fundamental assumption is that humans need some kind of external stimuli to regulate or extinguish undesirable behavior because they lack internal self-mastery, discipline, and free will. In exchange theory, people are said to be motivated by self-interest, to analyze human interactions in terms of the degree of costs they expend and the benefits they accrue. Last, Marxist theory presupposes that the ruling elite in any society is subject invariably to avarice and the insatiable need to monopolize material resources and power, thus limiting the possibility of "compassionate" leadership or rulership.

A common theme of the paradigms and theories that have gained prominence in Eurocentric human service and social science is an overemphasis on conflict. It is this conflict-oriented worldview that assumes, of tentimes implicitly, that antagonism is a normal attribute and outcome of human behavior, development, and social interaction. Though some paradigms within the Eurocentric tradition underscore a more optimistic picture of humans and their potential, these paradigms are often relegated to the margins of mainstream Eurocentric thought.

Cultural Values, People of Color, and Eurocentric Hegemony

The insufficient use of the cultural values of people of color as a theoretical base to construct new human service paradigms and theories also reflects the Eurocentric hegemony in the human services. Those who have given attention to cultural values of people of color have usually referred to their form of human service practice as "ethnic sensitive," "ethnic minority," or "cross-cultural." Although this attention represents an important step toward cultural sensitivity and political correctness, these models generally have fallen short in conceiving the cultural values of people of color as a legitimate foundation to establish new human service paradigms and theories (Schiele, 1996, 1997). These human service paradigms usually underscore the following: (1) how racial discrimination and minority status have blocked opportunities and caused disproportionate psychosocial pain for people of color; (2) how the human service practitioner should be aware of the cultural values and nuances of a consumer of a different racial/ethnic group; and (3) how the human service practitioner should be cognizant of his or her biases and preconceptions when working with someone of another racial/ethnic group (Schiele, 1997). These clearly are critical areas that need to be considered when delivering human services, but by not conceiving the cultural values of people of color as theoretical foundations for establishing additional human service paradigms, the significance of these values in helping to diversify and expand the human service knowledge base is attenuated. The lack of diversity also obviates the formation of innovative methods and strategies that might lead to greater and more effective success in bringing about human and societal transformation.

As it concerns more effective service, the Afrocentric paradigm maintains that since the consumers assisted by many human service practitioners are members of groups of color, it is imperative that human service paradigms reflect the cultural values and worldviews of these groups (Everett, Chipungu, and Leashore, 1991; Schiele, 1996). Because these groups, especially African Americans and Hispanics, disproportionately experience poverty, they are more likely to be the consumers that human service practitioners serve, especially in public settings or agencies. It is essential, therefore, that human service organizations employ the world-views of these groups as theoretical foundations to implement different interventive strategies that are more compatible with the particular cultural styles, experiences, traditions, and interpretations of these groups, which can lead to more effective human service practice. It has been demonstrated that when the cultural values of consumer groups of color are integrated into the helping process, the likelihood of achieving desired treatment objectives increases (Brisbane and Womble, 1991; Chau, 1991; Devore and Schlesinger, 1981; Green, 1982; Jeff, 1994; Lum, 1992; Phillips, 1990; Sue, 1977).

Another corollary of not using the cultural values of people of color to form new human service paradigms is that the values, norms, and visions inherent in European-American culture are perceived as the chief—if not exclusive—precepts through which human behavior can be explained and social problems eliminated. This reinforces the illusion of cultural universalism and promotes the idea that the cultural background and milieu of a social theorist is meaningless—that theorizing and the emergence of professional ideas is an objective activity, or at least a culturally devoid one (Akbar, 1984; Asante, 1987; Carruthers, 1972; Schiele, 1997).

In addition, by not conceding the cultural values of people of color as foundations for new paradigms and theories and by relying primarily on Eurocentric paradigms and theories, the misconception that the variance in perspectives within Eurocentric models is large enough to explain human behavior and solve social problems is perpetuated. Drawing on the critical theory wing of Marxist thinking, it can be suggested that the variability and competition among Eurocentric human service and social science paradigms is a means to camouflage the unity that exist among these paradigms so as to protect their hegemony in the marketplace of ideas. If this is true, the Afrocentric paradigm would advocate that the marketplace of ideas be viewed as the locus of change. This change should not be dependent on the capriciousness of the market or a "survival of the fittest or most acceptable ideas" framework, but, rather, in a multicultural society in which the participation of people from diverse cultural backgrounds is crucial, conscious and deliberate efforts should be aimed at rendering the marketplace of ideas culturally inclusive, at least inclusive of the cultures represented in that society. The relevance here for the human services is that each cultural perspective, represented in the human services by the ethnically diverse consumer and service provider populations, should have an equal opportunity to assert its own particular cultural truths concerning the causes of, and remedies for, social problems.

Definition and Objectives of Afrocentric Human Service

Afrocentric human service can be defined as methods of human service practice that arise from the sociocultural and philosophical concepts, traditions, and experiences of African Americans. Its fundamental philosophical thrust emanates from traditional African philosophical assumptions about human behavior and nature that have been documented to have survived among many African Americans (see Akbar, 1979; Asante, 1988; Daly et al., 1995; Dixon, 1976; Herskovits, 1941; Kambon, 1992; Martin and Martin, 1995), though modified by experiences of racial and cultural subjugation. The African root, American fruit metaphor discussed earlier can be applied to describe the philosophic bases of Afrocentric human service.

Similar to many other human service paradigms, Afrocentric human service seeks to describe, explain, solve, and prevent the problems that people face. Although it is especially concerned with the problems confronted by people of African descent living under conditions of cultural oppression, the focus of Afrocentric human service extends beyond the scope of people of African ancestry to address problems confronted by all people. From an Afrocentric framework, the problem of cultural oppression, for example, is believed to have adversely affected most people, the culturally dominant and the culturally oppressed. Thus, the Afrocentric paradigm of human service is both particularistic and universalistic: it endeavors to address the distinctive liberation needs of people of African descent and to foster the spiritual and moral development of the world (Akbar, 1984; Karenga, 1993; Kershaw, 1992; Schiele, 1996, 1997). This dual perspective is captured in the following major objectives of the Afrocentric paradigm, as discussed by Schiele (1996):

(1) it seeks to promote an alternative social science paradigm more reflective of the cultural and political reality of African Americans; (2) it seeks to dispel the negative distortions about people of African ancestry by legitimizing and disseminating a worldview that goes back thousands of years and that exists in the hearts and minds of many people of African descent today; and (3) it seeks to promote a worldview that will facilitate human and societal transformation toward spiritual, moral, and humanistic ends and that will persuade

people of different cultural and ethnic groups that they share a mutual interest in this regard. (p. 286) (Copyright 1996, National Association of Social Workers, Inc., *Social Work*)

It is the latter objective that is often omitted in contemporary debates on the Afrocentric paradigm. Too often, in some social science circles and in the popular media, Afrocentricity is associated erroneously with ethnocentrism. Afrocentricity is viewed by some as cultural chauvinism (see, for example, Chavez, 1994; Schlesinger, 1991). As Verharen (1995) observes, however, Afrocentricity is not cultural chauvinism because it is not ethnocentric. Ethnocentrism generally implies that one group views its cultural values as superior to other groups or as the center of the social universe and, therefore, believes that its values should be imposed or universalized. The Afrocentric paradigm acknowledges the importance of being grounded or centered in one's historical and cultural experience, but it does not promote the notion that the Afrocentric view is the only or superior view, as does ethnocentrism (Asante, 1988, 1990; Bekerie, 1994; Verharen, 1995). Instead, the Afrocentric paradigm acknowledges that it is only one component of an enormous human web of "polycenters" of culture and history that represent the assorted worldviews of divergent cultural groups who occupy the planet (Bekerie, 1994; Welsh-Asante, 1985; Verharen, 1995). Although it advocates that people of African descent, especially under conditions of cultural oppression, should be centered in their cultural experience and history, the Afrocentric paradigm does not suggest that people of African descent are at the center of humanity (Asante, 1988; Bekerie, 1994; Verharen, 1995).

The universalistic feature of the Afrocentric paradigm is important because it underscores the adverse consequences of cultural oppression on both the culturally dominant and the culturally oppressed. Both have been demoralized and dehumanized psychologically, and oppression, itself, as a political/economic and sociocultural entity, impedes social change that would assist all people to better elicit and fully actualize positive human potentiality. To maximize positive human potentiality, the Afrocentric paradigm of human service advocates for substantive change in the worldview that pervades the social institutions and the intricacies of the most intimate interpersonal relations in the United States. Discussed in more detail in Chapter 4, Afrocentric human service asserts that this worldview is characterized by oppression and spiritual alienation, which are viewed as primary sources of the human problems that human service practitioners address.

Assumptions of Cultural Differences

Because the Afrocentric paradigm has culture at the center of its paradigmatic thrust, it is important to briefly identify its ideas about cultural differences in a multicultural society, such as the United States, in which the human services exist. Fundamentally, the Afrocentric paradigm of human service endeavors to promote cultural pluralism in both the knowledge base of the human services and the wider society. Cultural pluralism can be defined as the belief in the equal affirmation and contribution of the various groups who constitute a multicultural society, in other words, equal cultural affirmation of all groups without political hierarchy. To this extent, the Afrocentric paradigm maintains that, although similarities exist between and among people of divergent cultural groups, important differences also should be acknowledged and celebrated (Asante, 1992; Bekerie, 1994; Karenga, 1993; Verharen, 1995). Afrocentrists believe that the concept of difference does not have to be construed as negative or antagonistic, and a focus on cultural similarities, though necessary, is not inherently better or more moral than a focus on cultural differences (Asante, 1988, 1992). From an Afrocentric framework, the greater test of one's humanity is the ability to tolerate the perspective of a person or group operating within a divergent cultural worldview.

Though the Afrocentric paradigm recognizes differences in the internalization and manifestation of a cultural ethos among members of a specific cultural group, it assumes that these within-group differences are not as great as the differences that exist between and among cultural groups (Swigonski, 1996). The Afrocentric paradigm, therefore, regards a cultural or ethnic group as distinctive, but not monolithic.* The problem in a multiethnic and multicultural society in which cultural oppression prevails is that, oftentimes, the cultural distinctiveness of the culturally oppressed is hidden or suppressed. The control the culturally dominant have over societal resources and institutions compels the culturally oppressed to adapt to the dominant group's lifestyle, at least publicly. But, cultural adaptation is not cultural adoption, and, thus, it is possible for a culturally oppressed group to maintain some degree of distinctiveness, especially if it takes on a bicultural or traditional ethnic identity (English, 1984, 1991; Hutnik, 1991; Schiele, 1993). Both the bicultural and traditional identities, as opposed to the assimilated and marginal ones, demonstrate high levels

---

*The phrase "distinctive but not monolithic" is borrowed from the Howard University School of Social Work Mission Statement, which uses the phrase to describe the "Black Experience" in America.

of participation and commitment of a person of color to his or her own culture (English, 1984, 1991; Hutnik, 1991; Schiele, 1993).

The major point here is that cultural oppression is inimical to the free-flowing expression of the culturally oppressed's worldview and ethos. The Afrocentric paradigm of human service attempts to eradicate the pernicious consequences of cultural oppression for human service providers, consumers, educators, scholars, and students by codifying the cultural values of people of African descent into a paradigm for explaining human behavior and solving societal problems.

OVERVIEW OF THE BOOK

This book is envisioned as a conceptual guide to provide a general overview of how the Afrocentric paradigm can be applied to explain human behavior, to solve social problems, and to explore social issues that are of concern to human service and social policy practitioners, social policy analysts, human service administrators, and students and educators in social work and the social sciences. It does not attempt to provide answers to, or give examples of, the sundry ways the Afrocentric paradigm can be employed in the human services. Rather, the book applies the Afrocentric paradigm to what the author sees as some important aspects of the human services' knowledge base. Its fundamental purpose is to expand and diversify the knowledge base of the human services by codifying the cultural values, traditions, and experiences of people of African ancestry, specifically African Americans, into a human service paradigm.

Each chapter highlights and explores issues and concepts raised by the Afrocentric paradigm for both descriptive and prescriptive purposes. Thus, the reader should view this book as a way to both conceive human problems and shape human services. In Chapter 2, a definition of the Afrocentric worldview, an explanation of its philosophical assumptions, and a discussion of its shortcomings are provided. With a spiritual and holistic cosmology and ontology as their base, these assumptions are shown to encourage equality and human liberation. Chapter 3 examines traditional helping assumptions and methods of West African societies and discusses how these assumptions and methods have influenced the traditional helping strategies of African Americans. This chapter also examines the evolution and shortcomings of some early African-American human service thinkers, especially in regard to their rejection of traditional African methods in favor of ideas based on Eurocentric notions of human behavior and scientific charity. Chapter 4 explains that, from an Afrocentric framework, oppression and spiritual alienation are viewed as the primary sources of human and societal problems that human service workers seek to eliminate. It further contends that spiritual alienation is the more important of the two because it is conceived as both a cause and an outcome of oppression in the United States.

Chapter 5 takes the theoretical, philosophical, and historical ideas in the previous chapters and applies them to demonstrate how the Afrocentric paradigm explains and would resolve problems related to youth violence. Chapter 6 takes these same ideas to show how the Afrocentric paradigm explains and would resolve problems associated with substance abuse. In Chapter 7, the Afrocentric paradigm is offered as a foundation for understanding social welfare philosophy, ideology, and policy. In this chapter, social welfare policy recommendations that flow from Afrocentric assumptions about resource distribution, morality, and societal relationships are discussed. Chapter 8 draws on ideas from Chapter 7 and some of the previous chapters to identify and discuss the characteristics of an Afrocentric, social welfare policy analytic framework. In this chapter, questions that would be important from an Afrocentric perspective are used as a foundation for evaluating and analyzing social welfare policies. Chapter 9 applies the Afrocentric paradigm to human service organizations. It does this by identifying some differences in the ways organizations are conceptualized from Eurocentric and Afrocentric viewpoints, and by showing how Afrocentric themes can be used to help human service organizations become more effective in enhancing positive organizational potentiality, workplace diversity, and organizational empowerment for people of color. In Chapter 10, the Afrocentric paradigm is used to describe characteristics of Afrocentric social work research. This chapter fundamentally describes some of the basic assumptions and methods appropriate for knowledge inquiry and development within an Afrocentric framework. Last, Chapter 11, the concluding chapter, discusses some current and future challenges facing the viability and survival of the Afrocentric human service paradigm.

Chapter 2

The Afrocentric Worldview

HISTORIC OVERVIEW

Several writers of African history contend that many of the horrific events occurring on the African continent today are a primary consequence of the many years of the colonization and enslavement of Africans by both Europeans and Arabs and do not mirror pivotal values and mores of traditional Africa (Clarke, 1991; Diop, 1991; Karenga, 1993a; Rodney, 1980; Williams, 1993; Zahan, 1979). These authors also suggest that, although diversity was present in traditional African values and cultural practices, some conspicuous commonalities existed in core philosophical assumptions across the various ethnic groups. These assumptions fundamentally validated an ontological and cosmological framework that underscored a collective and spiritual worldview.

It has been suggested that the civilizations of the Nile Valley in Africa are the origins of this worldview—some say of human civilization itself (see Cann, 1987; Diop, 1974; Dubois, 1965; Jackson, 1990; Montagu, 1958). The idea that Nile Valley civilizations should serve as the classical reference point for the study of other African civilizations emanates from the "Diopian" school of thought (Oyebade, 1990). Named after the eminent Sengalese scholar, Cheikh Anta Diop, the "Diopian" school's primary source is Diop's (1974) *The African Origin of Civilization*. In it, Diop maintains that just as Greek society serves as the reference point for European civilizations, the Nile Valley should serve as the reference point for African civilizations. The ancient civilizations of the Nile Valley consisted of Ethiopia, Kemet (Egypt), and Kush (Nubia), and Kemet is believed to have emerged about 8,000 years before the current era (B.C.E.)

Portions of this chapter originally appeared in "Afrocentricity As an Alternative World View for Equality," published in the *Journal of Progressive Human Services*, 1994, 5(1), pp. 5-25. Reprinted with permission from The Haworth Press, Inc.

(Karenga, 1993a). Some contend that the cultural themes prevalent in the Nile Valley were disseminated throughout Africa when groups began to migrate from the Nile Valley westward into what is now West Africa and southward into southern Africa (see Diop, 1991; Jackson, 1990). Because of the survival of many of these cultural themes, these authors maintain that the themes of the Nile Valley reemerged, although with modifications, in newer civilizations in Africa such as Ghana, Mali, and Songhai. With the legacy of the Arab invasion of Africa starting in the seventh century of the current era (C.E.) and the European slave trade beginning in the sixteenth century (C.E), some maintain that traditional African cultural themes were altered significantly (Serequeberhan, 1991). Several writers, however, acknowledge the tenacity and resiliency of these values in spite of the European and Arab influences (Mbiti, 1970; Nkrumah, 1970; Nyerere, 1968, Senghor, 1964). These values were maintained primarily by the continuation of extended kinship systems among Africans (see Fallers, 1964; Madu, 1978; Radcliffe-Brown and Forde, 1967), the lack of physical contact between traditional Africans and Arab and European colonizers (Cabral, 1973; Diop, 1978), the survival of the peasant economy as the predominate economic mode (see Hyden, 1983; Mazrui, 1986), the advocacy of socialism and its relation to African communalism by prominent African leaders (see Nkrumah, 1970; Nyerere, 1968), and the desire to maintain tradition (Mazrui, 1986).

It is important to note here that although the predominant perception among many African historians has been that Africa has been shaped by foreign influence and invasion, little attention has been devoted to studying how early African civilizations, especially those in the Nile Valley, have influenced the philosophy, theology, and scientific development of later-evolving civilizations such as Greece, Phoenicia, and China (Diop, 1991; Finch, 1982; Jackson, 1990; James, 1954; Williams, 1987). It has been intimated that much of the philosophical, theological, and scientific development of these latter civilizations were based on characteristics and achievements of Nile Valley civilizations (Diop, 1991; Jackson, 1990; James, 1954; Van Sertima, 1989; Williams, 1987).

Based on these assumptions regarding the historical development and persistence of traditional African cultural patterns, the Afrocentric worldview can be conceived as a set of philosophical assumptions that are believed to have emanated from common cultural themes of traditional Africa and to have survived the effects of European and Arab colonization and imperialism. Further, the worldview is assumed to be relevant to many people of African descent today, although to varying degrees. Several writers contend that people of African descent tend to function within the

Afrocentric worldview in spite of their geographical location (Akbar, 1979; Asante, 1988; Baldwin and Hopkins, 1990; Boykin, 1983; Boykin and Toms, 1985; Brisbane and Womble, 1991; Hale-Benson, 1982; Schiele, 1994; Sudarkasa, 1988). In the case of African Americans, several authors (see Akbar, 1979; Franklin, 1980; Herskovits, 1941; Martin and Martin, 1985; Nobles, 1980; Sudarkasa, 1988) contend that slavery and the defamation of African culture did not destroy all of the cultural vestiges of Africa for African Americans. These writers generally posit that the social isolation of African Americans, brought about by slavery and forced segregation, helped, rather than hindered, the preservation of traditional African values and customs among African Americans.

These writers believe that traditional Africa has survived enough to render African Americans a distinct cultural and ethnic group with a unique worldview, though they acknowledge that African Americans vary in the internalization and manifestation of this worldview. Several researchers have used the concept of "African self-consciousness" to connote the internalization of an Afrocentric worldview by African Americans. Originating from the works of Baldwin (1981) and Baldwin and Bell (1985), African self-consciousness can be succinctly defined as a state of awareness among African Americans that they are a cultural group and that their behavior should be aimed at fostering the collective survival, advancement, and prosperity of people of African ancestry. Several factors have been found to be positively correlated with African self-consciousness (see Baldwin, Duncan, and Bell, 1987; Baldwin, Brown, and Rackley, 1990; Bell, Bouie, and Baldwin, 1990; Cheatham, Tomilinson, and Ward, 1990; Stokes et al., 1994). Chief among these factors are (1) predominantly African elementary school experiences, (2) black studies curricula exposure, (3) race-oriented socialization and social experiences with racism, (4) feelings of comfort in African cultural environments, (5) educational level of the mother, (6) parental membership in black organizations, (7) attending a predominantly black college, (8) chronological age, and (9) social class, which also has been found to be negatively related to African self-consciousness (see Bell, Bouie, and Baldwin, 1990). Some, however, who promote the Afrocentric paradigm assert that if African Americans do not establish organizations and institutions that imbue traditional African cultural themes and that are independent of European-American culture in their organizational structure and behavior, the survival of the Afrocentric worldview is placed in significant jeopardy (Akbar, 1996; Karenga, 1993a; Schiele, 1999).

CRITICISMS OF AFROCENTRIC WORLDVIEW

Before moving on to discuss the specific characteristics of the Afrocentric worldview and their implications for equality and human liberation, it may be instructive to provide a brief examination of some of the major criticisms of the Afrocentric paradigm. The criticisms are as follows: (1) the definition of African philosophy is suspect; (2) it is inappropriate to impose a cultural unity among the diverse African societies and among the varied groupings of people of African descent; (3) the Afrocentric paradigm apes concepts from European/European-American social science and history; and (4) the Afrocentric paradigm lacks a "social class" analysis of Africa and people of African descent.

Concerning the criticism regarding the validity of the definition of African philosophy, the belief is that much of what is promoted as African philosophy is nothing more than "folk philosophy" or "ethnophilosophy." Appiah (1992) has been a prominent proponent of this notion. He asserts that for an observation to be truly philosophical in nature, it must include a critical discourse. For him, critical discourse is the very foundation of what he calls the formal discipline of philosophy. Appiah believes that those who have advanced African philosophy are uncritical of some of the basic ideas and values that form that philosophy. As has been conceptualized by others, African philosophy for Appiah is mere recitation or systematic delineation of what are assumed to be African traditions (i.e., folk philosophy or ethnophilosophy). Although he admits that folk philosophy or ethnophilosophy is a component of the discipline of philosophy, Appiah maintains that it cannot stand alone as true or "real" philosophy.

Second are those who critique the Afrocentric assumption that cultural unity exists among the diverse groupings of people of African descent (Appiah, 1992; Farrar, 1997; Lemelle, 1994; Serequeberhan, 1991). These writers suggest that to impose a cultural unity on people of African descent is to deny the complexity of culture and the uniqueness and integrity of the diverse groupings of people of African ancestry. Appiah (1992), for example, contends that Africa must be viewed as a geographical concept and not a cultural or metaphysical one. Lemelle (1994) agrees, in that he claims that the Afrocentric critique, especially as presented by Molefi Asante, one of its leading proponents, "is guilty of essentializing an entire people and constructing an abstract, nonexistent 'Africa' " (p. 335).

Third, the Afrocentric worldview is criticized because some say it emulates concepts from European-American social science and history. Lemelle (1994), in his critique of Molefi Asante, suggests that Afrocentricity is wedded to the European philosophical tradition of idealism and that it has no implications for the material lives of people of African descent and other oppressed people. Some maintain that Afrocentrists are nothing more than an elite group of black scholars who are more concerned with status and fame than with social change (Chavez, 1994; Crouch, 1996). Appiah (1992) notes that black nationalists, of which some from the Afrocentric camp can be included, rely heavily on concepts of race developed by white philosophers in the seventeenth and eighteenth centuries. These concepts of race, which are predicated on biological determinism, are said to have been used to promote racism. Further, the notion of a coherent biological concept of race, for Appiah, is bogus. Appiah believes that black thinkers who adhere to this concept of race are guilty of "intrinsic racism." He defines intrinsic racism as a system in which people of different races are differentiated by moral standards and are socially preferred simply because of their race. Appiah believes that the racial solidarity and preference that intrinsic racism generates, even if it is couched in terms such as community or cultural bonds, is problematic.

Finally, some contend that the Afrocentric paradigm lacks a social class analysis of Africa and African Americans (Akinyela, 1995; Lemelle, 1994). For these critics, Afrocentrists excessively glorify Africa and depict it as a place where there was perennial harmonious relations. Class domination, within traditional African societies, they say, is ignored or downplayed by Afrocentrists. To this extent, Akinyela (1995) intimates that the current Afrocentric movement is not a critical discourse and, as currently conceptualized, cannot play a significant role in changing political and economic institutions. Because of this flaw, Akinyela argues for a "critical Afrocentricity."

Although I appreciate the critical dialogue regarding the Afrocentric worldview, I believe these critics have a myopic and incomplete understanding of this worldview. Moreover, in their evaluation of the Afrocentric worldview, they tend to superimpose Eurocentric or Western concepts on a model that is based on a culturally different set of philosophical assumptions. For these reasons, it is important that I address each criticism. First, the notion that there is no African philosophy or an incomplete African philosophy because it does not subscribe to a critical tradition, supposedly characteristic of Western philosophy, is not only misleading but also reinforces Eurocentric cultural universalism and cultural universalism of any form, to which the Afrocentric paradigm is opposed. To suggest that the Eurocentric philosophical tradition is critical may be misleading. What may be interpreted as "critical" in the Eurocentric tradition may be the emphasis in the West on the competition of ideas. Horton (1993) maintains that knowledge development and theorizing in the Western tradition tends to be competitive, whereas in the African tradition it tends to be cooperative and integrative. It may be, then, that the Western tradition is not as critical of its worldview and assumptions as Appiah (1992) and others suggest. Instead, scholars of the Western tradition may have been more concerned with critiquing one another's work so that a dominant theory could emerge. So, the concern may have been less over a critique of Western values, norms, and mores, and more about defeating what is perceived as a rival theory or set of ideas.

Second, by relying on Western standards of defining what philosophy is or is not, Appiah (1992) demonstrates his own inability to transcend Western standards and to view the world as truly multicultural, and not unicultural. As with many African and African-American scholars, Appiah's training in Eurocentric interpretations of science and philosophy may be crippling his ability to conceive the world through lenses other than Eurocentric ones. The effects of Eurocentric cultural oppression, as manifested in academic training, have disconnected many people of African ancestry, even ones reared in Africa, as was Appiah, from concepts of science and philosophy prevalent in traditional Africa. These writers are unwilling to explore these concepts possibly because they view them as subordinate to what they see as more sophisticated and well-conceptualized epistemological methods of Western social science and philosophy.

The second critique, which maintains that there is no unified African experience or culture, is also problematic. The Afrocentric paradigm does not deny the diversity within the African diaspora and often celebrates that diversity, which is seemingly unknown to these critics. However, what these critics fail to admit is that what is often observed as diversity among the African diaspora is nothing more than the diverse ways both diasporic and continental Africans have responded to European and Arab colonization and slavery. The manifold manner in which people of African descent have integrated or rejected European and Arab cultural forms seems to evade these critics. In addition, although it is true that Africa before the influence of Europeans and Arabs included diverse groupings of people—and still does—many writers have identified important commonalities that should not be ignored and that are not a function of coincidence (see, for example, Asante, 1990; Davidson, 1969; Diop, 1978; Karenga, 1993a; Mbiti, 1970; Nobles, 1980; Williams, 1987). What many of these critics of African cultural commonality highlight, to demonstrate African diversity, are small details, not substantive themes. They appear to be overly concerned with the trees and unaware of the continuity of the forest. Further, these critics appear to assume that little or no social and cultural interaction took place among the diverse ethnic groups in Africa, as if each existed in social and geographical isolation.

The critique that Afrocentricity is not concerned with social change and that it is a form of reverse racism (intrinsic racism) incisively demonstrates these critics' severe misunderstanding of the Afrocentric paradigm. First, Lemelle's suggestion that Afrocentricity is wedded to idealism and not materialism evinces his allegiance to a dichotomized categorization of paradigms. Also, it is apparent that Lemelle misunderstands Molefi Asante's emphasis on value transformation, and it shows that Lemelle has not read others who promote the Afrocentric paradigm. Most Afrocentric scholars are clear about the connection of their ideas regarding cultural affirmation and their desire to effect political and economic liberation for people of African descent. The focus on transforming the consciousness of African Americans among Afrocentrists is not an end in itself. Ultimately, Afrocentrists desire material change in the lives of people of African descent but, admittedly, contend that material change must be preceded by a change in consciousness. The change in consciousness is underscored because although Afrocentrists believe that slavery, colonization, and general Eurocentric cultural oppression have caused significant material devastation and injustice for people of African descent, they assert that the most deleterious and insidious consequence of European/European-American slavery, imperialism, and oppression is the mental and cultural alienation among people of African descent. This alienation, Afrocentrists claim, is expressed by African people's depreciation of, and lack of knowledge about, African history, African cultural traditions, and Africa's role in contributing to the development of other civilizations. What Afrocentrists fundamentally imply here is that by depreciating and rejecting their ancestral homeland, people of African descent do not fully realize and affirm their humanity. Affirmation of a group's humanity, for Afrocentrists, is the most basic and essential step toward a group's transforming its material conditions.

What Lemelle and other critics fail to grasp is, by liberating one group, we help make the world a better place for all because the world becomes more inclusive of the optimal contributions of all. The contributions of people of African descent have been systematically suppressed and denied by Eurocentric cultural oppression. As a result, the world has suffered because achievements from a significant proportion of its population, both past and present, could have been employed to help eliminate the spiritual malaise that afflicts social relations. Lemelle and other critics want Afrocentrists and others to conform to a Marxist or neo-Marxist version of human and societal transformation. Although the Marxist analysis and method is important, and certainly worth considering and applying, it tends to assume that racial oppression is subordinate to class oppression, that racism's strength will be significantly diminished when capitalism is abolished, and that economic modes are the primary cause of human and societal relations (Asante, 1988, 1990), all of which run contrary to an Afrocentric perspective. What these critics fundamentally misunderstand is that there are many roads to making this world a better place, and by attempting to impose one method on all who are concerned with social change, they, perhaps unknowingly, participate in a form of implicit oppression and defeat the very objective of inclusion they purport to revere.

Consistent with the aforementioned, the criticism that Afrocentricity lacks a social class analysis suggests (1) that Afrocentrists do not include social class in their analyses and (2) that there is a universal concept of social class and, by extension, power that can be applied to all groups throughout history. Several Afrocentrists are mindful of the role that internal stratification plays in the oppression of people of African descent (Akbar, 1996; Karenga, 1993b). They recognize that corrupt power within any group will not serve the collective interests of that group. Afrocentrists acknowledge that an overemphasis on material acquisitions and material inequality can place people at risk of oppressing others and also keep them from better tapping the humanity that is within them. The Afrocentric thrust differs with analyses that underscore class as the prominent variable in that (1) it conceives culture and worldviews as the chief causative variables, with economic structures as primarily outcomes (Asante, 1990; Schiele, 1994); (2) it places more emphasis on the role of Eurocentric cultural oppression in the lives of people of African descent, despite their social, geographical, and educational backgrounds (Ani, 1994; Asante, 1988, 1990; Kambon, 1992); and (3) it does not adhere to a rigid, universal definition of class (Asante, 1988, 1990).

The allegiance to a universal notion of social class and power is especially problematic for Afrocentrists when analyzing traditional Africa. Although social hierarchy and stratification did exist in many traditional African societies, that stratification differed in some important aspects from the form found in many European societies. For example, the meaning of "king" and "queen" in many traditional African societies did not connote an autocratic ruler who was omnipotent (Diop, 1987; Farrar, 1997; Williams, 1987). Kings and queens in traditional African societies were obligated to show just as much esteem and deference to others as others were to show to them (Diop, 1987; Farrar, 1997; Williams, 1987). Additionally, since much of the class argument is associated with private land ownership, it would be inappropriate when applied to traditional Africa because the idea of private land ownership has been found to have been absent (Diop, 1987; Nyerere, 1968; Williams, 1987). There also were more natural resources in Africa, as compared to Europe, and Diop (1987) suggests that this influenced a more equitable distribution of material resources.

CHARACTERISTICS OF THIS WORLDVIEW

Those who assume the existence of common cultural themes of traditional African societies, especially West African societies from which African Americans are direct descendants, maintain that the cosmological and axiological attributes of the Afrocentric worldview underscore interdependency, collectivity, spirituality, and affect. It is important to note that these attributes are not exclusively African (Myers, 1985) and that they are found in other cultures, although to varying degrees. However, convincing evidence indicates that this worldview originated in Africa long before the emergence of other civilizations (Asante, 1988, 1990; Ben-Jochannon, 1971; Carruthers, 1972; Diop, 1974; James, 1954; Karenga and Carruthers 1986; Keita, 1978).

The cosmological perspective of Afrocentricity highlights the interdependency of all elements of the universe. All elements, whether animate or inanimate, are considered to be dependent on one another; they are, in essence, considered as one (Baldwin, 1985; Bell, Bouie, and Baldwin, 1990; Keita, 1978; Mbiti, 1970; Nobles, 1980; Schiele, 1994). There is no demarcation between that which is spiritual or material (Asante, 1980; Myers, 1985; Schiele, 1994); reality is assumed to be "both spiritual and material at once" (Meyers, 1985, p. 34). The depth of the emphasis on an interdependent cosmological view is discerned in the African belief that to destroy one part of the web of elements is to destroy the whole universe, even the Creator (Mbiti, 1970; Nobles, 1980).

The cosmological perspective of the Afrocentric worldview fosters an axiological perspective that centers on spirituality, collectivity, and affect. As it relates to spirituality, the Afrocentric perspective recognizes the centrality of the spiritual feature of all elements of the universe. Spirituality is taken here to mean the nonmaterial or invisible substance that connects all elements of the universe (Akbar, 1984; Schiele, 1996). Whether animate or inanimate, all elements are assumed to have a spiritual base and to have emanated from a similar universal source (Mbiti, 1970; Nobles, 1980; Schiele, 1994; Zahan, 1979). The emphasis on spirituality in the Afrocentric worldview supports and fosters the cosmological view of interdependency. For elements to be considered interconnected and interdependent, there must be a universal link, and, in African philosophy, that link is the nonmaterial spirit of the Creator (Akbar, 1984; Mbiti, 1970; Nobles, 1980).

Applying this perspective of spirituality to human behavior means that nonmaterial characteristics of people are just as important as other human qualities (Akbar, 1984; Bolling, 1990; Weems, 1974). Mind, body, and soul are given equal value and are believed to be interdependent and interrelated (Akbar, 1984; Asante, 1987; Mbiti, 1970; Nobles, 1980; Weems, 1974). While mind and body are viewed as temporary human attributes limited by time, the soul is believed to transcend time and represents the fundamental core of human beings (Mbiti, 1970; Zahan, 1979). To this end, the soul becomes just as much a target of individual development as does the mind and body.

A high value placed on morality also is an important feature of spirituality within the Afrocentric worldview (Akbar, 1979, 1984; Baldwin, 1981, 1985; Boykin, 1983; Nobles, 1980; Schiele, 1994), which reflects the paradigm's focus on humanistic values (Oyebade, 1990; Schiele, 1994). The concept of humanism should not be confused with the one associated with the humanistic school of Western psychology. Within that school, humanism tends to imply a secular humanism in which the relationship between God and humans is downplayed. Humans are conceived as being independent of God in that their capacity to behave morally has little or nothing to do with their relationship with, or connection to, a deity or creator. The African concept of humanism does not sever the relationship between God and humans (Gyekye, 1987). Humans' ability to be moral and caring is believed to be linked with God's model of morality and care. Since the soul is viewed as the core of the human being in African philosophy, it is the invisible, spiritual nexus between God and humans that generates the potential of humans to behave morally.

Akbar (1984) asserts that "morality and spirituality are inseparate" (p. 409) within the Afrocentric worldview. Spiritual development and moral development are tantamount. A major social implication of the Afrocentric worldview's emphasis on spiritual development and its relationship to morality is that social problems and human suffering would be assumed to diminish. As indicated in later chapters, social problems in the United States are linked with spiritual alienation, and to eliminate or reduce that alienation, focus should be placed on the spiritual development of humans.

Just as spirituality and morality were connected in traditional African societies, so too were spirituality and religion, and both were integrated thoroughly throughout these societies (Mbiti, 1970, 1991; Karenga, 1993b; Zahan, 1979). The rigid fragmentation of religion and spirituality from other institutions, as is found in the United States and some other Western societies, was not apparent in traditional Africa. The overarching cosmo-logical thrust on interdependency precluded issues of God and spirituality from being marginalized and dichotomized. Although there were special ceremonies and rituals, the emphasis on spiritual growth was not specific to any one event, day, or hour (Mbiti, 1991; Paris, 1995). The focus on enhancing spiritual development occurred in all institutions, and in most of the educational institutions, a primary objective was to become more like God, that is, to be able to emulate and tap the source of the Creator (Akbar, 1994; Hilliard, 1989). No ontological divide was believed to exist between God and humans (Karenga, 1993b), and self-knowledge was thought to be associated with knowledge of God (Zahan, 1979). This intimate and ontological nexus between God and humans in the Afrocen-tric worldview suggests that God is subjectified rather than objectified.

The emphasis on collectivity, especially in human relations, is also an essential value in Afrocentricity. Considerable emphasis is placed on a collective conceptualization of human beings and on collective survival. This is because, in the Afrocentric worldview, individual identity is con-ceived as collective identity (Akbar, 1984; Baldwin, 1981; Myers, 1985; Nobles, 1980). This model does not reject the notion of uniqueness (Ak-bar, 1984; Boykin, 1983; Boykin and Toms, 1985), but it does reject the idea that the individual can be understood separate from others in his or her social group (Akbar, 1984). This repudiation of an insular identity is predicated on the belief that there is no perceptual separation of the indi-vidual from other people (Dixon, 1976). The African adage "I am because we are and because we are, therefore I am" (Mbiti, 1970, p. 141) captures the essence of this belief. In this way, individual identity within the Afro-centric worldview is akin to a spiderweb. When one thinks of a spiderweb, one knows that its composition is a series of interconnected and inter-dependent strands, and if one strand is touched, the entire web shakes. Thus, the individual is never separated from his or her corporate identity and the influences of the broader and intimate social milieus. To under-stand the individual, one must understand the milieu in which the person is socialized. There is variance in the manner in which people internalize the stimuli of the environment, but the environment dictates the kind of stimu-li to which the person is exposed. In essence, the stimuli form what can be called the ethos of a group. Within this framework, "individual identity is only a unique way in which an individual expresses a common core ethos" (Schiele, 1997, p. 805).

The emphasis on collectivity also leads to a focus on detecting and highlighting commonalities of a people rather than detecting and high-lighting individual differences (Schiele, 1990, 1994). Instead of fostering an emphasis on difference and exclusiveness, the Afrocentric paradigm encourages a focus on similarity and inclusiveness. In this regard, a fundamental attribute of Afrocentricity is the preeminence given to the group: "the welfare of the group takes precedence over the welfare of the individual" (Schiele, 1990, p. 149). This is because the emphasis on the collective conceptualization of self fosters attention on group survival, oneness, and prosperity. However, as Gyekye (1992) posits, the focus on collective rights in traditional African thought does not imply that people are prohibited from rendering an evaluation of the social structure. Rather, it suggests that, in traditional African philosophy, an uncompromising and excessive orientation to individual rights—which compromises individual obligation, to and consideration of, the welfare of others—is dissuaded (Ani, 1994; Baldwin and Hopkins, 1990; Schiele, 1994).

Last, within the Afrocentric worldview, an affective epistemology is validated. One's emotions are deemed essential in self-exploration and in furthering knowledge generally. Indeed, a primary assumption of the Afrocentric worldview is that emotions are the most direct experience of self (Akbar, 1984). The focus on affect in the Afrocentric worldview does not preclude recognition of the rational. Rather, this worldview sees rationality and emotionality as two transparent and penetrable sides of the same coin: that coin being the ways in which people experience life. In this worldview, reasoning or thoughts do not occur within a vacuum but are filtered through the maze of emotions and values to which one holds (Schiele, 1996). Thus, thoughts do not occur independently of feelings, nor do feelings occur independently of thoughts. Thoughts are no more supreme to emotions as emotions are to thoughts. In this way, the Afrocentric worldview relies more on a holistic or diunital mode of understanding the relationship between feelings and thoughts and, by extension, interpreting the world generally (Bell, 1994; Dixon, 1976).

Another component of this affective and holistic epistemology is symbolic imagery. Dixon (1976) defines symbolic imagery as the use of phenomena, such as words, gestures, and objects, to convey multiple meanings. Kambon (1992) refers to this as "Affect-Symbolic Imagery Synthesis" and asserts that within this cognitive style, "the phenomenal world is not separated out of experience as an object to be known through measuring the conceptual space or distance between it and the self" (p. 91). Based on these observations, objectification would be an inappropriate method of knowing.

The Afrocentric worldview's cosmological and axiological focus on interdependency, collectivity, spirituality, and affect places it in an excellent position to promote equality and human liberation. This is primarily because of Afrocentricity's emphasis on similarity, inclusiveness, and appreciation of human differences, all of which can be conceived as cornerstones of equality and human liberation.

AFROCENTRICITY, EQUALITY, AND HUMAN LIBERATION

Equality and Afrocentric Assumptions

Social equality would be an appropriate outcome if the Afrocentric worldview were applied. Although there was social stratification in many traditional African societies, the focus on collective identity and spirituality, and the practice of extended kinship ties, precluded the kind of material despair that is often associated with political and social stratification in Western societies (Chazan, 1993; Diop, 1987). The focus on collective identity, spirituality, and the abundance of natural resources in traditional Africa encouraged greater sharing of wealth (Diop, 1987; Williams, 1987). The sharing of an individual's wealth generated considerable community reverence, prestige, and status for that person, and many African societies had built-in checks and balances to obviate the ostentatious display of affluence (Dei, 1994). Further, because the concept of private land ownership was absent in precolonial Africa (Biebuyck, 1964; Diop, 1987; Williams, 1987), most persons had access to land, the concept of land took on a more collective character, and kings and queens could not hoard property (Biebuyck, 1964; Diop, 1987; Williams, 1987).

It is my contention, however, that it is the African cosmological thrust of collectivity and spirituality that can provide a philosophical foundation of equality, which is a fundamental value of many human service practitioners and many of the national organizations that represent them. This is because, to achieve equality, focus must be placed on sameness or similarity. A focus on similarity can only emerge from an emphasis on inclusion. Generally speaking, a collective and spiritual worldview can facilitate this by viewing humans as one, with similarities underscored over differences and acknowledgment that all people emanate from a similar universal source.

Specifically, collective identity can foster equality because in collective identity, the emphasis is on group oneness. From this vantage point, one is encouraged to devote more time trying to discern how people are similar to one another rather than different. This is not to imply that differences are unimportant or that they should not be acknowledged. The problem arises when differences are ascribed normative values of good or bad, when difference is interpreted as inherently pejorative, and when there is an attempt by some to render everyone in their own image. From an Afrocentric viewpoint, differences (primarily group differences) should be recognized as a means to underscore appreciation of human diversity rather than to highlight negativity.

The emphasis on similarity in the Afrocentric worldview is related to the common experiences of human beings. More specifically, it reflects the shared experiences of a group. Nobles (1980) called this "experiential communality," and it is through this communal sharing of experiences that individuals take on a collective identity. Once individuals adopt a collective identity, they can then strive to work toward similar goals. This phenomenon is captured in Asante's (1988) concept of the "collective cognitive imperative," which is the full spiritual and intellectual commitment to a vision by a group. The key concept in Asante's definition is fullness. Fullness implies completeness or inclusiveness. Thus, the spiritual and intellectual commitment is viewed as inclusive because it incorporates the visions of all in the group, which are considered as one. The critical theme in both Nobles' (1980) and Asante's (1988) concepts is oneness. Combining the concepts of both would suggest that equality occurs when people coalesce their personal identities into a collective identity that then leads to establishing and defining common goals or visions.

Spirituality is the medium through which collective identity and oneness of vision are attained. This is accomplished through the dimensional nature of spirituality that incorporates concepts of interconnectedness and morality. The focus on interconnectedness recognizes that people are spiritual (i.e., nonmaterial) beings who are connected with one another through the spirit of the Creator. This simply means that all human beings stem from a similar source of creation, in spite of their material and physical differences. Spirituality mediates and attenuates these differences. This is because the spiritual aspect of human beings is recognized as the most indelible human attribute—one that permeates multiple spheres of time and space.

Applying the latter perspective to the notion of collective identity makes it possible for one's identity to be merged with the living (those in the present), with those who lived (those in the past), and with those who will live (those in the future). This transdimensional viewpoint, which is an important feature of African philosophy (Mbiti, 1970; Myers, 1985, 1988; Nobles, 1980; Zahan, 1979), significantly promotes inclusiveness, which was offered earlier as a fundamental prerequisite of equality.

As stated earlier, morality is a central feature of spirituality within the Afrocentric worldview. Similar to the dimension of interconnectedness, the moral dimension of spirituality also is important in fostering equality. Morality underscores humanistic values such as collective well-being and respect for all human life. Indeed, equality can only emerge through the exaltation and esteem of *all* human life, not just that of a few. This is why the Afrocentric view of the collective conceptualization of self (i.e., collective identity) is so important. It is through this process that people are able to develop universal esteem for all. Without it, the actualization of equality is improbable.

The latter discussion has important implications for intraracial and interracial/ethnic relations in the United States. For intragroup relations, the focus on collective identity and oneness of vision can help ethnic and racial groups that have been victims of cultural oppression to affirm the unique history and traditions of their group. Because these groups have often been separated from information that underscores their group's role in advancing the human family and that highlights their group's self-worth, there is a penchant for some within these groups to dissociate themselves from their group and identify with other groups, especially those which are revered in society. The desire of a member of a culturally oppressed group to psychologically dissociate himself or herself from that group could be considered a manifestation of internalization of negative messages about the group that are facilitated by, and germinate from, cultural oppression.

If members of these groups are exposed to a wider range of information, especially information that reconstructs the value and worth of their group, a collective identity and oneness of vision are likely to emerge or be enhanced. This could reduce much of the psychosocial behavior that some social scientists associate with group self-hatred and could help aggrandize the political and economic status of the group.

Once every racial/ethnic group in a multicultural society such as the United States receives the dignity and respect that should be afforded all racial/ethnic groups, then authentic intergroup relations can be forged. A collective, intergroup identity can guide these groups to establish visions that speak to the interests of all, especially when common space is shared. True and more inclusive debate and dialog can accrue about important concerns common to the diverse groups. The collective cognitive imperative that Asante speaks of can be one that does not marginalize the distinctive perspective of the many in order to impose a false universal one that reflects a few. All groups will be able to project their ideas and interpretations, and in doing so, the collective vision that is formed becomes one that all can own, even if time demonstrates the vision to be a mistake. The desire for the collective human identity that many people speak about can truly come about because each group will be able to optimally demonstrate its contribution to the advancement of humanity and to human history.

For those in the human services, this discussion implies that, to shape an authentic human service identity, it is critical to include the narratives and interpretations of all, even the consumers of service delivery. The assumptions of the Afrocentric worldview would foster relationships between deliverers and consumers of services that are based on reciprocity and consumer empowerment and that eschew professional elitism (Brisbane and Womble, 1991; Harvey and Rauch, 1997; Phillips, 1990; Schiele, 1996, 1997).

Human Liberation and Afrocentric Assumptions

The Afrocentric worldview encourages the belief that human beings have a proclivity toward goodness and construction rather than evil and destruction (Akbar, 1984; Asante, 1988; Schiele, 1990). Too often in Western philosophy and Western social science, the norm of human behavior is thought to be that of evil and destruction. A corollary of the perpetuation of this belief is that people begin to use it to justify decadent behavior and the practice of inequality. Thus, human liberation toward moral and spiritual ends is seen as impossible to come by because the human being's capacity for goodness and construction is considered to be inherently limited. The Afrocentric worldview does not restrict the human being's capacity for goodness and construction. Because the spiritual/nonmaterial aspect is so central within the Afrocentric perspective, the capabilities and positive transformative potential of human beings are considered to be vast (Schiele, 1994).

Since the Afrocentric worldview encourages an expansive concept of humans connected to their spiritual essence, the potential for human beings to be liberated from the restrictions placed by an excessive emphasis on material and physical development is immense. This is because of the Afrocentric worldview's focus on spiritual development, which is linked with material and physical development and which coalesces the three components of mind, body, and soul. The holistic conception of the human being enhances the likelihood of humans conceiving themselves as intimately connected with others and to the Creator, or God. It helps people recognize that there is more to them that meets the eye, that there are unseen forces perpetually at work, and that their self-worth extends beyond their material acquisitions. The basic assumption, therefore, is that a holistic and interconnected conception of humanity and nature helps one to acknowledge and tap into sources that can enhance human achievement aimed at collective compassion and advancement.

This form of human liberation increases the probability of spiritualizing a society's technological development. In ancient Kemet, or Egypt, for example, the shrines, temples, pyramids, and other indicators of material and technological development were viewed by the Kemites as material expressions of deeper spiritual concerns targeted at forging a greater oneness between people and God (Akbar, 1994; Ameen, 1990; Hilliard, 1989). This perspective can help obviate human technology from being exclusively associated with aggrandizing human pleasure and efficiency, and it can help preclude technology from being used as an instrument of human exploitation and for the rape of nature. Regarding nature, the value of "mastery over nature" can be replaced by the value of "harmony and coexistence with nature." With this conceptualization as a foundation, technological growth and achievement can be liberated from its association with human oppression and the genocide of the ecology, known as ecocide.

Another form of human liberation can be generated by the Afrocentric worldview, and that is liberation from negative notions of human differences. In the Afrocentric worldview, the value of xenophilia is encouraged (Diop, 1978; Kambon, 1992). Xenophilia is concisely the belief that strangers—those who are different or who have a different lifestyle—should be treated affably, and, by extension, that one's cultural or lifestyle biases should not be imposed on the stranger, or alternatively, the "culturally different other." This xenophilic tradition is examined by Diop (1978) in his two-cradle cultural theory. Diop suggests that two cultural cradles developed in antiquity: (1) the northern and (2) southern cradles. The northern cradle represented the Indo-European or Aryan culture, and the southern cradle represented the culture of Africa. Diop suggests that because Africa was abundant in physical space and natural resources, the African tendency was to not view strangers as a threat (xenophilia). In the northern cradle, where the physical environment was more harsh and barren, xenophobia was prevalent because the nomadic social style, along with the lack of physical resources, rendered competition as the primary behavioral adaptation. Diop's analysis indicates that the physical environment has a significant impact on cultural attributes.

Further, Karenga (1993b) offers a moral reason for the emergence of xenophilia within the African tradition. He underscores the pivotal role that Maatian ethics has played in the development of this affable view of the stranger. In ancient Kemet (Egypt), the symbol of Maat—the spread wings of a bird with the head of a woman—represented the values of truth, justice, and righteousness. Maatian ethics, which were developed between 4000 and 3500 B.C.E., provided the ancient inhabitants of the Nile Valley with moral guidance in their social and political conduct. An important component of Maatian literature is "The Instructions of the Prime Minister," which were used primarily as a guide for bureaucratic ethics (Karenga, 1993b). One quote from this document relevant to our discussion is "Treat equally the one you know and the one you do not know, the one who is near and the one who is far away" (Karenga, 1993b, p. 379). Interpreted another way, this quote can be seen as encouraging people to treat those who are different in a similar manner as they would treat those with whom they are familiar. It also could suggest that in treating equally the one who is different and the one who is similar, one becomes more willing to accept the stranger on his or her own terms. If so, this could prevent the practice of cultural universalism and cultural oppression, in that attempts at making others conform to one's own cultural standards could be eliminated or alleviated. What this emphasis can foster is an appreciation of the distinctiveness of diverse cultural groups and the idea that each group can make important contributions to world development and to human civilization.

For professionals in the human services, this focus on xenophilia can help create service technologies wherein consumers contribute to the design and application of those technologies. Too often in human service work, consumers are vilified and their viewpoints, experiences, and narratives are marginalized (Chapin, 1995; Saleebey, 1996). This practice can be viewed as a function of human service professionals lacking appreciation of the lives and experiences of consumers. Although lack of appreciation can be interpreted as an outcome of a lack of knowledge about these groups, it also can be considered a result of fear and cultural elitism on the part of human service professionals. It can be maintained that a form of xenophobia about some consumer groups has emerged, especially if those consumers are viewed as morally deficient and socially undesirable. If human service professionals employ Maatian ethics as their guide and practice it in an honest way, the likelihood of gaining greater appreciation of the consumer "other" is augmented.

A final way in which human liberation can be achieved through application of the Afrocentric worldview is liberation from the concept that the unseen or spiritual world is spooky and mystical. An unfortunate aspect of the separation of the secular from the sacred and the overemphasis on a material epistemology is that the spiritual world has been bastardized and made an object of comedy. Icons such as "Casper, the Friendly Ghost," and popular movies such as *The Exorcist* give one either a fictionalized idea of spirituality or a spooky one in which fear of the unseen or the spiritual world is taught.

This apprehension and bastardization of the spiritual world creates a cultural climate among mental health and human service professionals that conceives of 'the soul as something to avoid when planning social and mental health services. If human service professionals would comprehend the soul as a natural component of humans and as merely representing that unseen and transdimensional element that connects humans to one another and to a transcendental source or being, the possibility for positive human transformation can be enhanced. This is because service interventions could be designed to help people tap into an often unexplored source of power and self-affirmation. This topic will be examined in more detail in Chapters 5 and 6.

Chapter 3

The Evolution of Black Social Work
and Its Pitfalls

To gain a full appreciation and understanding of the Afrocentric paradigm of human services, it is necessary to examine and trace important themes of the helping process found in traditional Africa and among people of African descent in the United States. Before Africans were kidnapped and imported as slaves to the United States, they enjoyed and practiced a rich tradition of social welfare. This tradition is believed by some to have continued once Africans were imported to the United States as slaves (see Herskovits, 1941; Martin and Martin, 1985; Paris, 1995; Stuckey, 1987). Although slavery altered this tradition somewhat, in some ways it strengthened the tradition. Nonetheless, African Americans, in slavery and once free, developed self-help institutions to look after their own, to mitigate against the deleterious effects of racial oppression, and to instill hope for a better day. The self-help tradition among African Americans, although maintaining some of its original character, was altered significantly with the coming of scientific charity, the greater professionalization of social work, and the establishment of the National Urban League and the Atlanta School of Social Work. This chapter describes and examines the evolution of the helping process among people of African descent in the United States by underscoring major themes, practices, and pitfalls.

SOCIAL WELFARE IN TRADITIONAL AFRICA

Social welfare in traditional Africa ensured that people had access to needed material resources and that people felt a sense of group cohesiveness. Each person had the civil and, more important, the human right to

Portions of this chapter originally appeared in "An Afrocentric Perspective on Social Welfare Philosophy and Policy," *Journal of Sociology and Social Welfare,* 1997, 24(2), pp. 21-39. Reprinted with permission from Western Michigan University of Social Work.

work, decent housing, and sufficient food and clothing. Williams (1993) explains that in African economic philosophy, the concept of profits implies a surplus only after the human needs of all in society have been addressed. To more adequately describe the philosophy of social welfare from a traditional African standpoint, three tenets are discussed: (1) human identity is conceived through an extended kinship system; (2) poverty is unnecessary and intolerable; and (3) government and individual responsibility are mutually dependent and affirmed.

Extended Kinship

In traditional Africa, people did not view themselves as isolated entities with autonomous selves. Instead, a more fluid and holistic concept of identity that conceived the individual as embedded in his or her social group was practiced (Davidson, 1969; Horton, 1993; Mbiti, 1970). This holistic concept of identity was best manifested in the practice of the extended kinship system, better known as the extended family. As Martin and Martin (1985) note:

> Kinship bonds were so strong in traditional Africa that sometimes smaller family units (nuclear families) would become part of a larger extended family network, and the larger extended family network would often make up a clan, and several clans would make up the entire tribe or community. (p. 12)

Thus, in traditional Africa, extended families consisted of immense multigenerational clusters of relatives built around a central group referred to as a lineage (Madu, 1978; Radcliffe-Brown and Forde, 1967; Sudarkasa, 1997). These lineages could be traced through the "male" line, termed patrilineages, or the "female" line, termed matrilineages. In West Africa, extended families lived together in what were called compounds. Compounds were a series of individual dwellings that were clustered together to form a community of "blood-related" relatives (Radcliffe-Brown and Forde, 1967; Sudarkasa, 1997). Though these compounds included conjugal families that would consist of a husband, a wife, and their children, these families differed from the nuclear family form characteristic of European-American culture (Harvey, 1985; Nobles, 1974; Sudarkasa, 1997). Sudarkasa (1997) asserts that one important difference was that African extended families were far less rigid in the categorization of relatives. For example, children of a similar generation were treated more as sisters and brothers rather than adding the label of cousin. Nobles (1974) suggests that African extended families, besides the expansive lineage concept, also reflect "role elasticity" in that family roles allow for considerable flexibility and interchangeability. From this point of view, family expectations, unlike those in European-American culture, were not shaped so rigidly by gender, and there was greater latitude in legitimating family structures that were different from the nuclear style.

Part of what fostered this extended concept and practice of family was the belief in what some have called "fictive kinship" (Billingsley, 1994; Gutman, 1976; Martin and Martin, 1978). This form of kinship did not confine family formation along conjugal or blood lines but rather extended it to include anyone who belonged to the social group. Billingsley (1968) referred to this type of family as an "augmented family" because the family is expanded or augmented to accept or take in persons who are not blood related. What this form of kinship provided was a sense of belonging and group cohesiveness in that the likelihood of feeling alienated from the group was minimized (Gyekye, 1987, 1992; Williams, 1993). It also created a climate that emphasized the sharing of resources and encouraged a collective sense of land ownership (Diop, 1978; Fallers, 1964).

Poverty As Unnecessary and Intolerable

Because of the extensive amount of natural resources and land, as well as the emphasis on collective or extended identity, poverty was not prevalent in traditional Africa. A critical dimension of the collective or extended identity in traditional Africa was the focus on collective rights (Menkiti, 1984; Williams, 1987). Although individuals could voice their evaluation of the community structure and practice, the collective rights of the community were believed to be more vital than the rights of any one person (Gyekye, 1992; Menkiti, 1984; Williams, 1987). Another reason for the lack of poverty was the collective concept of land ownership that prevented anyone from hoarding large amounts of land and then compelling people to pay to either work or live on the land (Dei, 1994; Diop, 1987; Williams, 1987, 1993). In traditional Africa, everyone was afforded adequate food, clothing, and shelter; thus, there was little anxiety about where the next meal was coming from or whether one would be homeless (Biebuyck, 1964; Diop, 1987; Williams, 1987, 1993). The critical criterion was that each individual contribute to his or her fullest potential.

Although it is true that some people had fewer resources and less prestige than others in traditional Africa, they were not maligned or defamed because they had less. In traditional Africa, moral deficiencies or attributes were not associated with one's economic status (Diop, 1987; Gyekye, 1987). This can be partially ascribed to the absence of the value of individualism in traditional Africa, and to the spiritual ontology that cut across and characterized much of it. Regarding the deemphasis on individualism, both personal success and failure were thought to be shared in traditional Africa (Karenga, 1996; Williams, 1987, 1993). Traditional African philosophy reminds us that "the total results of one's efforts are due to aids, circumstances, and powers entirely beyond one's own control" (Williams, 1993, p. 156). This is not to suggest that the individual is completely absolved of personal responsibility; rather, it posits that the individual is embedded in, and is the result of, social networks and intercourse. The individual is never separated from these networks, and his or her behavior is a reflection of them. This is one reason why every effort was made in traditional Africa to provide nurturing social environments. When one person failed or engaged in behavior inconsistent with community norms and mores, the collective actions of the individual's immediate and wider social milieu were examined (Gyekye, 1987, 1992).

The presence of a spiritual ontology also explains why persons with less were not vilified in traditional Africa. A significant corollary of this spiritual ontology was that the concept of talents and abilities did not take on a rigid hierarchy (Carruthers, 1981; Williams, 1987). Just as each human being was seen as a critical component connected to other humans and the Creator, so too were all abilities and talents, if used toward good, conceived as important to the unity and collective survival of the group. This belief, therefore, validates the notion of the interconnectedness and mutual dependency of diverse talents and abilities (Schiele, 1997). Thus, in traditional Africa, those whose speciality was making pottery were thought to be just as vital to the community as those whose speciality was healing. What this more equalitarian affirmation of diverse talents obviated was the overglorification of skills that can cause some talents to gain overwhelming prestige to the devaluation of others.

Government and Individual Responsibility As Mutually Dependent

In traditional Africa, a mutually dependent and morally affirming idea of government and individual responsibility was perpetuated. The emphasis on mutual dependency was supported by the belief in "cooperative democracy" (see Williams, 1993). Unlike the dichotomous and antagonistic idea of government and individual responsibility found in European-American culture, cooperative democracy takes on a more unitary and reciprocal notion of government and individual responsibility. Within this framework, all units of people—individuals to very large aggregates and bureaucracies—play an equally important role in ensuring the welfare of the entire nation or community. With diunital logic (i.e., logic that emphasizes unity in polarity) as its foundation, cooperative democracy conceives that groupings of individuals are linked through social and spiritual intercourse. From this perspective, it is illogical to impose an insular and unilinear view of human behavior and social events because this view negates highly complex, subtle, and polydeterministic ways in which the actions and thoughts of people are interrelated. A call for individual responsibility in no way diminishes or cancels out a call for government responsibility, and vice versa. Rather, government and individual responsibility are considered to be obligations that are motivated less by self-interest—which is the basis of a conflict-oriented view of government and individual responsibility—than by the essential interdependency of humans as interactive "social" beings (Gyekye, 1992).

In traditional Africa, the concept of cooperative democracy was best manifested through the African "council of elders" (see Chazan, 1993; Gyekye, 1992; Williams, 1987). The council of elders served as the chief's cabinet or close advisors and decided on matters of community policy and adjudication. Public opinion and involvement were encouraged and did influence the decision making of the elders. When there was disagreement on an issue, the council or the other officials would allow debates until unanimity was achieved (Chazan, 1993; Gyekye, 1992; Williams, 1987). The tolerance for extensive debates was based on the idea that the objective of political debates was not to compete: factions attempted to obscure opposites so that a compromise could be attained (Chazen, 1993; Gyekye, 1992). In addition, the tolerance of lengthy debates was buttressed by the deemphasis on efficiency and the centrality of localized government (Chazen, 1993). The concept of time in traditional Africa was seen less as a quantitative and linear phenomenon and more as a holistic and cyclical occurrence that was intimately connected to human events (Kalu, 1991; Mbiti, 1970). This prevented time from being conceived as a commodity for exploitation and it obviated the practice of swift decision making, unless the decision concerned an immediate threat to the survival of the community. Decentralization also was a feature of many traditional African societies, and this helped to foster the practice of local self-government (Chazen, 1993; Stoeltje, 1994). The practice of localized rule allowed input from greater numbers of people and facilitated an enhanced participatory form of government.

Political participation and localized government help individuals to acknowledge that they have a stake in their community, which leads to better regulation of behavior. When people feel a sense of belonging to, and ownership of, the larger community, they are more likely to behave responsibly and take into consideration the effects of their behavior on others. Furthermore, in traditional Africa, consideration of others was supported by the belief that the proclivity, potential, and expectation of humans was to do good (Gyekye, 1992; Mbiti, 1970; Zahan, 1979). This belief helped to preclude xenophobia (Diop, 1978) and served as a catalyst for enhancing individuals' desire to be responsible (Karenga, 1996; Schiele, 1997).

Another critical component of cooperative democracy is the power and authority women wielded in traditional Africa. Unlike the traditional practices of many European cultures—including the United States—the female in traditional Africa played significant public roles that dealt with policy making and adjudication (Farrar, 1997; Stoeltje, 1994; Sudarkasa, 1989). Some of the titles given to women who held high status and assumed political responsibility were queenmother, queensister, chief, or princess (Stoeltje, 1994; Sudarkasa, 1989). In traditional Africa, many of the political systems were categorized as a "dual-sex" political system (Okonjo, 1976). In this dual-sex system, women presided over and made decisions about the affairs and conflicts that pertained to women, and men monitored those which were relevant to men. Although separate, these systems were parallel; thus, in one community, there could be two councils of elders, one for women and one for men. In addition, the decisions made by the female council were just as legitimate as the ones rendered by the male council (Farrar, 1997). Though the practice of the dual-sex political system varied in traditional Africa, the primary point here is that women were prominent in civic affairs, and this prominence can be attributed to at least three factors: (1) the validation of matrilineal kinship systems, (2) the concept of gender in traditional Africa, and (3) the presence of feminine concepts and images of God.

The validation of matrilineal kinship systems acknowledged that women's lineages were just as important as the men's. This not only enhanced the importance of a woman's familial history but also validated a more complete understanding of family history. Also, since wealth and power often followed a specific lineage, many African women in matrilineal societies were able to secure considerable resources and prestige (Stoeltje, 1994).

In traditional Africa, male and female were not conceived as opposing dualities (Carruthers, 1981; Sudarkasa, 1989); they were viewed as opposites which could be unified and which differed in degree and not in kind (Mbiti, 1970; Ray, 1976). There was also complexity in gender relations for "Women and men might be hierarchically related to each other in one or more of their reciprocal statuses, but not in others" (Sudarkasa, 1989, p. 153). Thus, many traditional African societies did not stratify consistently the categories of male and female. Furthermore, the language of many traditional African societies excluded pronouns that were gender specific, and distinctions between "public" and "domestic" domains did not follow closely along gender lines (Sudarkasa, 1989).

In many traditional African societies, masculine and feminine concepts and images of God were acknowledged and affirmed (Karenga, 1993; Mbiti, 1970; Ray, 1976). For example, in ancient Egypt, or Kemet, Isis was the feminine aspect of the God Trinity of Isis, Osiris, and Horus (Akbar, 1994; Day, 1997; Hilliard, 1989). Day (1997) maintains that the "religion of Isis" underscored the need for class and gender equality and that many of its converts in early Rome were disenfranchised persons who rejected the state religion of Rome, which emphasized male and class domination. Moreover, Amma, the name for God used by the Dogon, a West African ethnic group, is conceived as having female and male characteristics and is based on their belief that the origin of the universe, and by extension, God was characterized by the emergence of twins that included both feminine and masculine attributes (Griaule, 1978; Ray, 1976). In traditional Yoruba religion, the divinities of Obata'la' and Oduduwa' are deemed androgynous, "for the divine is neither male nor female, but both" (King, 1986, p. 10).

What the participation of traditional African women in public affairs indicates is that patriarchy may not be a universal concept, or it may not be a concept that can be applied monolithically. Diop (1978) maintains that patriarchy arose out of the nomadic cultures, such as the Teutons, of the Northern Hemisphere, and Day (1997) contends that it was patriarchy which influenced the oppression and eventual poverty and destitution of women, especially in Europe and the United States. The implication here, for our purposes, is that in traditional Africa, gender was less significant in determining the distribution of material resources. If one demographic characteristic in traditional Africa brought noticeable attention or additional status, it was chronological age. Both the very young (babies) and the very old were viewed as special because both were closer to the spiritual world of the ancestors, the former having just arrived and the latter being about to return (Mbiti, 1970; Paris, 1995).

BLACK SOCIAL WELFARE IN AMERICA

Traditional Methods Used in Slavery and During the Nineteenth Century

When Africans were brought to North America as captives and as slaves, there is evidence that some African relics survived and were maintained by the enslaved Africans despite the horrors of slavery (see Franklin, 1980; Herskovits, 1941; Martin and Martin, 1985; Nobles, 1980; Sudarkasa, 1988, 1997). There is disagreement, however, about the degree to which these relics survived, in that some maintain that they tenuously, if at all, survived, in the captives' speech, dance, music, folklore, and religion (Frazier, 1964; Stampp, 1956), while others contend that these relics have shown more substantive persistence in the areas of worldview, cognition, and behavioral styles (Azibo, 1991; Kambon, 1992; Khatib et al., 1979; Nobles, 1980).

Frazier (1939) was one of the most prominent scholars who argued that slavery destroyed African cultural relics in the Americas, generally, and in North America, specifically. His primary rationale for this was twofold: First, the enslaved Africans were not allowed to institutionalize their African culture because of their chattel status and because of the practice, especially in the United States, of breaking up the families of enslaved Africans. For Frazier, the family is the most conspicuous social institution through which cultural attributes are learned and kept alive. Without stable families, therefore, Frazier contended that African cultural vestiges' chances of survival were improbable. The second reason was the close physical proximity of enslaved Africans to European Americans in the United States brought about by the large dispersion of the population of enslaved Africans. Thus, the lack of population density among enslaved Africans enhanced their likelihood of being exposed and acculturated to the norms and mores of European-American culture.

Viewing the effects of slavery from a different lens, Nobles (1974, 1980), a major Afrocentric family theorist, maintains that the social isolation and insulation of enslaved Africans brought about by slavery encouraged, rather than hindered, the preservation of African cultural vestiges. Nobles' argument relies on the assumption that enslaved Africans did not have the degree of exposure to European-American culture that Frazier posited. Rather, the isolation created opportunities for enslaved Africans to insulate themselves from complete exposure and internalization of European-American culture, thus aiding in the protection of their African cultural traditions. Herskovits (1941) adds another dimension to support the survival of what he refers to as "Africanisms." He maintains that a primary theme of the literature on slavery is the acquiescence of the Africans to slavery, which he asserts is an erroneous concept of enslaved Africans and a critical factor used to explain why African traditions did not survive. Herskovits contends, by reviewing several studies, that a more correct story of enslaved Africans is that they resisted their slave status, as indicated by the many slave revolts and the narratives of enslaved Africans. If enslaved Africans were reluctant to accept their slave status, Herskovits states, then this could have motivated enslaved Africans to retain whatever African customs they could and to do their best to reject the imposition of European-American culture.

Clearly, based on the points covered in Chapter 1, the Afrocentric paradigm relies more heavily on the research and logic of Nobles (1974, 1980) and Herskovits (1941) than on that of Frazier (1939). Moreover, as it concerns the traditional methods used by enslaved Africans, free Africans before the abolition of slavery, and people of African descent following slavery's abolition, some maintain that these methods are quite similar to the ones used in the traditional West African societies from which African Americans are descended (Martin and Martin, 1985; Pollard, 1978; Ross, 1978). According to Martin and Martin (1985), during the years of slavery and the remainder of the nineteenth century, there were four institutions through which African Americans practiced self-help, and three of them can be said to reflect and validate traditional African cultural practices: (1) the extended family, (2) the black Church, and (3) mutual aid societies and benevolent organizations. In these institutions, African Americans merged traditional cultural practices and values of West Africa with European-American cultural values to shape ideas and methods of social welfare. Moreover, throughout these institutions, considerable status group cooperation between freed and enslaved African Americans led to a sense of collective consciousness and the belief that there were common problems, related to racial oppression, that all people of African descent faced (Jackson, Rhone, and Sanders, 1973; Martin and Martin, 1985; Pollard, 1978; Ross, 1978).

The extended family, previously discussed, was the prominent self-help institution among Africans in slavery and during the remainder of the nineteenth century. Through fictive-kin relations, African Americans were able to extend themselves in unlimited ways to offer support both financially and emotionally. Martin and Martin (1985) maintain that among enslaved Africans, the care of the elderly and the rearing of children were two prominent ways the spirit of mutual aid was demonstrated through the extended family. They suggest that since older slaves could not work as efficiently as younger slaves, often the younger slaves would assist the older slaves to accomplish their activities and would help the aged when they got sick. Additionally, similar to patterns in Africa, older slaves were designated as having special wisdom and were ascribed high status in the slave community (Gutman, 1976; Martin and Martin, 1985; Stuckey, 1987). The extended family worked on behalf of caring for children in that children did not have to fear lack of love or support if a parent died, got sick, or, in the case of many enslaved Africans, was sold to another planta-tion (Gutman, 1976; Martin and Martin, 1985). When these events oc-curred, the extendedness of family bonds and fictive kinship ensured that the children "would be absorbed naturally into existing households" (Mar-tin and Martin, 1985, p. 24).

The black church also was a primary institution of the black self-help tradition. The integration of spirituality throughout all aspects of society was a central feature of traditional African culture (Mbiti, 1970; Paris, 1995; Zahan, 1979) and affirmed a worldview that conceives the entire universe as interconnected and sacred (Lincoln and Mamiya, 1990; Mbiti, 1970; Paris, 1995). Although Christianity was not practiced in traditional West African culture before the European slave trade (Karenga, 1993; Mbiti, 1970), enslaved Africans were nonetheless able to use an alien religion, as imposed by slave masters and others, and adapt it to the spiritual ethos that characterized their worldview (Cone, 1969; Paris, 1995). In this sense, as Paris (1995) conveys, enslaved Africans relied on Eurocentric religious forms but integrated African-centered religious con-tent and style. The intense spirituality of the early African Americans fostered an emphasis on interconnectedness that helped them come togeth-er to pool their resources and talents to deal with the problems and pain of racial oppression. The black church then became a means through which the spirituality could be collectively expressed and a safe refuge to miti-gate the inimical effects of slavery and racial oppression (Billingsley and Caldwell, 1995; Cone, 1969; Frazier, 1964).

However, the black church was not only a place of refuge and emotion-al relief from the hardships of racial oppression; it also was the sponsor for the numerous mutual aid societies and benevolent organizations that were formed to provide services for African Americans. One of the first mutual aid societies was the *Free African Society,* established in 1787 in Philadel-phia. Through these mutual aid societies, a host of social services were provided, such as pensions for the elderly, widows, and children whose parents were dead; the operation of schools for children; burial services; sick dues to disabled persons; and companionship for incapacitated mem-bers (Davis, 1980; Martin and Martin, 1985). In addition, some of these societies, along with fraternal orders, operated insurance companies and other businesses (Davis, 1980). A good example of this was The True Reformers, founded by Reverend W. W. Browne, which operated a news-paper and a grocery chain (Davis, 1980). These mutual aid societies and fraternal orders emerged not only out of the need to provide services that were denied to African Americans in the broader white world but also from the survival of the traditional African cultural values of self-extendedness and group cohesiveness (Billingsley, 1994; Nobles, 1974; Martin and Martin, 1985).

Thus, the method of helping used by early African Americans centered on localized and personal assistance. Emphasis was placed on a sense of interdependency and collectivity that underscored the importance of religion and spirituality in the helping process. There was little or no opposition to providing social and human services through the auspices of the church, and the secular and the sacred were viewed as one. Although some emphasis was placed on individual responsibility and character building when attempting to explain individual failure, the belief was that individual failure could not be viewed in isolation but rather should be seen as collective failure, particularly racial oppression's failure to acknowledge the humanity of people of African ancestry.

The Change Toward Scientific Charity

During the late nineteenth century and early twentieth century, many African Americans began to adopt a new attitude about the provision of social and psychological support. This was due, in part, to the emergence and increasing professionalization of social work brought about by the precipitous rise in social problems and social instability resulting from the expansion of capitalism, urbanization, immigration, and migration (Lubove, 1983; Wenocur and Reisch, 1989). African Americans increasingly began to accept the ideas European Americans held about the resolution of poverty and the problems associated with it. To this extent, many African Americans began to relinquish and demean the traditional ways in which black people sought to provide one another with social and economic security (Martin and Martin, 1995). Grounded in a secular worldview, these new black "social workers" began to interpret the old methods used by African Americans as backward and unprofessional. This was attributed to their belief in the superiority of "scientific charity," which emphasized the secularization and bureaucratization of assistance that stressed the importance of a division of labor, efficiency, rationality, and nonduplication of services. Both the secularization and bureaucratization of services were results of the increasing legitimacy ascribed to the philosophy of positivism in the mid- to latter nineteenth century, which viewed religious and metaphysical interpretations and resolutions of social problems as invalid. These African-American reformers fell vulnerable to and internalized the dichotomy between the secular and the nonsecular and the seen and the unseen prevalent in European-American culture and Eurocentric social science. Any attention given to emotions, sentimentalization, or "mystical" powers of the metaphysical or unseen world was deemed as ludicrous and uncouth, and they concluded that the secular methods, with their focus on efficiency, rationality, and division of labor, were the best methods to address the problems that confronted blacks at that time (Martin and Martin, 1995).

It should be mentioned that the beliefs held by these early African-American social workers did not emerge in a vacuum. Several of them, such as George E. Haynes, Birdye Haynes, and Forrester B. Washington, were trained at white universities that were beginning to offer social work courses to blacks. Because the knowledge base was Eurocentric, affirming the ideas of leading European-American sociologists and psychologists of that time, early African-American social workers were indoctrinated with ideas that did not emerge from or validate traditional African concepts about human behavior and human society. Furthermore, once these workers graduated from these early training schools, many of them were employed in organizations, such as the National Urban League, or settlement houses that were financed by leading white philanthropists of that time, such as Julius Rosenwald. The Eurocentric indoctrination began in school, and its application was guaranteed by those who financed the activities of social workers because they did not fund programs that were inconsistent with their personal views on poverty and other social problems (Carlton-LaNey, 1994; Wenocur and Reisch, 1989).

It can be assumed, therefore, that many of these early African-American workers were "accommodationist" in the sense that they did not challenge the fundamental epistemological and ontological assumptions of Eurocentric social and behavioral science, but that they were "confrontationalist" in that they worked to eliminate racial discrimination and injustice. In not challenging the epistemological and ontological assumptions of Eurocentric social and behavioral science, as well as scientific charity, which is the practical manifestation of Eurocentric social science, these early African-American social workers either (1) adapted the Eurocentric knowledge base to explain and resolve racial discrimination, and/or (2) adapted or applied the Eurocentric knowledge base to describe or explain aspects of African-American life, such as family patterns, religious practices, or sociorecreational patterns. Thus, as will be argued in the remainder of the chapter, with some concrete examples, the knowledge base of early African-American social workers and reformers was an adaptation of Eurocentric epistemological and ontological assumptions to describe and explain phenomena that were specific to the African-American community and issues of concern, such as racism. Though this was important because it exploited Eurocentric paradigms for the purpose of advancing the African-American community within a European-American-dominated society, the strategy lacked a sense of intellectual autonomy. It did not affirm or acknowledge the possibility of applying traditional African philosophical assumptions as a foundation for developing alternative social science and social work models. The belief that probably undergirded the "knowledge base accomodationist stance" of these early African-American social workers and reformers was social science and scientific charity universalism: the belief that social science and scientific charity are culturally neutral, that they represent universal "truths" about human beings and human societies.

Evidence of Knowledge Base Accommodation

The evidence for the "knowledge base accomodationist stance" can be discerned in the writings of many of the early professional African-American social workers and social reformers. George Edmund Haynes, E. Franklin Frazier, Charles S. Johnson, and Forrester B. Washington, four leading giants in framing the knowledge base that would be used by professional African-American social workers, all embraced and advocated the superiority of the scientific method in describing, explaining, and solving the problems of African Americans, generally, and African-American families, specifically. All of these men were associated with the National Urban League, established in 1911. Known initially as the National League on Urban Conditions Among Negroes, the Urban League was founded to address, reduce, and eliminate the problems of increasing numbers of African Americans who were migrating to urban areas in the North and the South (Moore, 1981). The Urban League's philosophy and organizational aims affirmed the scientific method in two ways: (1) by conducting research that relied heavily on the emerging sociological research methods of that day and (2) by employing scientific charity methods, such as casework, to assist African-American families. The founders and proponents of Urban League philosophy believed in the superiority of the emerging scientific methods—as opposed to the traditional strategies of healing among African Americans—in bringing about positive social change for African Americans (Martin and Martin, 1995).

George Edmund Hayes was the Urban League's first executive director. Charles S. Johnson was editor of the Urban League's monthly periodical, *Opportunity*. Forrester B. Washington was the first executive director of the Detroit office of the Urban League and third director of the Atlanta School of Social Work, the first school of social work to specifically offer social work training to African Americans. Last, E. Franklin Frazier received a scholarship from the Urban League to study at the New York School of Social Work and was the second director of the Atlanta School of Social Work. All of these men published, and because they did, they can be said to have been among the first to lend a "black perspective" to professional social work's knowledge base.

Of the four, E. Franklin Frazier was perhaps the most prolific, and because he focused much of his writing on the African-American family, his ideas may have been more useful among social workers. In his five years (1922 to 1927) as director of the Atlanta School of Social Work, Frazier published twenty-eight articles (Edwards, 1968). Many of these articles were published in prominent black periodicals of the time, such as *Opportunity* and *The Crisis*. Even before Frazier published his renowned *The Negro Family in the United States* (1939), he had published on the African-American family (see Frazier, 1926, 1927). Two major themes in Frazier's work on the African-American family during his tenure as the director of the Atlanta School were (1) slavery had eliminated most—if not all—of the vestiges of African culture among African-American families, and (2) the adverse conditions of slavery were primary reasons for many of the psychological and social problems that afflicted African-American families. Frazier (1927) identified three factors that rendered the "Negro" family as a unique sociological unit. Two reasons are particularly important for the present discussion.

The first reason was the breach in cultural continuity from Africa. Frazier avouched that this cultural disconnect had demoralizing consequences for sex mores and for family control among enslaved Africans:

> While the Negro lived under institutionalized sex and family relations in Africa, . . . the African sex mores were thoroughly disorganized under the institution of slavery. . . . The slaves on the plantations lived in the demoralized condition that naturally followed the destruction of the African tribal and family controls. . . ." (Frazier, 1927, p. 165)

A second reason Frazier offered for why the African-American family should be considered a unique sociological unit was the African-American family's failure at assimilating Eurocentric cultural norms. Frazier (1927) again attributed this to "the total destruction of the African social heritage" (p. 166), which for him meant that the African-American family had no other cultural model than that of the European-American culture. The implications of Frazier's ideas, here, for the knowledge base accomodationist stance, are clear: since the African heritage was decimated by slavery, then cultural understanding of African-American families, specifically, and African Americans, generally, has its roots in slavery. Any attention given to Africa as a cultural foundation from which African

Americans could be understood, could advance themselves politically or economically, or could provide assistance to one another was considered inappropriate and invalid. Regarding the latter, Frazier was critical of the old "folk" ways African Americans used to help themselves and promoted the supremacy of the scientific method (see Frazier, 1924a). For Frazier, focusing on emotions, sentimentalization, or mystical powers of the metaphysical or spiritual world was crude and unscientific. For example, Frazier (1924b) believed that African Americans' attribution of their illnesses to magical or metaphysical factors, which is a critical component of traditional African culture (Appiah-Kubi, 1993; Ezeabasili, 1977), was a chief psychological barrier to the amelioration of their health.

Charles S. Johnson, the editor of *Opportunity* and graduate of the University of Chicago, was no less weak in his belief that slavery had destroyed the African cultural legacy among African Americans. He reflects this in the following statement:

> In the end, many of the distinguishing cultural traits [for blacks] disappeared under the necessity for prompt and complete accommodation to institutions of the new world . . . cultural differences among blacks . . . are not a matter of modifications of an African culture. . . . They represent progressive stages of adjustment to the accepted American standard. (Johnson, 1936, pp. 6, 56)

What both Johnson and Frazier seemingly validate is the acquiescence or accomodationist theory of enslaved Africans that Herskovits (1941) discusses as a major impediment among scholars in acknowledging the resiliency and persistency of African cultural forms among African Americans. In the end, for both men, Africa had nothing to do with explaining the behavior of African Americans and, certainly, could not be used as a cultural foundation for establishing different social service models.

Although Forrester B. Washington, director of the Atlanta School of Social Work from 1927 to 1954, seemingly did not spend much time musing over the survival of African culture, he, similar to Frazier and Johnson, believed in the superiority of the scientific method. Washington (1925) believed that one of the method's most important advantages was time efficiency. He felt the conservation and exploitation of time would preclude mistakes and make better use of financial support:

> First of all it [the scientific method] saves time. The scientific method also prevents waste. Waste always results by the old method of trial and error. . . . The saving of time means that a social worker can get more done for a given expenditure of money. (p. 166)

For Washington, the scientific method not only would save time and money; it also would preclude the use of impressions, or personal experience, as a professional means for determining reality. The reliance on impressions leads to "the circulation of considerable misinformation" (Washington, 1925, p. 168).

Probably, of the four men mentioned, Washington did the best at conceptualizing the need for including different content and ideas in social work education when examining and seeking to assist African Americans. In his article "The Need and Education of Negro Social Workers," Washington (1935) makes the case for specialized training for what he referred to as "social work among Negroes" (p. 88). He contended that social work among Negroes should be different in content from social work with whites. Two factors that should distinguish social work among Negroes from other forms of social work were that (1) attention should be given to the collective problems of African Americans rather than to "individual" problems, and (2) of the role race and racism play in contributing to the problems of African Americans should be acknowledged. Washington (1935) advocated that because of their intimate knowledge of the African-American community, African-American social workers "can accomplish more with Negro clients than white workers" (p. 78) and that historically black colleges and universities were the most appropriate setting for the training of African-American social workers. Expressing a view that was quite radical at that time, and even now, Washington felt that traditionally white colleges and universities were too generic in their approach to competently train social workers for practice with African Americans.

Although he affirmed that social work with African Americans should be different in content, Washington (1935) asserted that it should employ and incorporate the techniques basic to all social work practice. He especially promotes the view that these techniques should be used to mediate and eliminate the effects of racism on African Americans. Furthermore, although Washington highlights the need for a "survival strategy" among African Americans that should be a component of social work among "Negroes," he admonished that this survival strategy should not be confused with "a strategy for the survival of Negroes as a cultural entity" (p. 93). Washington does not provide any reasons for this but only says that he does not deny or affirm the value of "Negro" culture.

The latter comments from Washington provide evidence of the previous assertion that early professional African-American social workers and reformers were not (1) interested in affirming the cultural legacy of African Americans nor (2) using that legacy as a foundation to develop new social work techniques. Their focus, as reflected in Washington's views, appeared to be on assuaging and eliminating the effects of racial discrimination for African-Americans. Apparently, and from an Afrocentric viewpoint, they did not recognize the dimension of racism discussed earlier in the book, namely, cultural oppression. The question that arises is, for what reasons did they deny cultural oppression and the influence of traditional African culture on the African Americans they worked to serve and advance?

Reasons for Denial of Cultural Perspective

Martin and Martin (1995) maintain that there are two reasons for the omission of the cultural perspective among early African-American social workers and reformers: (1) the concern over appeasing their white funding sources and (2) their bourgeoisie mentality. It is interesting that, in their book, Martin and Martin cite one of E. Franklin Frazier's most popular books, *Black Bourgeoisie,* to support the latter reasons. This is remarkable because, although Frazier (1957) is critical of African-American social workers for being beholden to their white benefactors, for their inability "to engage in independent thinking" (p. 86), he did not see how his allegiance to the epistemological and ontological assumptions of Eurocentric social science incarcerated his thinking by preventing him from looking to traditional African culture as a means to obtain a new outlook on human behavior, generally, and African-American behavior, specifically. Nonetheless, the control that white philanthropic organizations had over the activities and services of pioneering African-American social workers did play a major role in restricting the perspectives of these social workers (Carlton-LaNey, 1994; Davis, 1980; Martin and Martin, 1995). Referring to it as a form of "indirect rule," Frazier (1957) maintained that the control of these organizations compelled African Americans to conform to European-American social philosophy, especially on race relations. In this way, the control of white philanthropic organizations helped to suppress a redefinition of the problems experienced by African Americans, as well as their causes and solutions (Davis, 1980).

Since many of the pioneering African-American social workers and social reformers were trained at white colleges and universities, as well as taught by white professors, it is important to examine the potential effects of this kind of training on the thinking of these early social workers and reformers. Jones (1974) presents an interesting analysis of the training of early African- American sociologists, who were likely to contribute to the knowledge base of social work since, at that time, social work and sociology were intimately connected. Jones (1974) contends that the white professors who trained the early African-American sociologists were paternalistic in their relationships with their African-American students and believed that they needed "external" direction in the shaping of their ideas. African-American students, it was thought, did not have the innate, internal drive to make appropriate decisions about areas of study and scholarship. Because these white professors controlled the access early African-American sociologists had to research grants, jobs, and publication in prestigious (white) academic journals, early African-American sociologists were well aware of the adverse corollaries of challenging or even straying from the precepts that their white professors and mentors held as proper scholarship (Jones, 1974).

To maintain more efficient control over these early African-American sociologists, white mentors selected and appointed an African-American protégé who they felt was especially acquiescent and accepting of what was deemed proper scholarship (Jones, 1974). Jones refers to these exceptional protégés as "overseers," whose subtle and sometimes manifest purpose was to monitor and criticize the ideas of other African-American sociologists who did not conform to the white sociological establishment's view of scholarship. In Chicago, Charles S. Johnson was selected for this position (Conyers, 1988; Jones, 1974; Martin and Martin, 1995). Johnson matriculated at the University of Chicago and studied under one of the most prominent white sociologists at that time, Robert E. Park (Conyers, 1988; Robbins, 1974). Park took special interest in Johnson and became a lifelong mentor of his. As a student of Park's, "Johnson . . . was, like Park, no radical, not even in race relations" (Conyers, 1988, p. 153). Park's influence in the African-American community, his perceived authority as the expert on race relations, and the location of the Julius Rosenwald Foundation in Chicago, a major financier of social reform activities during that time, rendered Charles Johnson a very likely and suitable choice as the gatekeeper of black sociology (Jones, 1974). In addition, his position as editor of *Opportunity* and his intimate relationship with powerful white philanthropists gave him immense influence over the direction and ideas of black social work (Martin and Martin, 1995).

A second possible reason for the denial of the cultural perspective was the bourgeoisie attitude of early African-American social workers. A critical dimension of this attitude is the unwillingness of professional African Americans to identify with, and emotionally connect to, the African-American masses, who lack formal education (Frazier, 1957; Martin and Martin, 1995). Feelings of resentment, embarrassment, and condescension of the African American elite toward the masses of African Americans are all conspicuous components of the bourgeoisie mentality. Some have suggested also that this bourgeoisie mentality reflects intense feelings of racial self-hatred brought about by the internalization of messages of African inferiority found in European-American culture and society (Atwell and Azibo, 1991; Kambon, 1992; Welsing, 1991). These feelings among the black bourgeoisie are heightened and reinforced by the rejection and contempt they experience from the white world, even when they have attained high socioeconomic status and have demonstrated their ability to conform to white, middle-class norms (Frazier, 1957).

Martin and Martin (1995) maintain that this bourgeoisie mentality among the early African-American reformers and social workers prevented them from respecting and validating the viewpoints and experiences of the masses of African Americans who were migrating rapidly to the North. Concluding that these migrants were uncouth and unrefined, early African-American social workers failed to consider the narratives, interpretations, and experiences of the migrants as legitimate sources from which to identify the problems of the migrants and to develop social work practice interventions (Martin and Martin, 1995). Since the strategies and techniques that the migrants used to identify their problems and to ease their pain were grounded in the validation of spirituality and affect (Martin and Martin, 1995), the failure of African-American social workers to integrate the interpretations and narratives of the African-American masses not only alienated them from the masses but also further alienated them from their African cultural origins, in which the spiritual and affective components of humans were affirmed and integrated in the healing process (see Appiah-Kubi, 1993; Brisbane and Womble, 1991). Regrettably, the opportunity, among early African-American social workers, to use traditional African philosophical assumptions as a foundation to construct social work practice models was squandered. This tradition and practice would continue into the present, as many contemporary African-American social workers, and social workers generally, do not recognize traditional African and African-American culture as cogent sources to anchor social work practice models and ideas.

Chapter 4

Oppression and Spiritual Alienation

THE RELATIONSHIP BETWEEN OPPRESSION
AND SPIRITUAL ALIENATION

Schiele (1996, 1997) maintains that for the Afrocentric paradigm of human service, oppression and spiritual alienation are the primary sources of many of the problems that afflict American society. Oppression can be described "as a systematic and deliberate strategy to suppress the power and potentiality of people by legitimizing and institutionalizing inhumanistic and person-delimiting values such as materialism, fragmentation, individualism, and inordinate competition" (Schiele, 1996, p. 288). Spiritual alienation, according to Schiele (1996), "is the disconnection of nonmaterial and morally affirming values from concepts of human self-worth and from the character of social relationships" (p. 289). For this book's purpose, both oppression and spiritual alienation are not conceived as universal concepts with static meanings that can be equally applied to all groups and all historic periods. Rather, the Afrocentric paradigm contextualizes oppression and spiritual alienation. Although common attributes of oppression and spiritual alienation are acknowledged, it is believed that both can be understood more precisely and appropriately if they are conceived within the cultural context that has produced them and in which they both occur.

The cultural context addressed in this book is that of the United States. Although the United States comprises varied ethnic and cultural groups, the worldviews of these groups are not given equal political status (Asante, 1992). Instead, the United States can be thought of as a society with many cultural groups but also with a hierarchy that ascribes more significance to some cultural groups and less importance to others. The significance of a cultural group in the United States parallels that group's degree of political and economic power. Since people of European descent historically in this country have possessed and wielded more power than other groups, it can be suggested that the various cultural perspectives of these descendents of Europe dominate the American cultural landscape. Increasingly, Afrocentrists have referred to the collective attributes of the diverse European perspectives represented in the United States as comprising a European-American culture that affirms and projects a Eurocentric worldview (Akbar, 1984; Asante, 1980, 1988, 1990; Baldwin, 1985; Baldwin and Hopkins, 1990; Bekerie, 1994; Bell, Bouie, and Baldwin 1990; Boykin, 1983; Karenga, 1993; Khatib et al., 1979; Schiele, 1996; Verharen, 1995). An Afrocentric viewpoint would exhort that oppression and spiritual alienation in the United States be understood within the context of the dominance of the Eurocentric worldview. This worldview can be defined succinctly as the unique and diverse manner in which European-American culture interprets events and defines reality.

In this discussion, oppression and spiritual alienation are viewed as interrelated and interdependent phenomena. Oppression drives and cultivates spiritual alienation, and spiritual alienation undergirds and nurtures oppression. A critical difference in distinguishing the roles of each is that oppression is viewed more as the conduit through which spiritual alienation is able to maximally express itself. Oppression provides spiritual alienation with a "structure" through which societal institutions and human relationships are formed and sustained. It can be said, therefore, that, of the two, spiritual alienation is the most robust in that it lays the foundation for, and is an outcome of, oppression in the United States. As foundation, spiritual alienation provides the philosophical justification for oppression as a normative activity needed to advance human societies materially. As outcome, spiritual alienation pervades the beliefs, behaviors, and relationships of people.

It must be noted that although spiritual alienation is conceived as a cause and an outcome of oppression, cause and effect are difficult to separate when temporal conditions in human thought and action are arduous to determine or when time itself is viewed holistically rather than linearly. In this regard, some of the content in the discussion of spiritual alienation as cause may mirror and be reinforced in the discussion of spiritual alienation as outcome. Every effort is made, however, to convey similar content differently, that is, to ensure that content on spiritual alienation is presented in its appropriate and hypothesized relationship to oppression.

SPIRITUAL ALIENATION AS PHILOSOPHICAL FOUNDATION OF OPPRESSION

To understand spiritual alienation as a philosophical foundation of oppression in the United States, it is important to examine some of the predominant philosophical themes of Western society. These themes can best be gleaned from some of the more prominent philosophers of the Western tradition. Ani (1994) maintains that the roots of what she refers to as the despiritualization of Western culture lie in the prominence of the ideas of Plato and Aristotle. These ideas, although dormant in much of Europe during the medieval era, were revitalized in the writings of people such as Francis Bacon and René Descartes during the seventeenth century (West, 1982) and have created, because of their persistence over time and their role in contributing to social malaise and psychic dismemberment, what Berman (1981) has identified as a "disenchanted world."

Plato is probably the most important Greek philosopher for the purpose of this discussion because it is he who is credited with transforming the relationship between knower and known from one of emotional connection to one in which the emotional link was severed (Ani, 1994; Havelock, 1963). By severing the emotional attachment or connection of knower from the known, the known became objectified, viewed as an object external to the knower. This provided the impetus for what is generally termed objectification. Not only did this process render the known an object; it also reconceptualized the self or knower from a cosmic spiritual being—one who relied on symbols and allegory as the basis of knowledge—to a thinking subject who relied on cognition and calculation (Ani, 1994; Havelock, 1963). In this reconceptualization, it can be suggested that both the knower and the known were stripped of a spiritual, transcendent essence.

The paucity of spiritual essence and emotional connection that characterized Plato's epistemology created considerable concern over control (Ani, 1994; Havelock, 1963; Plato, 1992). The concern over control had two connotations: (1) control over self and (2) control over others (Ani, 1994; Harris, 1997; Havelock, 1963; Plato, 1992). Control over self meant that the self should not be manipulated by its context or milieu and that the various components of the self should work harmoniously to execute the functions for which they were inherently designed. The best way to achieve this harmony and control was for the self to gain mastery over its emotions or appetites, which were deemed inferior and oppositional to reason, or what Plato called the "rational desires." Once one had control of self, and had emotionally separated self from others, then one could be in a better position to exercise control over others, especially when the others (i.e., the objects) were believed to not be in control of themselves, or, in other words, were governed by their emotions or appetites. In the *Republic,* for example, Plato maintains that the tripartite components of the psyche—appetitive, spirited, and rational desires—mirror the class divisions found in society in that the desires determined which occupational activities were more appropriate for which people (Plato, 1992). This conceptualization can foster oppression because critical to many concepts of oppression is the justification of the masses being regulated and controlled by the few (Turner, Singleton, and Musick, 1984; Young, 1990). Furthermore, oppression is not only based on the belief that the masses are unintelligent (e.g., lacking self-mastery over emotions) but also on the belief in the absence of an emotional connection between and among people (Burgest, 1981; Schiele, 1994). In this sense, Plato's objectification validates the notion of insular identity or an isolated self that is thought to be independent of others as well as nature and God (Harris, 1997; Lovejoy, 1966).

The focus on objectification found in Plato's theory of knowledge was undergirded and paralleled by dichotomous logic. Once humans and nature were separated from their organic oneness, the notion that phenomena could be understood fragmentarily led to a logical system that viewed both ideas and concrete events as being best understood through dichotomization (Ani, 1994; Burgest, 1981). Because of its emphasis on the laws of contradiction (Dixon, 1976), the implication for either/or logic in buttressing oppression is that it encourages focus to be placed on conflict, difference, and exclusion rather than on unity, similarity, and inclusion (Baldwin and Hopkins, 1990; Dixon, 1976). The emphasis on conflict reinforces the concern for control and domination. As a foundation of oppression, the focus on conflict assumes that the ability to survive and prosper hinges on one's ability to adapt to hardships and struggle. Human struggle is considered to be a natural and integral component of human existence. Those who survive and prosper, then, are thought to be better fit to handle hardships and more capable of exercising control over those who are deemed unfit. This thinking ultimately valorizes human strength and fortitude, and, in this sense, creates the political ideology of possessive individualism—the belief that all successes and failures are attributed to the lone individual who owes nothing to the larger society (MacPherson, 1962).

Although difference among humans should be acknowledged and can be appreciated, the either/or logical tradition in Western philosophy has often encouraged a view of difference that has been bastardized and imbued with pejorative meanings (Baldwin and Hopkins, 1990; Schiele, 1994; Swigonski, 1996). Human difference or diversity, in this worldview, denies the existence of unity in polarity and thus seeks to separate people into mutually exclusive categories that are conceived antagonistically and as contradictions. Once people are bifurcated into mutually exclusive categories that are believed to be in conflict, a sense of cynicism about the intentions of oneself and others can emerge. This can influence the rise in ideas which accentuate the inherent evil in humans or which validate the penchant for humans to behave mischievously, selfishly, and aggressively. Ideas that underscore the inherent potential of humans to behave morally, affably, or altruistically are suppressed and, in many human behavior theories emanating from the West, are disavowed (Wakefield, 1993). The concept of humans as inherently mischievous and selfish in the European intellectual tradition may be attributed to concepts of morality found in the *Republic*. In it, Plato (1992) suggests that all people are corruptible, and because they are corruptible, they must be compelled to behave morally. The corruptible nature of humans that Plato assumes prompts him to conclude that justice is practiced unwillingly. This penchant in European-American cultural and intellectual thought can engender oppression because the existence of oppression from an Afrocentric viewpoint is predicated on at least two beliefs: (1) an "I have to get him or her before he or she gets me" line of reasoning, which promotes cynicism, and (2) human malevolence cannot be prevented; it is a predetermined and presumed human trait (Schiele, 1996, 1997).

The separation of self from others and self from the cosmic and spiritual world and the application of dichotomous logic are supported further when there is a juxtaposition of hierarchical thinking. Hierarchical thinking can be thought of as an extension of dichotomous logic. At the core of its thrust is the notion that some ideas, groups, or individuals are better or more supreme than other ideas, groups, or individuals (Rothenberg, 1990; Schiele, 1994). Undergirding this assumption is the notion that universal standards or criteria can be used to assess all aspects of life for diverse groupings of people. Young (1990) maintains that this assumption is the foundation of cultural oppression, which justifies the use of one group's norms and mores as the basis for normative thought and behavior for all.

The notion of universalism, when combined with objectification and dichotomous logic, dissuades an appreciation of human diversity and relegates certain distinctions and variations in human values and behavior as inferior or superior. Thus, one can argue that the notions of inferiority and superiority germinate partly from the value of cultural universalism. Moreover, this notion and practice of universalism can be viewed as a corollary of Plato's objectification in that, for example, European Enlightenment concepts of universal truth were based heavily on the belief that one should have, and had, the ability to transcend his or her biases (i.e., values and emotions) so that reasoning could be promoted as a superior strategy to accurately obtain the truth (Berman, 1981; Hekman, 1986; Smith, 1993). Because it was undergirded by notions of universalism, this form of human epistemology was transformed into ideology and, in the sixteenth through nineteenth centuries, used to justify European exploitation and enslavement of nations and people of color (Clarke, 1991; Leonard, 1995; Mosse, 1978). The transatlantic slave trade that emerged from this ideology significantly helped to advance capitalism in the United States and throughout the world (Bailey, 1992; Blaut, 1993; Hobson, 1949; Williams, 1944). Thus, it can be maintained that the values often associated with capitalism—competition, efficiency, individualism, and greed—have their origins in an epistemology of rationality and objectification.

SPIRITUAL ALIENATION
AS OUTCOME OF OPPRESSION

Just as spiritual alienation can be grasped as a cause of oppression, it also can be viewed as a consequence of oppression. This is important to note because often in discussions and debates on oppression, attention tends to be given to the political and economic outcomes of oppression (Asante, 1987; Karenga, 1993; Schiele, 1993) that focus exclusively on the inequitable distribution of resources and wealth. Although this is significant, and certainly a component of understanding oppression from an Afrocentric viewpoint, it is not the only, or even may be the less critical, corollary of oppression. A crucial aspect of the definition of oppression noted earlier was the emphasis on suppressing the potentiality of people. If potentiality is conceptualized multidimensionally, then the nonmaterial aspects of one's potential should be recognized. When nonmaterial aspects of potentiality are marginalized, the material exploitation, deprivation, and avarice that accompany oppression are more likely to develop.

To speak of spiritual alienation as an outcome of oppression is to fundamentally recognize the existence, within a sociocultural milieu, of a disconnect among people and between people, nature, and God. This disconnect is expressed in behaviors that manifest themselves as social problems and in beliefs that may be thought of as the foundation for many of these problems. The beliefs that may facilitate this disconnect are as follows: (1) the belief in the unidimensional and conflict-driven human being; (2) the belief that human life and nature are disparate and antagonistic entities; (3) the belief that the material world is separate from, and more valid than, the spiritual world; and (4) the belief in the objectification of God.

The Unidimensional and Conflict-Driven Human Being

An unfortunate outcome of objectification is the belief in the unidimensional and conflict-driven human being. This unidimensional and conflict-driven perspective is manifested best in two beliefs: (1) humans lack a substantive core that transcends time and space, and (2) humans are innately prone to evil and mischief.

The belief that humans lack a core or essence that transcends time and space limits human potentiality because human potential is restricted to what one does in the current material plane. By confining one's perspective to this plane, the resources from which one can draw to maximize human achievement are diminished. This unidimensional outlook on the human being also tends to foster a starved notion of human existence, joy, and self-worth because these concepts often are exclusively associated with material and physical attributes, such as how much and what one owns, how one looks, and how fast or far one's career advances (Myers, 1988; Schiele, 1996). These material criteria of human self-worth are reinforced by the concern over, and energy expended in, demonstrating that one is a successful, individual competitor. Supported by the devaluation of dependency, some maintain that the concern about one's ability to successfully compete is a primary source of anxiety in Western culture (Fromm, 1941; May, 1977).

The repudiation that humans lack a core that transcends time and space also tends to isolate time as a material phenomenon. With the overlay of objectification and aggression, time becomes an object to compete against or overcome. The "rat race" many people speak of becomes the race against the finiteness of time, a futile race to defeat the future. The future as a source of competition, and finite time, can trigger severe and undue stress on human relations (1) because the quality and completeness of these relationships are compromised by the substantive emphasis on the material dimensions of these relationships, and (2) because individuals can become trapped in the notion that life is only a series of material battles that must be overcome and that those who are more effective in overcoming these battles are more efficient in their use of finite time.

The belief that humans have a proclivity toward evil and mischievousness is especially important in comprehending the notion of the conflict-driven human being. To perpetuate the belief that the essence of human nature is evil reduces human potential and robs humans of their inherent capability of self-regulation and moral behavior. In addition, excessive validity ascribed to the belief in the inherent inclination of humans toward evil inhibits people from viewing human life as sacred. There is little recognition that humans are partial manifestations of God or a Creator who has endowed all with the potential to be judicious and morally affir-ming. Within this framework, human fallacy and wrongdoings tend to be attributed to human nature or instincts rather than to human judgment and adverse social conditions (such as oppression) that frequently place people at risk of malevolence. The belief in the instinctual, mischievous human can dismiss decadent behavior and conflictual human relationships as normal outcomes of human interaction (Schiele, 1994). This can engender unnecessary social conflict and psychosocial pain that can bring about the destruction of a society from within.

Human Life and Nature As Separate and Antagonistic

This disconnect among people and between people, nature, and God also is facilitated by the belief that human life and nature are disparate and antagonistic entities. When humans are separated from and seen as opposi-tional to nature, the rise in the rape and exploitation of nature is justified and occurs (Capra, 1982; Cohen, 1996; Dixon, 1976). Nature becomes desacralized and viewed as a force to be shaped and controlled by humans for their pleasure and comfort (Cohen, 1996). Nature becomes something "out there" that can be a danger to humans if not properly managed and accurately predicted. Although nature can pose a threat to humans, this objectification of nature fails to allow humans to conceive nature as vener-able and intimately a part of humanity.

According to Cohen (1996), this disconnect from nature not only sup-ports the assumption that humans should dominate and exploit nature, but also influences two other assumptions: (1) material consumption is synon-ymous with human fulfillment, and (2) technological invention and eco-nomic growth are inherently favorable. The assumption that material con-sumption is akin to human fulfillment can reinforce and nurture a society in which consumerism takes precedence over the quality of interpersonal relations. Things, and their acquisition, become the primary goal of life and the basis on which people define themselves and, too often, their relationships. Although consumption of food and the use of natural re-sources are important to sustain human life, they do not have to be inter-preted as ends in themselves. The notion of consumption as an end in itself renders humans as mere instinctual entities whose sole life purpose is to physically survive and materially prosper. This leaves little or no room for spiritual and moral development because the idea of "human" is restricted to material and physical dimensions. Thus, consumerism and the view of humans as primarily material and physical beings reinforce each other and, when the public is sold on both concepts, suppress critiques of the defilement of nature, making it easier for the architects of environmental exploitation to continue their activities.

The belief that technological invention and economic growth are inherently and invariably favorable also fosters the disconnect between people and nature. The role of technology in environmental imperialism and resource depletion often is masked by the convenience and pleasure technology affords (Ladd, 1988; Marcuse, 1964). Considerable emphasis on material production, wealth, and efficiency can generate economic modes that rely on the abuse of natural resources (Capra, 1982; Ladd, 1988; Marcuse, 1964). Less attention within these economic modes, such as with capitalism, is given to the preservation and safety of nature because critical to the concern of these economies is the existence of material inequality, the maximization of efficiency, and the containment of production costs (Rose, 1989; Wayne, 1986). Nature, then, becomes the feeder, the source upon which inequality, efficiency, cost containment, and capital accumulation are maintained. In short, nature becomes synonymous with capital and economic growth for the owners and investors of corporations. The focus on economic growth and technological invention has become more apparent with more discussion of the effects of the global economy on restricting the already limited "polluting space" the planet can sustain (Barbosa, 1990).

It should be noted that although Cohen's (1996) assumptions regarding the relationships among material consumption, technological and economic growth, and the objectification of nature are important, the Afrocentric paradigm would maintain that an emphasis on materialism alone does not automatically lead to objectification of nature. Rather, as Akbar (1994) observes, the problem arises when material advancement is separated from spiritual development. If the two were merged, material development via economic and technological advancement would be understood as an extension, and as an affirmation, of a deeper spiritual concern. Guided by a profound sense of spirituality, a sense of the interconnectedness of all elements of the universe, *spiritual materialism* would prevent the exploitation of not only nature but also people. This is because (1) an economic surplus would only be achieved when everyone's material needs have been adequately satisfied, and (2) nature would be valued more since it would be internalized by people.

The Separation of the Material and Spiritual Worlds

In the preceding section, a connection between material and spiritual development was said to be valuable in preventing exploitation of humans and nature. This lack of association between material and spiritual development found in U.S. society is supported by a more fundamental belief that the material and spiritual worlds are separate. What is validated in U.S. society is what can be called an empiricist view of the world that primarily accentuates experiences tapped through the five senses and relegates paranormal experiences, or those which exist outside of the five senses, as less credible. By being less credible, issues of the unseen, or spirituality, are generally not given as much attention as are phenomena that can be seen. When applied to the human makeup, the soul, which some contend is a critical aspect of human beings, is downplayed in favor of concerns regarding the mind and body (Akbar, 1984; Bolling, 1990; Elkins, 1995; Myers, 1988; Sermabeikian, 1994). Further, in the human or social sciences, as well as in the human services, where one may think that issues of the soul or spirituality should be explored, there is a tendency to view the soul as the exclusive purview of theology and, in some cases, philosophy.

The fallout of this separation between the material and spiritual not only restricts the growth of the human sciences and human services but also has profound implications for an absence of what some called "spiritual wellness" (see Bensley, 1991; Chandler, Holden, and Kolander, 1992; McGuire, 1993; Westgate, 1996). Westgate (1996) defines spiritual wellness as "openness to the spiritual dimension that permits the integration of one's spirituality with the other dimensions of life, thus maximizing the potential for growth and self-actualization" (p. 27). Westgate further maintains that a paucity of spiritual wellness has been shown to contribute to depression in a number of studies. This is an important observation because, until recently, depression was the most prevalent psychiatric disorder among the U.S. population and, today, is only second in prevalence to anxiety disorders (Levenson, 1997). In addition, depression has been shown to be associated with a host of disorders, such as substance abuse, child abuse, unemployment, suicide, sleep disturbance, and violence (see Bazargan, 1996; Chaffin, Kelleher, and Hollenberg, 1996; Gary, 1985; Harvey et al., 1996; Malmquist, 1995; Wolk and Weissman, 1996).

For some, such as May (1975), the lack of spiritual wellness and the need for psychotherapy in U.S. society are associated with objectification, which has influenced the decline in this society's reliance and integration of symbols and myths. For May (1975), symbols and myth help orient people to the cosmos and give a more substantial meaning to their lives and their relationships. Without symbols and myths, or when they degenerate in a society, May believes people experience greater anxiety and alienation, which are primary reasons for the interpersonal problems in their lives. May's assessment fits well into the current analysis about spiritual alienation. However, similar to many writers from the humanistic school, May makes little or no connection between spiritual alienation and oppression. Most of May's attention is devoted to how an absence of spiritual wellness affects the intrapsychic aspects of the individual client or person or his or her intimate relations. Although there is recognition of the roles objectification and Western intellectual tradition have played in bringing about the spiritual malaise and other psychological problems prevalent in the United States (see Elkins, 1995; May, 1983), many in the humanistic school still rely on individualistic solutions, such as psychotherapy, to redress the problem. Although individualistic solutions are appropriate from an Afrocentric perspective, the Afrocentric paradigm's holistic framework would suggest that macrosolutions should also be employed to prevent and arrest spiritual alienation and its effects. Indeed, if the individual is viewed as being invariably influenced by his or her environment, which is an Afrocentric precept, both the individual and the environment must be targeted for change simultaneously.

Since the social environment comprises complex and interrelated aggregates of people and their behaviors, macrosolutions are aimed at altering the collective mind-set and behavior of people. The collective mind-set and behavior of people within a given society are affected best by the traditions of the society that become institutionalized via the various organizations in the society, both formal and informal. Macrosolutions aimed at eliminating the spiritual alienation that is assumed to imbue the organizations and relationships in the United States must address the need to reconceptualize the basic values underpinning the stated policies and unstated practices of the land. From an Afrocentric perspective, rethinking and altering social policies and social planning, for example, are two important strategies at the macrolevel. The issue of an Afrocentric social policy framework and social welfare philosophy is addressed in more detail in Chapters 7 and 8.

An additional problem with the literature on spiritual wellness and spirituality from an Afrocentric framework is that contributions from the traditions of Africa are usually omitted or downplayed in favor of an accentuation of Eastern (i.e., Chinese and Indian) and Western (i.e., American and European) traditions. The omission of the contributions of Africa in understanding and explaining spirituality is problematic for at least two reasons. First, several scholars maintain that Africa is the cradle of human civilization (see Ben-Jochannon, 1971; Cann, 1987; Diop, 1974; Montagu, 1958). Several scholars who have acknowledged this and who have studied early African civilizations, especially in the Nile Valley, assert that spirituality was at the core of ancient African philosophical and scientific endeavors and was integrated throughout these societies (Akbar, 1994; Ameen, 1990; Asante, 1990; Diop, 1991; Finch, 1982; James, 1954; Van Sertima, 1989). Omitting the intellectual and philosophical traditions of what some refer to as the cradle of humanity is to be oblivious of the foundations upon which later civilizations may have based their concepts of spirituality and spiritual wellness.

Second, not recognizing the intellectual and philosophical traditions of Africa reinforces the notion, born of the transatlantic slave trade, that Africans were without a culture or, if they had one, that it was savage and undeveloped. These notions, which are deeply embedded in the American psyche, can preclude social scientists and others interested in advancing spiritual wellness in the United States from drawing upon the ideas and contributions that have emerged from Africa.

Objectification of God

The last belief that facilitates spiritual alienation in U.S. society is the objectification of God, that God is an external entity, an object that is separate from human beings. Since discussions about God and the soul have been relegated mostly to religion in the United States, concepts of God in the United States are best discerned by perusing the Judeo-Christian tradition. Religion is a powerful force in the United States, as indicated by data revealing that the majority of Americans not only believe in a God or Supreme Being but also attend religious services regularly (National Opinion Research Center, 1994). Further, as noted by Elkins (1995), "the religion or mythology of a culture is probably the best reflection of its values" (p. 88).

The goal here is not to provide a detailed explication of if or why the Judeo-Christian tradition does or may objectify God. Rather, the objective of this analysis is to identify some possible consequences of a society's supporting the view that God is external to human beings. This analysis relies on the assumption that religion and philosophy are inseparable and interrelated entities. If this is so, and if, as Ani (1994) maintains, the religion of Europe and the United States reflects the despiritualization and rationalization characteristic of much of Western philosophy, then the value placed on objectification could have permeated, or at least influenced, ideas about God.

There are at least two adverse consequences of social relations when God is objectified: (1) objectification tends to marginalize God's majesty and role in human achievement, and (2) it can influence people to more easily justify their roles in unfavorable deeds against others. When God is objectified, there is a proclivity to marginalize the role that God plays in enabling human achievement. When God is subjectified, however, the notion that human achievement is more than the mere coalescence of opportunity, training, and hard work is upheld. It adds to the idea that all humans have great inherent potential that is a function of being partial manifestations of a Creator. It further assumes that the things we often attribute success to, such as perseverance, talent, hard work, and patience, are all characteristics of God. If humans are viewed as partial manifestations of God, it can be maintained that all human achievement has been modeled after the achievement of God. This then places human achievement within the overall achievement of creation, which stretches into the depths of time. Objectifying God severs human achievement from the timeless achievement of the creation of all things and elements of the universe and renders human achievement the result of human activity only.

The fallout of this for human beings is that it can nurture a bland form of humanism that rejects a spiritual essence and reduces achievement to an inducement to maximize human competition. As such, achievement is transformed into an unsacred commodity that can be socially bought and sold, as necessary, to surpass and defeat others. Although some degree of competition is accepted within the Afrocentric paradigm, the problem with achievement being separated from its spiritual essence and being primarily associated with competition is that it can become a means to demonstrate the superiority of one over another. This situation can encourage a society to become preoccupied with competition and to associate self-worth with the defeat of others and of time. The preoccupation with competition and with the defeat of others and time can engender shallow relationships, at both the micro- and macrolevels of social existence, that are starved for mutual respect, consideration of differences, the virtue of patience, and the comfort of security. Indeed, competition has been said to engender feelings of insecurity that can lead to anxiety (Fromm, 1941; May, 1977).

Second, objectifying God can render the justification of unfavorable acts toward others more acceptable. Broadly speaking, objectification of God can increase the chances of immorality and selfishness. More specifically, the justification of inimical acts, brought on by God objectification, can nurture the likelihood of at least two phenomena: (1) the injudicious use of power and (2) the intellectualization of morality.

Objectifying God can bring about the injudicious use of power because, by not internalizing God, power, which is assumed to be a production of God, can take on a meaning conducive to exploitation. The meaning of power, therefore, becomes desacralized. Despite arguments that maintain that power absolutely corrupts all people all the time, power does not have to be conceived this way when God is internalized or when the concept of

God assumes new meaning. In large part, the origins of the concept of negative power can be attributed to the doctrine of the Judeo-Christian ethic in which one is taught that God is to be feared and obeyed, and, if not, he (a male God) will employ his massive powers to punish and exert calamity on humanity (see Harkness, 1957). This concept of God engenders an antagonistic relationship between people and God and, when applied to human relations, can shape a definition of human power that underscores conflict and punitive control.

The belief that power is inherently evil also has additional consequences. First, it obviates power from being conceived positively or as a means to bring about social justice. Second, it can prevent oppressed groups, especially those which adhere to concepts of power as evil, from using and coalescing their power to fight against the oppression that afflicts them. Third, it facilitates the belief that power must be seized by a few to efficiently control the inferior or injudicious "others" so as to expedite human progress or to promote the unequal distribution of resources. That power must be seized by a few to control the inferior masses and to justify a disparate distribution of resources creates an arrogant power elite and can render the masses of people invariably suspicious of concentrated power. For example, suspiciousness of concentrated power lies at the cornerstone of the thinking of those who established the U.S. Constitution (see Jansson, 1993; Kohl, 1989).

Suspiciousness of concentrated power, even in its representative form, can generate problems in human relations. Since concentrated power is usually held by those who are considered leaders of the society, the distrust that citizens have of their civic leaders also may trickle down to their intimate relationships. The logic is that if civic leaders are supposed to represent models of excellence and are distrusted by the general citizenry, then ordinary citizens may not expect human excellence and trust among themselves.

If God is subjectified or internalized, which is consistent with traditional African philosophical thought, as discussed in Chapter 2, a different view of power could prevail. This concept would promote the belief that, although there is always a chance of humans abusing power, power can be conceived and employed constructively. Here, the notion of "compassionate power" replaces the idea of "sinister power," or concentrated power aimed at exploitation. In compassionate power, the purpose and expectation is not to harm or hoard; rather, its aim is to make the best use of human ingenuity to maximize human morality and collective human well-being. Instead of using fear or seduction to uphold it, compassionate power relies on support, honesty, and love.

The justification of pernicious acts toward others, viewed as a function of God objectification, also can foster the intellectualization of morality. The intellectualization of morality is the cultural process through which morality is disconnected from behavior and becomes exclusively or primarily linked with ideas. In essence, morality becomes an abstraction, and, as an abstraction, it has often, in Western thought, become associated with one's ability to reason (Akbar, 1994; Ani, 1994). Some say this emphasis on ideas over concrete behavior is based on the belief that the idea or abstraction is more real than the behavior (Ani, 1994; Havelock, 1963; Lovejoy, 1966). This was justified because it was thought that the idea was timeless and more permanent than concrete behavior (Havelock, 1963; Lovejoy, 1966).

The consequence this has for enhancing the likelihood of defending unfavorable acts against others is that people can be deemed moral without their behavior being critically evaluated. Deleterious behavior toward others loses significance, and its contradiction to what may be considered moral beliefs is accepted or at least tolerated. In this sense, morality becomes despiritualized because pivotal to the definition of spirituality offered in this chapter was the notion of interconnectedness. This notion is not confined to the interdependence of elements of the universe; it also should extend to the interconnectedness between human thought and human action. Moreover, the rationalization of morality generates and nurtures deceit in that moral ideas may not translate into moral deeds (Ani, 1994).

The deceit and contradiction brought on by the intellectualization of morality has important implications for furthering oppression and social problems in the United States. If too much disparity exists between what is said and what is done in a given culture, cynicism is likely to emerge as an acceptable and core component of that culture. As an accepted and important component, cynicism becomes a central element in shaping societal relations that are characterized by aggression and excessive competition. This then validates the negative concept and injudicious use of power discussed previously, perpetuates the psychological need to oppress, and popularizes the idea of humans as innately sinister, mischievous, and selfish.

Chapter 5

Youth Violence
and the Afrocentric Paradigm

This chapter and the next will apply the theoretical and historical ideas found in the previous chapters to provide an explanation for, and solutions to, two significant social and public health problems of contemporary times: (1) youth violence and (2) substance abuse. Both problems are interrelated in that researchers have found youth violence to contribute to substance abuse (Zimmerman and Maton, 1992) and substance abuse to influence youth violence (Lowry et al., 1995; Webber, 1997). In explaining these problems, it is important to mention that the Afrocentric paradigm does not assert universality: its explanations may not be appropriate for all young persons who commit violence or for all drug abusers. However, some broad assumptions will be presented, and these assumptions will be grounded in the Afrocentric paradigm.

OVERVIEW OF YOUTH VIOLENCE

The type of youth violence that is referred to in this chapter is youth street violence or youth violent crime. The specific crimes are (1) homicide, (2) aggravated assault, (3) rape, and (4) robbery. In addition, youth violence will be conceptualized more broadly to connote what some refer to as *interpersonal violence*, which is a form of individual aggression

Portions of this chapter originally appeared in "Cultural Alignment, African-American Male Youths, and Violent Crime," *Journal of Human Behavior in the Social Environment*, 1998, 1(2/3), pp. 165-181; "Afrocentricity: An Emerging Paradigm in Social Work Practice," *Social Work*, 1996, 41(3), pp. 284-294. Reprinted with permission from The Haworth Press, Inc., and the National Association of Social Workers.

perpetrated against another that may or may not lead to criminal arrest and prosecution (Hilton, Harris, and Rice, 1998; Lowry et al., 1995). It is, however, youth violent crime that generally receives more attention, primarily because of the severity of the aggression and its grave criminal consequences for the youths themselves as well as the social consequences to society at large. During the early 1990s, youth violent crime increased, rising from 95,677 arrests in 1991 to 125,141 arrests in 1994 (U.S. Bureau of the Census, 1998). However, youth arrests for violent crimes declined between 1994 and 1996 from 125,141 arrests to 104,598 arrests (U.S. Bureau of the Census, 1998). This decline does not negate the years of devastation youth violence has had on these youths, their families, and the broader society. Furthermore, although youth violent crime has declined overall, some segments of youths, such as young African-American males, continue to show high arrest and victimization rates (U.S. Department of Justice, Federal Bureau of Investigation, 1998).

The response of many governmental officials to the increase in, and devastation caused by, youth violent crime is to get tougher on punishment. The "three strikes and you're out" campaign, mandatory drug sentences, and, more recently, the U.S. House of Representatives' passage of HR3 (the Juvenile Crime Control Act) and the U.S. Senate's consideration of S10 (the Violent and Repeat Juvenile Offender Act)—both policies include provisions to increase youth placements in adult correctional facilities—indicate a growing intolerance and frustration with youth crime among the general American public. Although Senate Bill S10 was defeated in 1998, the "get tough trend" also suggests a serious lack of critical reflection, among many politicians and the general public, of how dominant European-American cultural values and historic and contemporary practices of political and economic oppression underlie and contribute not only to youth violence but also to a society with the reputation of being the most violent nation in the industrialized and modern world.

The paucity of critical reflection nurtures and reinforces several unfortunate consequences. First, it fosters the reliance on individual deficit models, whether moral or biological, to explain violence. Second, and undergirded by the individual deficit model, scapegoating of society's most vulnerable members is justified and encouraged. Third, prevention strategies that require substantive resources for implementation and successful effectiveness are eliminated or are never given a chance to show their worth. Last, the role of official governmental and extragovernmental forces in fostering and furthering socioeconomic conditions that enhance the likelihood of youth violence is rarely explored and revealed.

Thus, what is needed to better explain and prevent youth violence, as well as substance abuse (to be addressed in the next chapter), is a critical perspective that draws on a sociocultural and political economic framework to analyze and investigate the emergence and continuation of social problems in the United States. The Afrocentric paradigm embraces this framework, which Oliver (1989) has called *structural-cultural*. Borrowing from the works of Oliver (1989), Schiele (1996, 1998), King (1997), Wilson (1990, 1992), and Kambon (1992), three important themes of this framework can be distinguished: (1) political/economic oppression, (2) spiritual alienation, and (3) cultural misorientation. This framework assumes that these factors, separately and together, can exert direct and indirect effects on many youths and can place them at risk of committing violent acts.

POLITICAL ECONOMIC OPPRESSION AND YOUTH VIOLENCE

Political economic oppression, for this chapter's purpose, is defined as institutionalized impediments, placed in motion by governmental and extragovernmental entities to ensure that power, wealth, and other resources are distributed unequally and that significant numbers of people, while maintaining their loyalty to the values and visions of the power elite, are placed in conditions that facilitate self-destructive behaviors. The major objective of this form, and perhaps all forms, of oppression is to suppress the power and positive potentiality of a copious number of people so as to maintain a secure and unchallenged power elite. One of the most important ways in which political economic oppression manifests is through the occurrence of massive poverty, underemployment, and unemployment. Indeed, some have found poverty to be the strongest predictor of youth violence (Centerwall, 1984; Hill et al., 1994; Sampson, 1993). Because much of youth street violence is associated with participation in illegal activities, and because youth participation in illegal activities often is associated with lower socioeconomic status (Myers and Drescher, 1994), the Afrocentric paradigm highlights the need to reveal the role that poverty—which is engendered by the U.S. political economy—plays in generating youth violence.

Some of the most devastating consequences of poverty are as follows: (1) it causes extreme material deprivation for people; (2) it significantly restricts options and choices people have to legitimately advance themselves economically; (3) it provides a real and persistent example of how unfair society is to many of its members; and (4) it can foster hopelessness, despair, and depression. From an Afrocentric perspective, youths who are born and reared in communities wherein there is significant material deprivation or in communities of lower socioeconomic status realize that the United States clearly does not support the positive potentiality of all. They, rightfully so, have an unfavorable concept of the "system," one that affirms and reinforces a cynical and critical view of the society. Although this cynicism often is mitigated by the overt and covert messages of meritocracy they see on television, hear on the radio, and receive from their caretakers and schoolteachers, the material realities of lower-income youths poignantly contradict these messages.

The Afrocentric paradigm maintains that the discrepancy between the messages of meritocracy and youths' material conditions, and the sense of cynicism and despair that accompany this discrepancy, serve as the primary motivations for lower-income youths to commit violent crimes. In other words, the cynicism created by the discrepancy can lead to rational, though self-destructive, choices to join the ranks of the street life, and the despair can bring about powerful feelings of anger that too often are expressed in perilous and petty acts of aggression. Thus, from an Afrocentric viewpoint, violence among lower-socioeconomic-status youths represents a strange marriage between rationality and emotionality: (1) rational choices lead them to seek their economic livelihood in the street economy, and (2) their immense anger and frustration can cause them to explode with little provocation.

For many lower-income youths, entering the street economy becomes a rational choice they make. These youths are sophisticated and politically mature enough to know there are substantive impediments to legitimate economic success and mobility in the United States. The current U.S. economy, characterized by falling or stagnant wages, layoffs, the need for more education in an increasingly competitive job market, and the relocation of many U.S. industries to countries in which wages are significantly lower and corporate regulations almost nonexistent, does not present much hope for increasing numbers of poor and working families and individuals. In addition, many lower-income youths become turned off by school early in their education, which prevents them from gaining an appreciation for academic learning and the value of delayed gratification (Kunjufu, 1984; Shujaa, 1994). Faced with these circumstances, and the wide availability of alternative and illicit modes of making a living, these youths consciously decide to engage in lifestyles that place them in jeopardy of committing violent street crimes (Lemelle, 1991; Schiele, 1996). Although their behavior has detrimental corollaries for both themselves and others, an Afrocentric analysis would suggest that these youths' decisions to engage in the street life represents "a logical means for them to cope with, and protest against, a society that practices pervasive employment discrimination" (Schiele, 1996, p. 289). Furthermore, the money these youths can generate from the street economy, with little or no requirement to delay gratification, is far more attractive than the alternative of attending college or graduate school for prolonged periods and still possibly being unable to command an income that is desirable or commensurate with the training thus acquired (Lemelle, 1991; Majors and Billson, 1992).

From an Afrocentric perspective, the political and economic oppression experienced by lower-income youths is especially revealed in the anger they feel toward others, and even perhaps themselves. The anger can be interpreted as a function of the wretched living conditions they have been reared in, which, conspicuously, are not conducive to the development of a "happy" and wholesome self. The anger also can be indirectly gained through adverse family relations and dynamics that depict too many lower-income families in the United States. Because of the devastating effects that years of intergenerational political and economic oppression have had on the caretakers of these youths, many have been crippled in their capacity to optimally nurture their children and are unable to instill in them a sense of hope (Carten and Dumpson, 1998; Ogbu, 1978, 1988). One salient indication of this in many inner-city communities is the large number of single-parent, mother-only households in which the father is absent, whose participation in family life is episodic and marginal, and wherein the extended family network is missing or significantly attenuated.

The observation about the weakening extended family structure, especially in some African-American communities over the last thirty years or so has prevented many African-American families from functioning optimally. Sudarkasa (1997) notes that although the absence or marginal participation of black fathers is important to acknowledge, it may not be the primary problem facing many African-American families today. Instead, she maintains that the more alarming issue is the large numbers of single African-American mothers who live alone with their children. In the past, single African-American mothers would reside in multigenerational homes that would include both fictive and blood relatives of different generations and age groups. These relatives would provide emotional and financial support to one another that compensated for the lack of assistance from the biological fathers. In this way, Sudarkasa (1997) admonishes that, traditionally, in the African-American family, marital instability was not inherently synonymous with family instability but that family stability was associated with a viable and cohesive extended family. Sudarkasa's (1997) observations are supported by findings from Thomas, Farrell, and Barnes (1996) that show the delinquency rate of black male adolescents from single-mother families was only slightly higher than that of black male adolescents from two-biological-parent families.

Although Sudarkasa's observation and Thomas, Farrell, and Barnes' finding are important, the absence and marginal participation of many fathers in home life can be a critical obstacle to optimal black family functioning (Akbar, 1991; Billingsley, 1994; Madhubuti, 1990). Many factors have been attributed to the absence and marginal participation of fathers, especially African-American fathers, in the family. For African-American men, unemployment, episodic employment, incarceration, and a lack of educational and training opportunities have been found to be some of the primary factors contributing to marginal family participation (Billingsley, 1994; Bowman, 1995; King, 1997; Madhubuti, 1990; Wilson, 1996). Some, such as Jewell (1988), contend that social welfare policies, such as the former Aid to Families with Dependent Children (AFDC) program, are responsible because of the requirement that the male be absent for the mother and family to be eligible for public assistance. Because of the substantial reliance in European-American culture on individualism, many attribute a male's inability or unwillingness to secure stable employment and to support his family to intrinsic deficits within himself. An Afrocentric analysis would suggest examining the effects of intergenerational and persistent political and economic oppression on the man's attitudes, hopes, and dreams. In this regard, the inimical behaviors and attitudes that obviate the man from attempting to support his family are not decontextualized. As Billingsley (1968, 1970) reminds us, the family and its structure should not be conceived as the independent variable for the problems experienced by the family. Instead, families, in this case black families, must be contextualized, perceived as an integral component of a larger historical and political web of institutional racism and oppression. Within this conceptualization, family weaknesses are the result of larger, hostile societal forces.

The fallout of this societal victimization for many lower-income youths is that they do not have the opportunity to benefit from the love, nurture, and wisdom of a male parent. This can be especially harmful to male children, and some have found, and maintained, that the absence of a positive male role model and provider is a chief reason why too many lower-income, especially African-American male, youths end up engaged in delinquent and self-destructive acts (Akbar, 1991; Kunjufu, 1984; Madhubuti, 1990; Zimmerman, Salem, and Maton, 1995). In addition, even when a nonresident father is involved with his son who lives only with the mother, conflict can ensue and may have adverse consequences for the male child (Amato and Rezac, 1994; King, 1994; Thomas, Farrell, and

Barnes, 1996). Some of this conflict may be a result of the father's participation in socially deviant activities (Thomas, Farrell, and Barnes, 1996) or over issues regarding custody and visitation rights (Dudley, 1991). Youths who witness and are deleteriously affected by this type of conflict may experience feelings of remorse and anger, first directed at their parents but later at the entire community and society. The conflict between the custodial mother and nonresident father can also exacerbate the existing problems experienced by the mothers, as they struggle, often with restricted resources, to successfully raise their children (Jackson, 1999).

The tension these single mothers endure is revealed in studies that indicate that single parents, particularly if they are young and poor, or both, abuse their children more than two-parent or multigenerational families (Gelles, 1989; Gelles and Conte, 1990; Vosler and Proctor, 1991). Moreover, the lack of parental supervision in many of these homes is associated with the economic necessity of female caretakers having to work full-time or multiple jobs (Jung, 1996). Youths reared in families such as these, wherein there is excessive abuse and lack of supervision, can learn very early that life is not a full bed of sweet roses, that life is gloomy and tough. This early socialization, unfortunately, can create a psychic atmosphere that is bursting with anger and pain, as these youths perhaps begin to realize that they have not received the kind of nurture, love, and guidance that they should have received, and that they deserve. This realization, though perhaps suppressed, may intensify their anger because they may feel "dissed" (disrespected) and that they have been handed the short end of the stick. The anger, fundamentally, then can be said to be an expression of feelings of injustice, and, so, to attain some degree of justice or retribution, these youths may use violence as their exercise of law, as their courtroom, and as their constitution.

Although youth violence can be random and often overtly senseless, the suggestion here is that its motivation is not unlike that which forms the basis of criminal prosecution and the practice of capital punishment: the need to ensure justice through the use of state-supported violence. From an Afrocentric framework, therefore, some forms of youth street violence can be interpreted as a more personalized expression of a larger societal ethic that legitimates violence as a logical way to battle injustice.

Intervention and Prevention Strategies

From an Afrocentric perspective, the best means to attack, assuage, and obviate political and economic oppression is to critically reexamine and eliminate social policies and economic practices that place large numbers of the population in jeopardy of undergoing superfluous psychosocial stress.

First should be an acknowledgment of the significant interplay between politics and economics, especially in a capitalist society such as the United States. It should be recognized that elected politicians are, in large part, supporting policies that are sanctioned by the corporate or capitalist elite. If this is true, then the form of government characterizing the United States may be more properly described as a plutocracy than a democracy. In this vein, one way to alleviate political and economic oppression, which is assumed to be a primary source of youth violent crime, is for human service workers to advocate for substantive campaign finance reform to prevent those who run for elective office from being almost exclusively beholden to corporations and others who render large financial gifts.

A second strategy that can be applied to assuage and eliminate political and economic oppression is for human service professionals to support and advance government social policies and corporate workplace policies that offer greater opportunities for people to maximize their abilities to express positive human potentiality. This implies that human service professions ought to advocate for government social policies that endeavor (1) to expand educational and training opportunities, (2) to provide health care coverage to all citizens, (3) to provide tax and other incentives for inner-city residents and others in low-income communities to start and maintain businesses, (4) to improve the public school system, (5) to expand and protect civil rights, (6) to provide greater employment opportunities, and (7) to either repeal and/or significantly alter the provisions of the Personal Responsibility Act of 1996, which abolished the federal program known as Aid to Families with Dependent Children. For human service professionals to more effectively advocate for progressive social policies at the national, state, and local levels, they should assume the role of policy practitioner, as delineated by Jansson (1994).

Changes also are needed in the workplace. These changes should focus on (1) providing employees with more work autonomy and decision making, (2) ensuring ample family leave and vacation time, and (3) offering child care services at the workplace. The latter two recommendations would be especially helpful for single parents, strengthening their ability to provide more direct guidance and supervision of their children's behavior.

A third method that should be employed to combat political and economic oppression is for human service professionals to call for a different system to elect public officials. The current two-party, single-member district system places significant constraints on the formation and potential of additional political parties and does not adequately represent the diverse interests of the U.S. population (Amy, 1993). As alternate or additional routes, human service professionals should take advantage of the growing displeasure the general American electorate has with the two major political parties by aligning themselves with alternate third or "green" political parties or by helping to establish alternate political parties themselves. The advantage of a multiple-party system, along with proportional representation, is that such a system would provide diverse political options and would ensure that the interests of a smaller party or minority group are adequately represented in, and infused into, policy formulations (Amy, 1993). This kind of political radicalism was found among the early social reformers, who, in the early part of the twentieth century, aligned themselves with progressives and socialists alike (see Day, 1997; Jansson, 1997; Trattner, 1994).

Last, although an Afrocentric analysis conceives the expansion of business opportunities in lower-income communities as an important and necessary step to prevent and arrest youth violence in those communities, it also encourages human service professionals to critically examine the nature of capitalism and how it has fostered and relied on labor exploitation, capital accumulation, and excessive economic stratification. With the emergence of "market socialism" (see Kotz, 1995; Steele, 1996), however, a few critical questions that human service professionals should pose are as follows: (1) Can a happy medium be established between state-sponsored socialism and free-market capitalism? (2) Is capitalism inherently evil, or can it be reformed in some way that can elicit more humanistic features and results? (3) Just as there is a minimum wage, should there also be a maximum wage or salary? In Chapters 7 and 8, these questions will be further explored in relation to some of the core values and assumptions of the Afrocentric worldview. For now, suffice it to say that human service professionals should not only critique and change the political system but also the economic system from which all in the human services receive their economic livelihood, benefits, and prestige.

SPIRITUAL ALIENATION AND YOUTH VIOLENCE

Consistent with the notion of spiritual alienation discussed in Chapter 4, the Afrocentric paradigm conceives youth violence as being significantly influenced by the level and extent of spiritual alienation nurtured by the culture pervasive in the United States. Spiritual alienation can be defined as "the disconnection of nonmaterial and morally affirming values from concepts of human self-worth and from the character of social relationships" (Schiele, 1996, p. 289). It emerges out of a sociocultural ethic that validates the material over the unseen, that defines human relationships as a conduit through which material objects can be acquired, that glorifies aggression as a normative value in human interaction, and, last, that advances xenophobia as an appropriate mind-set to relate to the "stranger." Although attention to spirituality has emerged recently in the social work and general social science literature (Bensley, 1991; Canda, 1998; Cohen, 1996; Sermabeikian, 1994), little attention has been devoted to the application of spiritual knowledge to explicating and preventing youth violence.

In one exception to the literature, Ward (1995), in her discussion of youth violence among African Americans, contends that "Violence destroys the underlying interrelatedness and interdependence not only of its perpetrators and victims, but of the community at large" (p. 179). She continues by observing that the increase in youth violence is a reflection of the "me" generation and the overemphasis that society places on individualism and the acquisition of material possessions. The value placed on excessive individualism and materialism, she observes, contributes to a "cutthroat morality" that extols and engenders a callous social milieu. For Ward, it is out of this callous social climate that youths learn that indifference and human disconnection are appropriate aspects of human relations and that youth violence, which stems from this kind of socialization, is too often the result of the relational breakdowns that occur in an uncaring sociocultural environment such as the United States. The assumptions in Ward's (1995) analysis are (1) that the United States fosters a sociocultural ethic that legitimates indifference and human disconnection and (2) that youths learn and internalize these cultural prescriptions.

Mass Media and Youth Violence

An increasingly significant mode through which youths learn and internalize these prescriptions is through the media, especially the visual media (Charren, 1995; Schooler and Flora, 1996; Ward, 1995; Zimmerman, 1996). More attention, recently, is being given to the role of the media in producing violent acts among youths (see Lowry et al., 1995; Price and Everett, 1997; Schooler and Flora, 1996; Zimmerman, 1996), and these writers have begun to connect these media images and messages to a larger sociocultural ethic. The relationship between youth violence, the media and other modes of information dissemination, and the broader sociocultural context is acknowledged and deemed an important trilogy in explaining youth violence from an Afrocentric perspective.

An Afrocentric viewpoint would maintain that the media, and many other information dissemination conduits found in U.S. culture, reflect and affirm not only the extremities and bizarre fantasies of a Hollywood elite but also the cultural values to which many ordinary persons in the United States adhere. These cultural values accentuate materialism and individualism and, significantly, emerge from the vestiges of social relationships found in precapitalistic Europe and from aspects of the Judeo-Christian ethic that substantially shape the philosophical scene in the United States (Ani, 1994; Baldwin, 1985; Bradley, 1991; Diop, 1978; Schiele, 1996). Within this ethic, considerable attention is given to the belief in original sin; that is, when all is said and done, the core of the human being is thought to be characterized by mischief, aggression, and selfishness. Destruction and evil are projected as normative attributes of humans, and, as inherent qualities, the best that humans can do is to monitor them (Akbar, 1984; Ani, 1994). Since egoism and selfishness are normal, the ability of humans to self-extend and connect to others in both altruistic and spiritual ways is circumscribed. And, because this ability is viewed as inherently limited, objectification of humans becomes more possible and can serve as a contributing factor in youth violence.

In other words, from an Afrocentric viewpoint, youth violence, and by extension all violence, becomes a "process of reciprocal objectification of human beings in which physical aggression is the primary method of expression" (Schiele, 1996, p. 289). Physical aggression is legitimated because central to understanding this reciprocal objectification is the belief in a pessimistic vision of human behavior, one that underscores the value that human nature is innately mischievous. This belief, which is considered an essential component of human survival within a Eurocentric cultural context (Baldwin, 1985; Kambon, 1992), is assumed to be internalized by most persons in the society, especially those who wield tremendous control over the knowledge validation and information dissemination process, such as media executives, producers, and editors.

An Afrocentric framework would suggest that persons in the media are subcomponents or subsystems of the overall sociocultural system that encourages reciprocal objectification, which stems from the values that undergird spiritual alienation. However, consistent with the emphasis in the Afrocentric literature on holistic logic, it would be appropriate to view those media personnel as not only products of spiritual alienation but also as producers of it. In addition, since the survival of media sectors in the United States depends heavily on responses from the public, the creations of those in the media, in large part, also reveal and mirror the values of the larger citizenry. Furthermore, because those in the media, particularly major media outlets, are owned and financed by the advertisements of the corporate elite, the spiritual alienation projected in the media reinforces the financial interests of this elite. In this regard, the dramatization of violence in the media can serve to titillate a public already prone to notions of the inherent evil and destructive nature of humans. Susceptibility to this cultural value manifests as profits for the corporate elite.

Media images that glorify violence by inculcating spiritual alienation are important when speaking of youths who spend an inordinate amount of time consuming visual media images. Youths spend more time watching television than they do engaging in other leisure activities and than they do in school (Strasburger, 1995). It has been estimated that by the time youths complete high school, they will have watched 15,000 to 18,000 hours of television (Strasburger, 1995). Low-income and at-risk children have the highest average television viewing time, particularly of violent material, (Schooler and Flora, 1996; Zimmerman, 1996) and perhaps this is attributed to their need to live out their fantasies to be affluent through media projections. Teen youths can be extremely susceptible to visual images of the "good life" and its associations with group acceptance because these youths are, consistent with psychosocial theory, grappling with issues of peer acceptance (Newman and Newman, 1991).

The problem with the pervasiveness of violence in the visual media for youths is the media not only arouse youths by appealing to a wide range of human emotions and perceptions but also are considered by many as the legitimate and ultimate source of information or "truth" about the world (Schooler and Flora, 1996; Wass, Raup, and Sisler, 1989). Within American culture, youth, especially the teen years, is a time when people begin questioning and wondering about the core values that society upholds and abhors (Longres, 1995; Newman and Newman, 1991; Zastrow and Kirst-Ashman, 1997). It is an impressionistic time, one in which people are simultaneously seeking personal mastery and external guidance (Longres, 1995; Newman and Newman, 1991; Zastrow and Kirst-Ashman, 1997). The visual media, with all their shortcomings, provide an enormous source of guidance for youths. Because of the expansive range of human interactions, emotions, and experiences projected, visual media allow youths to have experiences that they otherwise would not have. In other words, through virtual and vicarious experience, the visual media offer youths opportunities to extend beyond the confines of their personal experiences and milieu, thus providing them with a set of prescriptions for appropriate and inappropriate behavior and thoughts. The ubiquity of violence in the visual media sends the message to youths that violence is both an appropriate and effective method to resolve human conflict and to protect and advance one's self-interest (Schooler and Flora, 1996; Zimmerman, 1996). Whether depicted in the extreme by movies such as *The Terminator* or through subtle displays of aggression in verbal interactions, the visual media's message to youths is that aggression is a normal and necessary part of daily living and human interaction (Schooler and Flora, 1996; Zimmerman, 1996). From an Afrocentric perspective, at the center of this message are values that support and reinforce spiritual alienation and reciprocal objectification.

Although the effects of media messages and images of violence are potent, they do not affect all youths similarly. Other factors, such as socio-economic status, parental involvement in the home and school, academic achievement, spousal divorce and separation, and parental and youth drug abuse, also place youths at risk of violence (Lowry et al., 1995; Schooler and Flora, 1996; Webber, 1997). The point here, through an Afrocentric lens, is that the pervasiveness of violence in a seductive, authoritative, and societal sanctioning instrument such as the visual media places all youths who are exposed to it at risk of accepting aggression as normal for human intercourse. It places the young person who never commits a violent act at risk of possibly committing his or her first, and a young individual who consistently participates in violence in jeopardy of participating even more. With the increase and expansion of mass, visual media outlets, especially interactive video games, the "at-risk" status of youths is likely to increase, placing many more in jeopardy of internalizing the edicts of spiritual alienation and reciprocal objectification.

Prevention Recommendations

The fundamental recommendation that ensues from the latter discussion is to alleviate and eliminate spiritual alienation from the sociocultural fabric of the United States. Most of these activities would have to occur in the macroarenas of human service work, but there is an important role for microlevel human service interventions as well. First, major knowledge validation and information dissemination institutions in the United States should reexamine concepts of the inherent nature of human beings. Institutions such as religious organizations, schools, and the media need to re-explore the value in promoting the pessimistic, inherently mischievous image of humans and the implications it has for fostering unfavorable and antagonistic human relationships. This, of course, requires these institutions to reevaluate some of the core values of Eurocentric culture and their contribution to an extraordinarily violent society.

In regard to young people, these institutions must be particularly sensitive to youths because they are impressionistic and because they represent the hope of improving society. One strategy that might be used to alleviate spiritual alienation in these institutions is to encourage a more holistic, spiritual, and optimistic concept of human beings and for adults to serve as greater behavioral models of this notion. This can be achieved by promoting and teaching holistic reasoning among youths to offset the focus on fragmented or analytic reasoning, which some say lays the foundation for the objectification and, ultimately, the exploitation of human beings (see Ani, 1994; Burgest, 1981; Schiele, 1994).

Holistic reasoning or logic is thinking predicated on at least two properties: the first is the union of affect (feeling) and thought (Ani, 1994; Bell, 1994), and the second is the spiritualization of human beings. The union of affect and thought recognizes the epistemological importance of both feelings and thoughts and that both can be seen as two transparent and penetrable sides of the same coin. Acknowledging the interconnectedness of feelings and thought allows youths to make decisions that more completely tap the multidimensional makeup of their being. This allows young persons to get in touch with latent aspects of themselves that can serve as new avenues through which to achieve a greater capacity for positive potentiality and change.

The spiritualization of human beings is the belief that at the core of the human being is a spiritual essence that releases vast capabilities for interconnectedness, or what Nobles (1980) calls "spiritual oneness." Bringing youths into spiritual oneness helps them (1) to understand that they are spiritually, socially, and mutually connected to others; (2) to acknowledge the sacredness of all human life; and (3) to appreciate the many shades and variations of human beings and human experiences. This transformation from materialistic/individualistic thinking to spiritual/holistic thinking among those who seek professional help can be brought about by a therapeutic process known as the Belief Systems Analysis (see Myers, 1988). Although this helping/healing process can be conducted through direct, one-on-one practice, it should be noted that the Afrocentric paradigm of human services invariably views the broader society, in which the individual exists and in which the Eurocentric worldview prevails, as being the primary target for change.

There also is a role for human service workers who are policy practitioners. The government, at the federal, state, and local levels, can promote holistic logic and spiritual wellness by supporting and enacting legislation that speaks more to meeting the holistic and spiritual needs of citizens as well as their material needs. One of the reasons for the existence of spiritual alienation is the downplaying or repudiation of a holistic concept of humans by governmental agencies that place substantive emphasis on material and physical needs. Although these needs are certainly important, this predominant focus communicates, though subtly, to the citizen that needs of the soul and interpersonal relationships are less critical. The domain of social welfare policy has been too restricted, and social welfare policy analysts and practitioners should work more to reconceptualize the meaning of "welfare" to highlight human needs that speak more to spiritual and interpersonal development. Using their skills as analysts and practitioners, these human service professionals should then endeavor to interject this conceptualization into public and social legislation by influencing the thinking of elected officials, executives, and the larger citizenry. The roles discussed by Jansson (1994) can be applied to achieve this objective.

Special efforts need to be targeted at the mass media to change the images and messages they project. Afrocentric human services would support activities initiated by such groups as Action for Children's Television (ACT) who seek to eliminate gratuitous violence and deceptive advertising in children's television programming and who endeavor to place pressure on the Federal Communication Commission (FCC) to improve and strengthen its oversight responsibilities. Human service professionals must become more knowledgeable of the role of the FCC and involve themselves more in developing strategies that will affect new FCC guidelines for television. Afrocentric human service professionals also should establish greater links with major players in Hollywood and the entertainment community. These bonds should be aimed at (1) providing more information and evidence that the messages of violence are pernicious to fostering the optimal potential in youths, (2) demonstrating the important responsibility the entertainment industry has in socializing youths, and (3) threatening the entertainment industry with boycotts and public protests. However, as with most defenders of the media, the constitutional provision of free speech likely will be invoked, which reinforces the value of individualism so central to the Eurocentric worldview.

Afrocentric human services also recommends that media strategies, such as public service announcements, be used and increased to enhance the prosocial behavior of youths. These public service announcements have been found to be effective particularly if youths perceive these announcements as authentic (Zimmerman, 1996). The involvement of youths in the design and creation of these media announcements also has been shown to aggrandize the interests of young people and their likelihood of engendering greater prosocial behavior (Zimmerman, 1996).

CULTURAL MISORIENTATION AND YOUTH VIOLENCE

The contributing factors to youth violence heretofore discussed—political economic oppression and spiritual alienation—can be applied to youths of diverse ethnic and racial backgrounds. Cultural misorientation, as a contributing factor to youth violence, is more specific to youths belonging to ethnic/racial groups who experience, and who suffer from, the consequences of cultural oppression. Young (1990) views cultural oppression as cultural imperialism and defines it as "the universalization of a dominant group's experience and culture and its establishment as the norm" (p. 59). Cultural oppression, therefore, imposes the traditions, history, and interpretations of the dominant cultural group onto less powerful cultural groups in a manner that suppresses and marginalizes the traditions, history, and interpretations of these less powerful groups.

One corollary of cultural oppression for the culturally oppressed is what Kambon (1992) calls *cultural misorientation*. Referring to the effects of cultural oppression on African Americans, Kambon maintains that cultural misorientation occurs when African Americans adopt definitions of reality imposed by Eurocentric culture without any regard for, or consideration of, an African-centered concept of reality. The person is conceptually and philosophically incarcerated and operates within an alien definitional system that does not validate his or her traditional cultural values and worldview (Kambon, 1992; Nobles, 1974). In this way, cultural misorientation is a form of cultural alienation for the culturally oppressed. This alienation fundamentally manifests as a form of anti-self-expression or cultural self-hatred (Akbar, 1981; Azibo, 1991; Fanon, 1961; Welsing, 1991). Specifically, Akbar (1981) and Azibo (1991) have even suggested that this form of misorientation for African Americans can be conceived as a mental disorder or *dis*ease.

Akbar (1981), one of the most prominent Afrocentric psychologists, offers three categories of what he referred to as African-American mental disorders: (1) alien self disorders, (2) antiself disorders, and (3) self-destructive disorders. Briefly, alien self disorders are revealed in African Americans who consciously reject their African cultural traditions and history and who internalize central values of the Eurocentric worldview, such as materialism, individualism, and white supremacy. African Americans suffering from antiself disorders possess the mind-set and value orientation found in the alien self disorder with an additional dimension: the person harbors antagonism, whether covertly or overtly, toward people of African descent, their history, and their traditions. African Americans who exhibit self-destructive disorders are those who participate in behaviors that represent their faulty and unsuccessful attempts to cope with the conditions of Eurocentric domination. These behaviors reveal how cultural oppression can victimize the culturally oppressed so severely that they will engage in behaviors that are psychologically and physically detrimental to themselves and others in their cultural group. Welsing (1991) maintains that these deleterious behaviors are a result of what she refers to as the *inferiorization process,* which is when African Americans become psychologically stressed out from the brunt of the historical, intergenerational, and institutional effects of what she calls the system of white supremacy. The consequence, Welsing concludes, are feelings of low racial and cultural self-worth.

Within this conceptual framework, youth violence is conceived, at least among those who are victims of cultural oppression, as a maladaptive self-destructive act that reflects youths' intense level of cultural misorientation and alienation. What follows is a discussion of this process using young African-American males as the population of study. Regarding one of the most severe acts of violence, homicide, African-American males between the ages of fourteen to twenty-four are disproportionately the victims and perpetrators of homicide in the United States (U.S. Department of Justice, Federal Bureau of Investigation, 1998). Their rate of victimization from, and perpetration of, homicide is the highest of any other population, and, when African-American males commit murder, they usually kill other African-American males (U.S. Department of Justice, Federal Bureau of Investigation, 1998).

Cultural Misorientation, African-American Male Youths, and Violence

For African-American male youths, cultural misorientation is a result of European-American or Eurocentric cultural oppression (Kambon, 1992; Oliver, 1989; Schiele, 1998). African-American male youths, specifically, and African Americans, generally, have most often been the victims of Eurocentric cultural oppression (Ani, 1994; King, 1997; Wilson, 1992). This can be primarily attributed to the experience and vestiges of American slavery.

The effects of slavery and its legacy have been particularly damaging for African Americans because, in slavery, the cultural legacy and practices of Africans were suppressed. This was done to exercise more efficient control over the African captives because it was believed that, to keep the captives acquiescent and passive, there was a need to vilify their culture, their homeland, and their language (Akbar, 1996). The goal was to destroy the African's humanity by defaming his culture and history (Asante, 1988). African captives, such as griots, who were caught communicating the culture and history of Africa to other captives were publicly beaten or murdered or their tongues were cut out of their mouths (Akbar, 1996).

The major consequences of this kind of cultural vilification and institutionalized brutality for African-American males, in regard to violence, were (1) the internalization that violence is an appropriate component of social relations and (2) the concept of manhood that overemphasizes the importance of physical prowess and abilities. King (1997) and Wilson (1990, 1992) contend that in order to comprehensively explain African-American adolescent male violence, one must acknowledge and examine the impact of years of white-on-black violence. These authors argue that the violence perpetuated by whites against African Americans during slavery and the years thereafter has affected the psyche of African Americans adversely and has placed many of them at risk of accepting and using violence as a sanctioned method to interact socially with other African Americans. For Wilson (1990, 1992), this has been a calculated strategy used to continue Eurocentric domination and supremacy. By being victims of intergenerational violence themselves, Wilson suggests that the political and historic abuse suffered by African Americans has caused severe psychological trauma for them, preventing African Americans from achieving optimal psychosocial development and political and economic progress.

Psychosocial development is impeded because African Americans have been robbed of ample opportunities to trust, and have faith, that the American system strives to protect them and promote their psychoemotional interests. This lack of trust is converted into cynicism targeted at anyone, especially those in the individual's immediate environment. When exacerbated by political and economic oppression and deprivation, this cynicism can manifest in unnecessary acts of violence, aimed too often at other victims of intergenerational violence and abuse (Gary, 1981; Madhubuti, 1990; Wilson, 1990, 1992). Wilson (1990, 1992) asserts that the tragedy of all of this is that (1) the African-American community is unable to elicit the vast potential and resources it has to fight against Eurocentric domination, and (2) the intergenerational, white-on-black violence is denied and, because of this disavowal, African-American male youths are frequently scapegoated and their character and culture impugned for being morally degenerative. Ultimately, this denial justifies the continued political, economic, and physical victimization and oppression of African Americans, generally, and African-American male youths, specifically (King, 1997; Wilson, 1990, 1992).

It is interesting to note that the same logic used by King (1997) and Wilson (1990, 1992) also is found in the literature on the effects of childhood physical abuse on later adulthood functioning. Several of the studies indicate that the trauma of early childhood physical abuse, for many adults, is never resolved and that it places these adults at risk of physically abusing their own children or others' children (DuCharme, Koverola, and Battle, 1997; Fergusson and Lynskey, 1997; Litty, Kowalski, and Minor,

1996; Rodriguez et al., 1997). King and Wilson merely apply this same logic to the political and historical nature of race relations in the United States. Last, although these authors' ideas are appropriate for African-American women, African-American males more often receive the brunt of violence and aggression from slavery and institutional racism (Gary and Leashore, 1982; Hall, 1981). Some say this can be imputed to the fear, in a patriarchal and racist society, that privileged and powerful men have toward the men whom they oppress, believing that these oppressed men may one day rise to avenge themselves (Akbar, 1991; Madhubuti, 1990).

Another corollary of Eurocentric cultural oppression as it concerns African-American male youth violence is the internalization of Eurocentric standards of manhood (Akbar, 1991; Ghee, 1990; Oliver, 1989). In American society, in which European-American cultural standards prevail, concepts of manhood generally center on values of individualism, aggression, and emotional inexpressiveness (Ghee, 1990; Oliver, 1989). These values are contrary to an African-centered cultural worldview that underscores collectivity, spirituality, and emotional expressiveness (Baldwin and Hopkins, 1990; Bell, Bouie, and Baldwin, 1990; Daly et al., 1995; Myers, 1988). Eurocentric values of individualism, aggression, and emotional inexpressiveness can effectuate the "tough guy" mentality or syndrome in males (Ghee, 1990; Oliver, 1989). The institution of slavery and its vestiges have placed African-American men in particular jeopardy of internalizing the tough-guy orientation. Because African captives were defined by slaveholders as exclusively "physical" beings, images of African-American manhood and womanhood have been tarnished by exaggerating the physical prowess of African-American men and accentuating the sexual promiscuity of African-American women (Akbar, 1996). Due to the intergenerational transmission of these concepts and images, advanced by white racism, African-American males are at risk of exclusively defining themselves in terms of their physical/sexual abilities, which confines their potential to comprehend the totality of their manhood (Akbar, 1991; Oliver, 1989; Wilson, 1992). Thus, aspirations of African-American male youths to become athletic superstars and their participation in acts of violence can be attributed in part to intergenerational indoctrination that, though implicit at times, suggests that African-American males are at their best when they exhibit physical ability and strength.

Another point about the adoption of Eurocentric values of manhood by African-American male youths is that some maintain that the values endemic to the European-American worldview (i.e., individualism, materialism, and rugged competition) represent the very basis for political and economic oppression in the United States (Ani, 1994; Baldwin, 1985;

Schiele, 1994). The logic is that since the cornerstone of political and economic oppression is inequality and exploitation, the values of individualism, materialism, and competition are quite appropriate. They are appropriate because, collectively, these values highlight and conceptually exhalt a human ontology that thrives on avarice, material things, and aggression. Thus, the ability of a more collective and spiritual human ontology to emerge is significantly restricted within the parameters of this worldview (Myers, 1988; Schiele, 1994). It can be said, therefore, that when African-American male youths internalize Eurocentric definitions of manhood, wherein the latter values prevail, not only do they become culturally alienated; they also legitimate the very values that create and continue their political and economic oppression.

Cultural Solutions and African-American Male Youths

Enhancing African Self-Consciousness

From an Afrocentric framework, the primary solution to the problem of African-American male youth violence is to bring African-American male youths in line with Afrocentric values. Afrocentric values underscore a collective and spiritual orientation to life that is consistent with traditional African philosophy (Daly et al., 1995; Dixon, 1976; Karenga, 1996; Myers, 1988). It has been shown that African-American children and adolescents who internalize Afrocentric values tend to participate less in, or think less about, violent and destructive behaviors (Jagers and Owens-Mock, 1993; Belgrave et al., 1994). Based on these findings and the underlying assumptions of cultural alignment, a comprehensive strategy of Afrocentric socialization needs to occur to increase what Baldwin and Bell (1985) call *African self-consciousness* (ASC). Afrocentric socialization is the dissemination and internalization of values that stem from traditional African philosophical assumptions that emphasize collectivity, spirituality, and social responsibility. African self-consciousness is the desired outcome of Afrocentric socialization and can be succinctly defined as a state of awareness among African Americans that they are a cultural group and that their behavior should be aimed at fostering the collective survival, advancement, and prosperity of people of African descent.

It is believed that the cultivation of African self-consciousness will aid in the development of a more culturally centered male and foster the ability in that male to more constructively contribute to the entire society and world. A critical objective of the Afrocentric worldview, upon which ASC is based, is to "facilitate human and societal transformation toward spiritual, moral, and humanistic ends" (Schiele, 1996, p. 286) and to persuade people of divergent cultural and ethnic groups that they share a mutual interest in this regard. To this extent, the Afrocentric worldview is both particularistic and universalistic, in that it underscores the need for African Americans to liberate themselves from Eurocentric cultural oppression and promotes the spiritual and moral development of the world (Karenga, 1993; Kershaw, 1992).

Manhood-Training and Rites-of-Passage Programs

Afrocentric socialization should occur within all areas of the African-American community, such as the family, churches, civic and recreational organizations, and schools. Within these realms of community life, emphasis should be placed on manhood-training and rites-of-passage programs that can help the boy transform into a socially and personally responsible man who is conscious of his cultural heritage.

Manhood-training programs are programs that help African-American male youths to reconstruct and internalize a definition of manhood that stems from the sociocultural and philosophical traditions of African Americans. Within this definition, manhood is conceived as a process through which the male regulates and transcends biological drives and pleasures to fulfill obligations needed for the perpetuation of the community to which he belongs (Akbar, 1991). This understanding of manhood affirms Afrocentric values of interdependency and reciprocity that help the African-American male recognize that he is not in opposition to womanhood but is its complement (Baldwin, 1991; Bell, Bouie, and Baldwin, 1990; Kunjufu, 1984), just one component of a very essential whole. In addition, acknowledging the complementary duality of manhood and womanhood allows the man to develop and appreciate aspects of self that are unknown and helps prevent the rigid dichotomy in emotional and behavioral expectations between men and women found in European-American culture.

Rites-of-passage programs are critical ingredients in manhood training for African-American male youths. Employed in many African-American organizations and schools today, these programs implement ritual ceremonies that signify a change in a youth's social status and that are assumed to facilitate successful transition into that new status (Brookins, 1996; Warfield-Coppock, 1992). In these programs, successful transition is predicated on assisting African-American youths in developing positive cultural self-esteem (Warfield-Coppock, 1992). Generating positive cultural self-esteem in African-American youths is assumed to help them meet life challenges, to achieve, and to successfully assume community obligations (Warfield-Coppock, 1992). For the African-American male youth, the major thrust of these ceremonies is to render him conscious of Afrocentric cultural values, community obligations, and manhood themes that are specific to a life stage and essential in the preservation of African life (Baldwin, 1991; Harvey and Rauch, 1997). Because many traditional African societies included rites-of-passage in their cultural lives, proponents of rites-of-passage programs maintain that these programs not only bring to consciousness concepts and expectations of manhood for African-American male youths but also help them to reconstruct and perpetuate traditional African cultural practices.

The Role of Human Service Professionals

Afrocentric human services recognizes that although the African-American community should play a pivotal role in preventing and reducing violent crimes among African-American male youths, human service professionals, who are likely to come in contact with African-American male youths, also bear responsibility. Human service professionals can help by (1) familiarizing themselves with organizations that sponsor manhood-training and rites-of-passage programs for African-American male youths and (2) ensuring that schools are made more user friendly and culturally appropriate for these youths.

Human service professionals working with African-American male youths should familiarize themselves with literature on, and programs that sponsor, manhood-training and rites-of-passage programs so that they may work with these programs or integrate them into existing service delivery models. The Louis Armstrong Manhood Development Program (LAMDP) in New Orleans, discussed by Jeff (1994), is a prime example of a manhood program that could be replicated and integrated into services to African-American male youths. Sponsored by the welfare department of the city of New Orleans, the program's purpose is to provide African-American male youths with a structure through which they can enhance their social functioning and responsibility in several areas of life, such as religion, education, economics, politics, culture, recreation, and sex. Program components are named after African countries, and the youths are required to learn about the unique qualities of each nation. In addition, the youths are required to learn about broader traditional African rituals and values. With cultural affirmation as its base, the program offers a range of sessions that focus on (1) antidrug education; (2) antiviolence seminars, (3) educational development skills, (4) group counseling, (5) mentorship/ self-esteem, (6) recreation, (7) rites-of-passage, (8) teen parenting skills, and (9) vocational education. Last, the LAMDP conducts three process evaluations a year, and the results reveal that the program interventions are having a positive effect on the social conduct of participants.

It has been shown that school is where many African-American males begin to evince signs of boredom and destructive behavior (Ghee, 1990; Hale-Benson, 1982; Kunjufu, 1984). To this extent, schools must be made more user friendly and culturally appropriate for African-American male youths. To render schools more user friendly and culturally appropriate for African-American students, some have called for the establishment of all-black-male schools or academies (Kunjufu, 1984; Wilson, 1992), black independent schools with an Afrocentric thrust (Dove, 1996; Shujaa, 1994), and the infusion of multicultural content and pedagogical styles into existing public schools (Asante, 1991; Gary and Booker, 1992; Hale-Benson, 1982). The basic idea is that because schools are primary socializing institutions, it is imperative that African-American students receive educational services that validate who they are culturally and historically.

Research has demonstrated that educational level and personal income, which are related, are salient correlates of depression in African-American men (Gary, 1985; Brown et al., 1992). If depression is conceived as an outcome of cultural oppression and a precursor to violent crime, then primary focus should be given to enhancing educational opportunities for African-American male youths. These educational opportunities can help African-American male youths to become professionals in adulthood, and, with African self-consciousness, these adult males can employ their skills to advance the African-American community. It is essential, therefore, that teachers, administrators, and school social workers help render schools more user friendly and culturally appropriate for African-American male youths so that their motivation to learn and aspirations toward academic and career excellence are not interrupted. The motivation to learn may be increased by doing the following:

1. Exposing black boys to knowledge that affirms the contributions of black people, generally, and black men, specifically
2. Building on and identifying black boys' academic strengths, no matter how scant they may appear to be
3. Making learning a fun activity rather than a sterile and monotonous one
4. Establishing a warm relationship with black boys (Much of enhancing the motivation to learn in black boys is directly related to whether the boys perceive that the teacher loves and cares for them.)
5. Helping black boys develop a sense of African self-consciousness
6. Reinforcing the resiliency of black men, specifically, and black people, generally

7. Teaching black boys how to cope with the realities of a racist society
8. Helping black boys to channel their anger at the system in more constructive ways, especially ways that will help uplift the black community
9. Emphasizing the relationship between their achievement as individuals and the survival, advancement, and prosperity of black people collectively
10. Reinforcing the importance of discipline in academic excellence

If these steps are taken, the likelihood of African-American males ending up in the criminal justice system may be reduced substantially. Perhaps the latter recommendations that center on Afrocentric socialization, manhood-training programs, and user-friendly schools also can enhance the probability of more African-American men being able and willing to manage the responsibility of being dependable fathers and husbands. If so, the problems of violence among young African-American males that may be attributed to family structure, marital instability, and conflict between former mates might be abated.

Chapter 6

Substance Abuse
and the Afrocentric Paradigm

The use of drugs and other mood-altering substances has characterized most societies throughout human history (Goodman, Lovejoy, and Sherratt, 1995; Westermeyer, 1995). The Afrocentric paradigm of human service does not view the use of drugs as inherently disruptive to human and societal relationships (Christmon, 1995; Schiele, 1996). It does, however, conceive the excessive use or abuse of drugs as problematic and as a destructive force not only for the individual but also for the individual's immediate and wider social environment. But, the Afrocentric paradigm would tolerate and recognize the importance of using mood-altering substances for significant social events, such as rituals, ceremonies, or other important social occasions. The point here is that given the Afrocentric paradigm's holistic viewpoint, and its acknowledgment of the multiple sources that shape human behavior, it would not assume or promote a hard-line view on drug use. Both Christmon (1995) and Lusane (1991) maintain that drug use in many traditional African societies was sanctioned if it did not compromise the individual's capacity to optimally function socially and contribute to the collective survival and advancement of the community.

Similar to many other paradigms used to explain substance abuse, the Afrocentric paradigm is concerned with the excessive and abusive use of drugs in society and attempts to offer explanations and solutions to the problem. This chapter again uses the tripartite framework of (1) political economic oppression, (2) spiritual alienation, and (3) cultural misorientation as the basis to explain, and offer some possible remedies for, substance abuse in the United States from an Afrocentric perspective.

As in the previous chapter, the concept of *structural-cultural* is used to suggest that the problem of substance abuse in the United States is primarily a function of the political economic institutions and sociocultural values that characterize and pervade the American landscape. In addition, and consistent with the Afrocentric paradigm, this chapter endeavors to apply the attributes of the structural-cultural framework to explain and provide remedies for the problem of drug abuse for Americans, generally, and African Americans, especially, keeping in mind that its explanations and recommendations may not be universally appropriate for all drug abusers, both African American and non–African American.

POLITICAL ECONOMIC OPPRESSION AND SUBSTANCE ABUSE

From an Afrocentric viewpoint, much of drug abuse in the United States is a response to the injustices that emanate from the political economy of capitalism and its relationship to other forms of oppression, such as white supremacy and patriarchy. The effects of oppression, as it concerns drug abuse, can influence both the victims of oppression and the beneficiaries and/or perpetrators of oppression. In other words, although political economic oppression may indeed place greater stress and pain on those who are the targets of oppression, an Afrocentric analysis would also suggest that the beneficiaries of oppression can experience stress and anxiety related to their concerns over maintaining control and privilege and any guilt that may be associated with that privilege. Central, then, to this discussion is the notion that oppression can victimize both the oppressed and the oppressor, that both can be placed at risk of abusing drugs as an avenue to manage the stress, anxiety, and guilt associated with oppression. For the victims of oppression, the stress and anxiety can be related to coping with the daily trials and tribulations caused by oppression and to not allow these stressful life events to rob them of a positive sense of self and a sense of purpose. The devastation of drug abuse has been most conspicuous in this latter group, so the discussion turns to it first.

Substance Abuse and Victims of Political Economic Oppression

The victims or targets of political economic oppression, generally speaking, are those groups in society whose physical, mental (i.e., value orientations), or behavioral attributes are used to construct barriers to the degree of power and wealth they can attain in society. For these groups, political-economic oppression places them at significant risk of abusing drugs by ensuring that they experience poverty or material deprivation disproportionately, as well as the hopelessness and despair that accompanies that deprivation.

As with youth violence, poverty also can contribute to substance abuse. However, to better understand poverty's role in placing those who experience it in jeopardy of abusing drugs, it is necessary to examine the function that drug abuse serves for those who benefit from and perpetuate economic inequality. For these beneficiaries and perpetrators, the abuse of drugs by the oppressed is just one more weapon to ensure that the oppressed are effectively contained and controlled. Hall (1997), for example, contends that since African-American families are disproportionately the victims of drug abuse-related crime, recent drug control policies and mandatory drug sentences have replaced the old slave codes as a means to socially monitor and contain the threat African Americans may pose to the stability and continuation of European-American hegemony. The Afrocentric perspective builds on Hall's contention and suggests that those in power recognize and calculate the risks for those who experience poverty or economic crises disproportionately. It is understood by the power elite that poverty and economic deprivation can function as a catalyst for potential insurrection, rebellion, and incisive critiques of the social system, an organizing theme around which the oppressed can unify. What is needed to counterbalance the misery of poverty are behavioral patterns that can distract the victims of poverty and economic deprivation from concentrating on the inhumanities of their material conditions in the face of pervasive opulence, experienced virtually on television or personally when traveling to another part of town. Drugs, whether licit or illicit, can produce pattens of behavior that serve this end. The abuse of drugs is powerful in this regard for at least two reasons: (1) it provides immediate biopsychological relief and transformation that relaxes the person by engendering an illusory—though real while experiencing a high—state of euphoria; and (2) it heightens the emotional sensitivities of individuals so that they can more readily displace the frustrations caused by the intricacies of political economic oppression onto persons in their immediate social environment. In short, from an Afrocentric perspective, drug abuse in poverty-stricken communities serves political economic functions aimed at preventing those who experience the brunt of society's atrocities from organizing politically to critique, successfully cope with, and eradicate the system that oppresses them.

Some evidence supports this theory, especially when many inner-city communities across the United States are examined. The first piece of evidence is alcohol consumption patterns and problems that result from this consumption. Lower socioeconomic status and unemployment have been found to contribute to higher alcohol consumption (Caetano and Clark, 1998a, 1998b), and African and Hispanic Americans are disproportionately unemployed and found in the lower economic strata (U.S. Bureau of the Census, 1998). While trends in alcohol consumption have remained stable or have declined slightly for most groups (Caetano and Clark, 1998b), frequent heavy drinking is slightly higher among African and Hispanic Americans compared to European Americans, and these ethnic differences are greater among men (Caetano and Clark, 1998b). In addition, African- and Hispanic-American men report more problems with alcohol and tend to have more alcohol-related emergency visits than other groups (Caetano and Clark, 1998a; Li et al. 1998). African-American men also have been found to have the highest rates of psychoactive drug-related deaths (Kallan, 1998). What these latter figures show is not only does substance abuse obviate victims of oppression from organizing politically but also can enhance their morbidity and lessen their life expectancy, thus limiting the amount of time they can exploit to develop and advance a collective, political consciousness.

A second piece of evidence supporting the notion that drug abuse serves political objectives is the disproportionate distribution of illicit drugs, such as crack cocaine, heroin, and marijuana, in inner-city communities of color. Although most of the major distributors of these substances do not reside in the inner-city, their products end up disproportionately in these communities (Lusane, 1991; Webb, 1996). Indicators of this phenomenon can be revealed in arrest rates for those selling and buying illicit substances. For example, whereas African Americans constituted about 12 percent of the U.S. population in 1995, they constituted almost two-fifths (39.1 percent) of those arrested on drug abuse violations that year (U.S. Department of Justice, Federal Bureau of Investigation, 1996). Moreover, in 1994, of the total number of serious offenses that resulted in imprisonment, drug offenses were the most common offense for African Americans, whereas they were the third most common offense for European Americans (U.S. Department of Justice, Federal Bureau of Investigation, 1995a).

Related to arrest rates is the racial inequality in conviction rates. Not only are African Americans arrested more frequently than are European Americans for drug-related charges, but when they are arrested, African Americans are convicted more often of the crime and receive harsher penalties and more jail time (Barnes and Kingsnorth, 1996; Free, 1997; Mauer, 1997). This disparity is conspicuously revealed by data indicating that although African Americans represented 13 percent of all monthly drug users in 1995, they constituted 35 percent of arrests for drug posses-sion, 55 percent of those convicted, and 74 percent of all drug prison sentences (Mauer and Huling, 1995). These statistics take on more mean-ing when considering that drug offenders increasingly constitute larger percentages of those incarcerated. For example, in 1983, one in eleven inmates nationally was either serving time or awaiting trial for a drug offense; by 1993, the ratio was one in four (Shine and Mauer, 1993). For federal prisoners, the increase has been greater: in 1996, 59.6 percent of all federal inmates were in jail for drug offenses (Mauer, 1999). Also signifi-cant in this discussion is the sentencing disparity between being arrested for powder cocaine and crack cocaine. The present law requires a mini-mum five-year federal prison sentence for possession of five grams of crack cocaine, whereas such a penalty is not mandated for powder cocaine possession of under 500 grams (The Sentencing Project, 1997). Thus, a person having 100 times less crack cocaine than powder cocaine receives a stiffer conviction. The importance of this sentencing disparity for African Americans is that whereas approximately two-thirds of crack cocaine us-ers are European and Hispanic Americans, the persons more likely to be convicted of possession of crack cocaine in 1994 in federal courts were African Americans (U.S. Sentencing Commission, 1995). Almost 90 per-cent (88.3 percent) of those convicted of trafficking crack cocaine in 1994 were African Americans (U.S. Sentencing Commission, 1995). These data are significant for the present discussion because (1) African and Hispanic Americans are more likely to reside in inner-city communities and experi-ence economic deprivation; and (2) because of this, they are less likely to have the political power and wealth to retain attorneys who have resources that can result in less or no jail time.

A last indicator that may underscore the role of political economic oppression in substance abuse is the increase of more illicit substances in inner cities following the civil unrest of the 1960s. Lusane (1991) con-tends that substantial historical evidence demonstrates a correlation be-tween high levels of black political protests and the increase of illicit substances in the African-American community. He notes that prior to the contemporary drug crisis in the African-American community, "the great-est amount of heroin use in Black American history occurred between 1965 and 1970" (Lusane, 1991, p. 13). Many people, especially in the African-American community and in inner-city neighborhoods, believe that the Central Intelligence Agency (CIA) has been involved in the dis-tribution of illicit drugs into inner-city communities. Webb's (1996) series documented possible CIA involvement in crack cocaine distribution, and the subsequent congressional hearings on the topic fostered more suspicion about the role the CIA may have played in the illicit drug trade in African-American communities.

In addition, many of the black youth gangs of the 1960s were involved in the African-American protest movement. For example, the acronym CRIPS, for the now notorious Los Angeles-based street gang, originally stood for "Continuing Revolution in Progress," which indicates that its original purpose was political mobilization, not violent self-perpetuation (Henderson, 1997). Other 1960s black youth gangs, such as the Businessmen and the Gladiators of Los Angeles and the Blackstone Rangers of Chicago, also were engaged in black protest and political agitation (Henderson, 1997; Lusane, 1991; O'Reilly, 1989). The Blackstone Rangers of Chicago, for instance, were a critical force against the political hegemony of former mayor Richard Daley's Chicago machine (Lusane, 1991).

Some believe that one strategy used by the CIA and the Federal Bureau of Investigation (FBI) to undermine black political mobilization among the 1960s youth gangs was to infiltrate these gangs and lure them into the illicit drug trade by exploiting their frustrations related to material deprivation and racism (Henderson, 1997; Lusane, 1991). The contenders of this perspective suggest this was a primary objective of J. Edgar Hoover's COINTEL (Counterintelligence) program of the 1960s that helped not only to enhance drug trade by youth gangs but also to instigate conflict between and among black protest organizations (Henderson, 1997; Karenga, 1993; Lusane, 1991; O'Reilly, 1989). One of the best-known and most-discussed conflicts in the African-American community was between Maulauna Karenga's—the creator of the holiday Kwanza—"US" organization and the Black Panthers. Some believe that this conflict was encouraged by J. Edgar Hoover's FBI to preclude the two organizations from unifying and becoming a potent force in the black protest movement (Henderson, 1997; Ngozi-Brown, 1997; O'Reilly, 1989).

Those who believe in the political function of illicit drugs in inner cities claim that one need only examine the social disorganization and alienation that has occurred in these communities since the 1960s. They maintain that the despair in these communities has become more regnant and that the greater infiltration of illicit drugs is a primary causative factor (Abdullah, 1998; Bourgois, 1995; Lusane, 1991). The corollaries that this despair has had on family functioning in the inner city are the greater availability and distribution of illicit substances in these communities as well as the risk this poses for many members of these families to use, abuse, and sell drugs (Bourgois, 1995).

Several people maintain that the risk of substance abuse, and other social problems, among inner-city families today is related to the transformation of the U.S. economy and the relocation of higher-wage/salary industries to the suburbs (Franklin, 1997; Rifkin, 1995; Wilson, 1987, 1996). These writers intimate that changes in the U.S. economy from a manufacturing economy to a service and high technology one has been inimical to many traditionally low-skill and blue-collar workers, but especially to inhabitants of inner cities, such as African Americans. Advanced technology, such as roboticism, and the corporate trend of downsizing and outsourcing compels Rifkin (1995) to conclude that we are experiencing the "end of work" and the wake of a new postmarket era. Indeed, for African Americans who began to make strides in industry at the same time when mechanization was emerging in U.S. industries, Willhelm (1970) observes that the issue for these increasingly displaced workers may not have been economic exploitation but rather *economic irrelevance*. For many inner-city residents, this end of legitimate work and economic irrelevance phenomenon has been paralleled by the expansion of an illicit job market in which the sale and distribution of illegal drugs are major employment activities. This trend can be gleaned in the previous data on the increase in the number of persons arrested for drug-related crimes, and may be especially detrimental for young African-American males. This is because although African-American males between the ages of fourteen and twenty-four constituted only 1 percent of the U.S. population in 1994, they represented 31 percent of all homicide offenders that year (U.S. Department of Justice, Federal Bureau of Investigation, 1995b). Since these males tend to be disproportionately arrested for drug-related offenses (Mauer and Huling, 1995), many offenders and victims of drug-related homicides are probably young black men.

Moreover, real wages for working families have not increased, have declined, or have remained flat since the late 1970s (Gordon, 1996), and social welfare expenditures have been diminishing since the 1981 Omnibus Budget Reconciliation Act, which created the federal block grant system of funding welfare programs and services (Day, 1997; Jansson, 1997). This retrenchment in federal social welfare spending culminated with the passage and signing into law by President Bill Clinton of The Personal Responsibility and Work Opportunity and Reconciliation Act of 1996, which, among other things, eliminated the federal Aid to Families with Dependent Children program. From an Afrocentric perspective, these economic and social welfare spending patterns have caused its victims to experience increasingly more precariousness, indeterminancy, and despair. Feelings of despair, uncertainty, and alienation are major contributing factors in substance abuse (Carroll, 1993; Foulks and Pena, 1995; Johnson, 1994; Nobles, 1984; Schiele, 1996). Although these feelings are clearly not endemic to the poor or to those on the economic and political margins of society, poverty and material deprivation can exacerbate feelings of hopelessness and alienation (Franklin, 1997; Lewis, 1969).

It can be assumed then that those in the worst economic circumstances are at greater risk of substance abuse because they may have more anxiety over securing the necessities of life: food, clothing, and shelter. In regard to those in the inner cities, substance abuse, from an Afrocentric lens, reflects (1) a response to what can be described as despair and anxiety associated with a radically changing economy that, among other things, is constricting the control of capital into fewer and fewer hands and (2) an enhanced opportunity to use and abuse drugs that has been created by the increasing availability of drugs in inner-city communities. At the heart of these occurrences, from an Afrocentric viewpoint, are diabolical and calculated decisions made by the white power elite who benefit both economically and psychologically from the hardships of others (Rowe and Grills, 1993; Schiele, 1996; Wilson, 1990).

Substance Abuse and Beneficiaries of Political Economic Oppression

White Racial Identity Development

Since substance use and abuse are pervasive in the United States, it is important, from an Afrocentric perspective, to examine how oppression also can place those in power, or those who benefit from oppression, in jeopardy of abusing drugs. In this sense, substance abuse can be seen as a function of anxiety, anger, or guilt associated with being a beneficiary of political and economic oppression.

Although oppression is manifested in many ways, racial oppression is one of the most conspicuous, regnant, and perpetual forms of oppression in the history of the United States. Most of the literature on race relations and racial oppression, however, focuses on the damaging consequences of racism on the targets, or victims, of oppression, whereas scant attention has been devoted to understanding and exploring the effects of racial oppression on its beneficiaries (Akbar, 1996; Asante, 1987; Helms, 1990a; Welsing, 1991). In recent years, some social scientists have begun to examine the corollaries of racism on the identity formation and development of European Americans (see Block and Carter, 1996, 1998; Helms, 1990a, 1990b; Rowe, Bennett, and Atkinson, 1994). These models are generally referred to as White Racial Identity Development Models (WRIDM), and Helms' (1990a) seminal book is credited for much of the advancement of these models. In the book, Helms (1990b) presents her

WRIDM, which is based on the linear assumptions of stage/developmental paradigms. Helms posits that white identity development has six stages, but that the six stages represent essentially two phases: (1) the abandonment of racism and (2) defining a positive white identity. Before discussing the potential relevance of Helm's model to substance abuse among European Americans, it is instructive to provide a brief overview of Helm's stages of white identity development: (1) the contact stage, (2) the disintegration stage, (3) the reintegration stage, (4) the pseudoindependent stage, (5) the immersion/emersion stage, and (6) the autonomy stage.

The contact stage is the beginning stage of racial consciousness. However, this awareness is a naive one and the white individual is frequently unaware of how he or she benefits from institutional and cultural racism. Fundamentally, in the contact stage, one begins to become inquisitive about racial differences, possessing "a superficial and inconsistent awareness of being white" (Helms, 1990b, p. 55).

In the second stage, disintegration, the white person becomes more conscious of the social meaning of whiteness and begins to experience moral dilemmas associated with that consciousness. During this stage, the individual begins to understand that, socially, a racial hierarchy exists and that whites are considered to be at the apex. Helms notes that, in this stage, the white person can experience considerable cognitive and moral dissonance that, on one hand, affirms the values of universal love for humanity and, on the other, affirms the values that blacks are inferior, should be viewed with suspicion, and should be kept in their place. In this way, whites begin to become aware of the racial "us" and "them" phenomenon, that, as Bell (1992) observes, is synonymous with feelings of closeness and loyalty tantamount to that of a family. Furthermore, this racial us/them dichotomy renders one conscious of the firm social control sanctions, such as ostracism, in place for those who violate the code of racial loyalty.

In the third stage of reintegration, the white individual is assumed to resolve the moral dilemmas and dissonance associated with the disintegration stage and to consciously validate and accept the value of white supremacy and black inferiority. Fear and anger are assumed to dominate the white person's feelings toward blacks during this stage. The guilt of the latter stage which was associated with moral dilemmas, has now been resolved, and the person wholeheartedly accepts the value of race as family. Helms notes that, given the values and institutional structures of U.S. society, it is quite feasible for whites to remain fixed at this stage.

For whites to overcome the belief in white supremacy, Helms suggests that they must question the notion of whiteness and its interconnectedness with racial and cultural superiority. The pseudoindependent stage is the first step toward this more positive redefinition of whiteness. More specif-ically, it is suggested that the white person in this stage begins to acknowl-edge white culpability for racism and "how he or she wittingly and unwit-tingly perpetuates racism" (Helms, 1990b, p. 61). However, although the person at this stage rejects a negative conception of whiteness, he or she has not yet developed a positive understanding of whiteness. At this point, the person is assumed to have a marginal racial identity.

The refinement of a more positive concept of whiteness continues in the immersion/emersion stage. In this stage, one becomes immersed in biogra-phies, autobiographies, and other stories of how whites who have been in similar circumstances have overcome racial stereotypes to adopt a more favorable understanding of racial differences. Often, the person will par-ticipate in white consciousness-raising groups to help explore and unearth his or her self-interest and the benefits of eliminating racist ideology from the mind. To this extent, and unlike the pseudoindependent phase, the person no longer focuses her or his attention on liberal activities of helping and changing blacks but rather redirects that attention by helping to alter the mind-sets of racist whites.

The autonomy stage is when the white person is assumed to achieve an authentically positive white racial identity. The individual's feelings and thoughts regarding white supremacy and his or her need to denigrate and oppress people based on racial characteristics are completely eliminated. This abandonment of racism is not only personal but also cultural and institutional. Thus, the person begins to realize that European-American cultural attributes are not, and should not be, universal and that he or she can learn from and appreciate other cultures.

The Stress of Racial Privilege and Substance Abuse

Throughout the discussion, Helms acknowledges that feelings—which can have stress-producing effects—are associated with each stage of white racial identity development. For example, Helms (1990b) maintains that feelings of anxiety and guilt are prevalent for whites in the disintegration stage. The anxiety and guilt are associated with becoming aware of the racial privilege whiteness affords as well as the moral dilemmas that accompany this awareness and the social pressures that compel one to be loyal to one's race. Race-related dissonance, Helms (1990b) contends, similar to other forms of psychological conflict, can cause immense dis-comfort for the individual. To reduce the discomfort, white persons who are experiencing race-related dissonance could, according to Helms (1990b), do three things: (1) avoid contact with blacks, (2) endeavor to convince other whites that blacks are not inferior, and (3) explore information that exonerates whites from racial inequities or that suggests that racism does not exist.

All three strategies, though potentially reducing race-related dissonance for whites, also can present stress for the individual. Attempts at avoiding blacks, especially for one who lives in a area where a significant number of blacks reside, may be futile and produce further anxiety about one's culpability in racial inequities. Striving to convince one's peers or significant others that blacks are not inferior can also be futile and frustrating, if indeed race loyalty and beliefs regarding black inferiority and moral deficiencies are regnant in the individual's personal milieu. The negative outcome for the white individual could be ostracism and stigmatization, both potentially stress-producing events. Last, striving to locate information which exonerates whites from racial oppression and which suggests that racism does not exist only reinforces the degree of guilt the individual may be experiencing and may cause further race-related dissonance if the information found does not completely relieve the person of guilty feelings, particularly if one is simultaneously exposed to contrary information. The point here is that the anxiety and guilt associated with race-related dissonance at the disintegration stage can place whites at risk of using drugs and other substances as an avenue to reduce anxiety and guilt. One can hypothesize, then, that to the extent that whites at the disintegration stage experience greater guilt and anxiety related to race-specific moral and cognitive dissonance, the greater their chances of relying on drugs to cope with and assuage feelings of race-related guilt and anxiety.

Likewise, Rowe, Bennett, and Atkinson (1994) discuss guilt and shame as feelings connected to whites who have developed what they refer to as the reactive type of *achieved white racial consciousness*. Unlike Helms, Rowe and colleagues contend that not all whites experience race awareness by progressing through a series of linear and universally assumed stages of development. They argue that not all whites achieve white racial consciousness, defined by them as a white person's willingness to explore his or her own ethnicity and "commitment to some position about racial/ethnic minority matters" (Rowe, Bennett, Atkinson, 1994, p. 136). They refer to whites who do not acquire racial consciousness as having a status of *unachieved white racial consciousness*. Those who explore and become committed to issues and positions regarding racial and ethnic minority matters have the status of *achieved white racial consciousness* (AWRC). Persons in the reactive type of AWRC, according to Rowe, Bennett, and Atkinson, "are likely to hold views based on the premise that white Americans benefit from and are responsible for the existence of discriminatory attitudes and practices" (1994, p. 139). These persons hold reactive attitudes against the white community and work, often futilely, to be accepted by people of color. Because of the ostracism they may confront from other whites and suspicion from people of color, these whites run the risk of becoming culturally marginal, and this marginality can lead to feelings of anger toward the white status quo and feelings of guilt and shame toward themselves for having unknowingly participated in, and validated, the behaviors and ideas of white supremacy (Rowe, Bennett, and Atkinson, 1994). An Afrocentric analysis suggests, similar to those in Helms' disintegration stage (1990b), that reactive-type whites are placed at risk of abusing drugs to ease the discomfort of personal feelings of guilt and shame related to achieving white racial consciousness.

Not only can feelings of guilt and shame place beneficiaries of oppression at risk of abusing drugs but also feelings of anger and hostility targeted at the victims of oppression, perhaps engendered by fear of losing power and privilege. For example, Helms' (1990b) reintegration stage assumes that a white identity is cemented by the acceptance of the belief in the inherent superiority of whites over nonwhites. And, Helms contends, that feelings of guilt and anxiety for individuals in the disintegration stage are transformed into fear and anger toward blacks in the reintegration stage. Although Helms does not specify the source of the fear and anger in this stage, it might be that both fear and anger are associated with concerns about sustaining a superior political, social, and economic position. Belief in white superiority could produce the fear that, one day, nonwhites might elevate and advance themselves and, therefore, reduce the privileges and status associated with being white in the United States (Welsing, 1991; Wilson, 1990). The same belief might foster anger, in that the victims of white privilege are often viewed as a burden to society and as the primary sources of social and moral degeneration (see Walters, 1995; Karenga, 1986; Quadagno, 1994). Thus, nonwhites, especially African and Hispanic Americans, are assumed to lower the moral quality of the presumed superior white culture and society.

The same feelings of fear and anger are said to characterize Rowe and colleagues' (1994) *dominative type of achieved white racial consciousness*. Those who adopt this type of consciousness hold the view that whites are justified in their dominance over people of color because of the superiority of the white majority culture. Rowe and colleagues posit that, in part, anger and fear for this type of person is a result of forced contact or competition with people of color. For whites who fit Helms' (1990b) reintegration phase and Rowe, Bennett, and Atkinson's (1994) dominative type of AWRC, the abuse of drugs might ease the pain associated with increasing concerns over losing privilege as white persons in America.

The euphoria induced by substance abuse may help to repress the social and economic consequences of the increasing "browning" of the American workplace.

The anger and fear associated with forced competition with nonwhites and concerns over reductions in power and privilege are perhaps especially poignant among blue-collar, non-college-educated white men. Pfeil (1997) contends that fear and anger among many blue-collar white men is fundamentally resentment toward the collapse of psychosocial power, or what Dubois (1935) called the *psychological wage.* The collapse is associated with the disconnections, according to Pfeil, between blue-collar white men and the factories and industries that formerly employed them. Pfeil asserts that these men no longer feel they are organically connected to the power elite or the company bosses of industry because much of industry has shut down, has relocated to nations that have fewer business regulations and lower-wage labor, or, if remaining in the local community, has become excessively bureaucratic and impersonal, to the point that the old intimacies of labor and management have all but dissolved. In essence, what Pfeil may be describing is psychosocial stress related to the perceived and real—when one considers how real wages for blue-collar workers have been declining or stagnant since the late 1970s—reduction in privilege and status associated with being white and male in society. As Pfeil (1997) states, the source of blue-collar white men's pain is their "bafflement, grief, and rage at the breakdown and/or removal of a profoundly undemocratic patriarchal and neofeudal hierarchy into which they once believed they fit organically, with their own zones of autonomy and . . . privilege, no matter how small" (p. 30).

Some evidence indicates the toll that this fear and anger may be having on white men in this category, if one extrapolates from drug usage trends. Caetano and Clark (1998b), in their national study of alcohol consumption patterns among whites, blacks, and Hispanics, found that education and income were significantly associated with alcohol consumption among white men in both 1984 and 1995. Their findings indicate that white men with less education and lower incomes (who are more likely to be blue-collar workers) consumed significantly more alcohol than white men with more education and higher incomes. In addition, educational attainment was a significant predictor of frequent heavy drinking (defined as having five or more drinks at a sitting at least once a week or more often), with less educated white men engaged more in frequent heavy drinking. Although there are many interpretations of these patterns among white men, Pfeil's analysis of the declining economic conditions and emotional trauma of blue-collar white men should be considered.

Recommendations to Reduce the Effects
of Political Economic Factors

There are several ways to reduce and eliminate the political and economic circumstances that support substance abuse in the United States. First, the recommendations identified in the chapter on youth violence that focus on restricting the excesses of a capitalist society and the questions raised are also relevant for substance abuse. Second, public health policies need to be more thoroughly integrated with economic policies. Although some research underscores the role of economic factors in substance abuse (see Bourgois, 1995; Hall, 1997; Riley, 1997; Zimmerman and Maton, 1992), policymakers appear to be lagging in the integration of this research in the formulation of public policy. Economic policies, such as the North American Free Trade Agreement (NAFTA) and the Personal Responsibility Act of 1996, should be analyzed for their potential to enhance substance abuse among targeted populations. When economic policies are formulated, every effort should be made to consider the policy's broader public health consequences, such as substance abuse. Questions such as the following might be asked and addressed in economic policies: (1) To what extent will an economic policy that displaces workers, if only ephemerally, contribute to greater alcohol and illicit drug consumption among those, and their families, affected by the displacement? (2) To what extent will the relocation of a plant or production facility place the workers who reside in the old location at risk of substance abuse? (3) To what extent will an economic policy that does not have adequate employment training, and thus results in trainees being placed in dead-end, nongrowth jobs, engender psychosocial pain for the trainees and render them vulnerable to substance abuse to assuage the stress? The Afrocentric paradigm encourages social policy formulation that coalesces concerns for the material, psychological, and physical well-being of people.

Since much of the discussion of the effects of political and economic oppression on substance abuse focus on racial oppression, the Afrocentric paradigm supports social policies and community activities which foster healing of the inimical effects of institutional racism and which atone for the injustices that people of color, particularly African Americans, have had to endure across generations. President Clinton's Council On Race Relations is a right step in this direction from an Afrocentric viewpoint. However, the Afrocentric paradigm would maintain that discussions and findings generated by the council should lead to specific and concrete policy recommendations that serve to redistribute resources to those who have been most victimized by institutional racism. Often, discussions on redistributive polices regarding institutional racism focus on affirmative action. Although there are several interpretations of affirmative action, the critical points of these debates, from an Afrocentric perspective, are two-fold: (1) Since the U.S. government has sponsored and supported institutional racism practices that provide preferential treatment to European Americans, especially European-American men, in its polity and economic realms since its inception, it would be fair for the federal government to support activities that create and expand educational and employment opportunities for African Americans and other people of color. (2) Although much is made over the point that some affirmative-action policies punish contemporary European-American males who had nothing to do with slavery and past institutional racism, and thus represent a "two wrongs don't make a right" policy agenda, less attention is devoted to the innocent victims of historic institutional racism and slavery and the adverse corollaries this victimization has had for generations of families of color. This is why the Afrocentric paradigm recommends that more research be funded for, and devoted to, unraveling, identifying, and analyzing the long-term, intergenerational effects of slavery and institutional racism on not only the economic conditions of African-American families but also the psychosocial functioning and well-being of these families. If substance abuse is viewed partly as a reaction to severe psychosocial stress and economic albatrosses, the opportunities provided by affirmative-action policies might help to diminish substance abuse in the African-American community. Hence, future research should examine the impact of enhanced educational and employment opportunities on African Americans' level of substance use and abuse.

The latter recommendations focus on the victims of racial oppression, but what about the political and economic beneficiaries of racial oppression? Since it was argued that their privileged status can place them at risk of substance abuse, what can be done to alleviate the fear, anger, and guilt associated with this privilege that can contribute to substance abuse? Fundamentally, the system of racial oppression has to be eliminated to completely destroy these feelings. Although the abolition of racial oppression may take just as long as its creation and evolution, a few steps can be taken that might help ease, but perhaps not eliminate, these feelings, particularly those of fear (i.e., anxiety) and guilt.

The feeling of anxiety or fear could be attenuated if more efforts were aimed at casting African Americans positively by providing greater opportunities for European Americans to experience the more favorable aspects of African Americans. Too often, African Americans are portrayed and projected as persons to be feared, such as street criminals, or other images that present them to be excessively violent, sensitive, and impulsive. Media images of African Americans are changing to project a more diversified African-American community (see Jhally and Lewis, 1992), and this trend should continue. Second, European Americans need to be exposed to more information about African-American culture, history, and traditions. Narratives which emanate from African Americans and which validate their experiences and interpretations should be given more coverage in the media and in schools. Although many of these narratives might demonstrate the frustrations many African Americans have toward America, which may enhance the fear in European Americans, many African Americans do not seek physical retaliation, but only social, political, and economic justice. This basic understanding among European Americans might help to diminish the feeling of fear many have toward African Americans.

Of course, another dimension of fear exists that deals with the fear of losing one's racial privilege. African Americans can do very little to ease this dimension; rather, social policies and societal practices will have to be aimed at convincing European Americans of the human and collective advantages of eliminating racial oppression and at helping many to acknowledge and honestly explore the need for the fear in the first place. A critical component of this exploration, from an Afrocentric perspective, is the necessity of many European Americans to reexamine the extent to which they may harbor feelings of racial and cultural superiority and to examine and apply techniques to overcome these feelings.

From an Afrocentric perspective, the best way for European Americans who experience race-related guilt to assuage that feeling is to participate more in efforts to alter the mind-set of other European Americans and to work to undermine practices of institutional racism and white supremacy. These endeavors, however, might place European Americans who engage in these activities at risk of being construed as "race traitors" and being socially ostracized by other European Americans. However, if these efforts are sincere and effective in bringing about concrete change, no matter how incremental, they can help reduce feelings of European-American guilt because African Americans and other people of color will be able to identify and benefit from these efforts and will extol those European Americans who participate in such activities. In essence, feelings of race-related guilt can be attenuated when European Americans engage in concrete and authentic social change activities that produce tangible improvements for African Americans and other people of color. In some ways, President Bill Clinton is an example of this kind of engagement. One of the reasons for the overwhelming support President Clinton received from the African-American electorate is that, despite some of his policy decisions, such as signing the Personal Responsibility Act of 1996, that may be devastating to the

African-American community (see Schiele, 1998), he participates in concrete activities that help to ameliorate the status and to promote the positive
visibility of African Americans. Two such activities are his unprecedented
appointment of large numbers of African Americans and other people of
color to cabinet and other high-level administrative positions, and his continued support of what he refers to as "effective and fair" affirmative-action
policies. Activities such as these might help to prevent and eliminate race-
related guilt and fear that, as argued earlier, are possible factors for placing
the beneficiaries of racial oppression at risk of substance abuse.

SPIRITUAL ALIENATION AND SUBSTANCE ABUSE

Several writers have found spirituality to be an important factor in
explaining substance abuse and in assisting persons toward recovery (see
Brisbane and Womble, 1985; Carroll, 1993; Chickerneo, 1993; Maton and
Zimmerman, 1992; Philleo, Brisbane, and Epstein, 1997; Watkins, 1997).
Much of the emphasis on spirituality in substance abuse springs from
Alcoholics Anonymous (AA) and Narcotics Anonymous (NA) and their
twelve-step programs of recovery. The twelve-step programs' concept of
spirituality primarily embraces the belief in a higher power and the notion
that one's trials and tribulations should be turned over to this higher power
for intervention and remediation. Although these are important beliefs that
clearly are consonant with an Afrocentric view of substance abuse,
twelve-step programs fall short in three important ways: (1) they tend to
restrict the concept of spirituality to the belief in a higher power; (2) they
tend to be oblivious to the belief in God subjectification, opting instead for
a belief that objectifies God; and (3) they do not provide a sociospiritual
critique of U.S. society; that is, they do not identify how a lack of individual purpose and meaning can be connected to a paucity of spiritual consciousness in the core institutions of U.S. society. The Afrocentric paradigm addresses each of these shortcomings found in the twelve-step model
by explaining and offering solutions to substance abuse in the United
States with a focus on spiritual alienation.

The Concept of Spirituality

First, the Afrocentric paradigm's concept of spirituality, as expressed in
Chapter 2, does not limit spirituality to the belief or acknowledgment of a
deity, as do many twelve-step programs. Albeit the belief in a Creator is
clearly a critical component of the Afrocentric model's vision of spirituali-

ty, as examined Chapter 2, the model also embraces the idea of interconnectedness and the belief that the soul is at the core of a human being's existence. The dimension of interconnectedness validates the belief that all human beings and world elements are intimately intertwined through a similar universal source and that everything in the universe possesses a spiritual base. Spiritual alienation, in this sense, is alienation from *connectedness*, from both human and nature connectedness. In this way, substance abuse can be attributed to "the disconnection that allows people to take on an insular, detached identity of self" (Schiele, 1996, p. 289), one that reinforces an extreme individualism which asserts that the individual alone is and/or should be responsible for her or his failures and successes (Nobles, 1984; Rowe and Grills, 1993). Thus, from an Afrocentric perspective, considerable stress can result from this insular identity because pressure is placed on the person to succeed and to overcome life's hurdles with very little—if any—psychosocial and economic assistance from others. There is a tendency for one to become ashamed when he or she has not lived up to the expectations of the strong, self-sufficient, and autonomous individual who should be able to exclusively or primarily solve problems on his or her own. Nobles (1984) postulates that this individualistic thrust reflects "a society whose philosophical heritage reinforces loneliness, separateness, and irrelevancy" (p. 249). He further notes that youth substance abuse, and substance abuse generally, is expected and inevitable in the United States because people are in search of meaning in their lives that is attenuated by pervasive societal alienation brought on partly by the chasm between signifier and signified found in Western culture.

Accompanying this view of the lone individual is the notion that, when all is said and done, the individual is primarily a material and physical being. The acknowledgment that the individual is also a spiritual being with a vibrant entity called the soul is deemphasized, or at best only recognized when one observes his or her religious Sabbath. The component of the human being known as the soul is marginalized, and, thus, its development is not well attended to. This lack of recognition and development of the soul is conceived as a major, contributing factor to substance abuse from an Afrocentric viewpoint.

To better understand the meaning of the soul in traditional African societies, a brief discussion that identifies how the soul was conceptualized in ancient Africa is needed. Many Afrocentric writers draw on the knowledge of the soul that emanated in what is referred to as ancient Kemetic (Egyptian) society. Ameen (1990) presents a comprehensive analysis of how ancient Kemites understood the soul, and both Akbar

(1994) and Nobles (1986) provide a digest of some of the analyses offered by Ameen and others. What is interesting about the observations of these writers is that the examination of the soul for the Kemites was akin to understanding the potential of the human being. To illuminate the soul was to underscore the human's potential for peace, happiness, and achievement.

For the ancients, the soul was believed to have seven components: (1) Ka, (2) Ba, (3) Khaba, (4) Akhu, (5) Seb, (6) Putah, and (7) Atmu (Akbar, 1994; Ameen, 1990; Nobles, 1986). The Ka was believed to be the physical manifestation of the soul. Akbar (1994) states that Ka actually means "blood," and it is the blood that interpenetrates and has been passed down to all living entities, including humans. Thus, the physical manifestation of the soul is blood, and it is blood (Ka) that connects all living entities, human and nonhuman. Akbar (1994) maintains that the Ba is what people traditionally think of as the soul. It represents the convergence of spirit and intelligence and is deemed the original creative energy that has been given to humans by the Creator. To this extent, the Ba is called the "breath of life," in that the avenue via which the Creator transfers the creative energy to all living entities is through breath or air. The third component of the soul, the Khaba, deals with emotion and motion (Akbar, 1994; Ameen, 1990). Both human emotion and motion were thought to be produced by the Khaba (Akbar, 1994; Nobles, 1986). The Khaba fundamentally is responsible for human sensory perception, that is, sight, hearing, and other physical perceptions. The fourth aspect of the soul in ancient Kemet was the Akhu or Ab, which was thought to be the source of intelligence and mental perception (Akbar, 1994; Ameen, 1990; Nobles, 1986). This is what Eurocentric social science considers to be the mind. The Akhu was considered the navigator of the human spirit, and the function of its entity, intelligence, was to direct the human being toward the wisdom of the Creator or God. The fifth element of the soul was the Seb. The Seb was the part of the soul that allowed the human being to reproduce biologically. It can be said to be the "regenerative spirit" (Akbar, 1994). The Putah was the sixth component of the Kemetic concept of soul, and it represented mental maturity and led to the establishment of the human identity (Akbar, 1994; Ameen, 1990; Nobles, 1986). The mental maturity of the Putah also was believed to bring about wisdom, which was the ability to provide guidance and tutelage to others (Akbar, 1994). Last, the Atmu was believed to be the divine and eternal soul, that dimension which transcended the human body, time, and space (Akbar, 1994; Ameen, 1990).

What was fundamental about this ancient conceptualization of the soul was that virtually all aspects of the human being were collapsed under the rubric of "soul." The human being's mission was thought to be a divine one that certainly was not devoid of meaning and purpose. A recurring theme in much of the substance abuse literature is that an absence of purpose and meaning in one's life contributes significantly to drug abuse in the United States. If this is so, then the acquisition and internalization of the concept of soul used by the ancients might prevent one from feeling his or her life has no meaning and may obviate one from relying heavily on drugs as a substitute for a life perceived as empty and worthless.

God Subjectification

The Afrocentric paradigm also fills the void in the twelve-step programs' view that God is external, that the human being is powerless, and that only through the acknowledgment of an external God can one's recovery be achieved. The Afrocentric model, although recognizing that God is external, omnipotent, and omnipresent, does not suggest that the human being is powerless over alcohol and other substances. Instead, the Afrocentric paradigm posits that humans can exercise considerable control over their lives if they would subjectify, rather than objectify, God. Subjectification of God, for this discussion, means conceiving (1) that the totality of oneself is spiritual and is divinely inspired, (2) that one has the potential to tap into the power, sagacity, and creative genius of the Creator, and (3) that one is a manifestation, though a small part, of the whole of the Creator. In succinct terms, God subjectification repudiates a sterile and spiritually alienated concept of humans and instead adopts and applies the seven components of the soul, discussed earlier, to an understanding of oneself. This notion of God and the human being is assumed to empower the individual in a way that provides him or her with greater self-confidence and a sense of internal vitality. One can gain greater self-confidence when one feels intimately connected to God because one can become aware of the vast and perhaps unrevealed possibility to excel and achieve. These aspects can play a critical role in substance abuse, as studies have found that feelings of low self-worth and esteem, which are associated with feelings of self-confidence, can contribute to substance abuse (Grant, Martinez, and White, 1998; Kasee, 1995; Maton and Zimmerman, 1992).

Greater internal vitality simply means the potential to have a greater sense of internal purpose. When the soul is not viewed as the core existence or essence of the human being, the meaning of life can be reduced to a materialistic understanding that lacks a sense of permanency and deeper acknowledgment of human interconnectedness (Akbar, 1994; Chandler

Holden, and Kolander, 1992; Elkins, 1995). Anxiety can be the consequence when people perceive their existence is not everlasting and when they perceive others and their world as fragmented and disjointed (Fromm, 1941; May, 1977; Myers, 1988). From this line of reasoning, fear can be said to be associated with the belief that humans have an inherent proclivity to be destructive and to doubt the spiritual or unseen. Thus, Nobles (1984) uses pieces of this argument to suggest that substance abuse in the United States is a function of antagonistic and external concepts of God, characteristic of Western culture, that help create and continue a psychospiritual gap between people and God. From an Afrocentric perspective, substance abuse can be a corollary of these cultural beliefs, which are assumed to diminish if people take on a more subjective notion and feeling of God. The adoption of this subjective idea of God could engender a greater desire among people to exist and to positively contribute to the human family.

Sociospiritual Critique

Another difference between the Afrocentric paradigm's view of spirituality and that of the twelve-step programs' is that the Afrocentric paradigm offers what can be called a sociospiritual critique of U.S. culture. Spiritual alienation is not only viewed as an individual's inability or lack of motivation to tap into the creative genius of the Creator but also the extent to which the broader social, political, and economic forces of a society facilitate or hinder spiritual development. In this regard, the Afrocentric paradigm demands that the institutions and values of a society be examined to determine how compatible they are in fostering spirituality among people.

Although not identifying herself as Afrocentric, Morell (1996) offers an analysis of recovery and addiction that reinforces Afrocentric principles. She maintains that although addiction occurs across social class, gender, and racial lines, a significant number of people who become addicted to substances are from disempowered groups, such as people of color, women, the unemployed and underemployed, and the extremely poor. To better understand and explain this phenomenon, Morell (1996) calls for a "sociospiritual approach." This approach combines a spiritual with a political worldview to underscore the social problems that can emerge when a sense of human interconnectedness is discouraged in society. The sources of this human disconnectedness for Morell are political and economic exploitation, and its consequences are separating people into mutually exclusive categories and then devaluating certain categories or groups. This can influence a sense of personal separation for devalued groups that can place them at risk for addictive behaviors (Morell, 1996). Rowe and

Grills (1993) maintain that the lack of a sociocultural and sociospiritual critique of the United States in explaining substance abuse stems from an overemphasis on an individual deficit model. This model, they assert, functions to detract attention away from systemic forces whose purpose may be to more effectively control those least valued in society, and the model is devoid of a cultural critique of the United States that demonstrates how cultural values of European-American society place little emphasis on nurturing the value of interconnectedness.

Schiele (1996) reinforces the ideas of the latter authors by stating that the disconnection of nonmaterial and morally affirming values, found in a society that promotes spiritual alienation, compels people to take on an extreme or exclusive "materialistic" view of themselves and social reality. Materialistic here implies (1) a view of reality that validates sensory perception over extrasensory perception as a means of knowing, (2) a view that exclusively associates self-worth with the acquisition and hoarding of material items, and (3) a finite and competitive concept of time. Especially relevant here to substance abuse are the latter points. Some suggest that drug abuse is a response to the stress associated with the need to successfully compete in an extremely competitive society (Eckersley, 1993; Linsky, Colby, and Straus, 1987; Moore, 1995). One of the primary indicators of successful competition in U.S. culture is the number and quality of material items one has acquired and, related, the speed at which one's career advances. Although the Afrocentric paradigm clearly is not adverse to the advancement of careers or to the necessity of acquiring material items, it does contend that overemphasis on these phenomena, and the value of rugged competition that undergirds them both, can cause unnecessary stress and can diminish the likelihood of nurturing human values such as collectivity, compassion, patience, and equality, all needed for the fruition of a spiritually mature society.

The same can be said of a finite and competitive concept of time. One of the accompanying features of the Eurocentric worldview is a materialistic and rigidly linear concept of time (Ani, 1994; Hall, 1997). An important corollary of this understanding of time is that, as with everything else within an overly materialistic worldview, time becomes a source of competition, a potential enemy to compete against (Schiele, 1996, 1997). This can be especially so in regard to the future because, congruent with the progressivistic orientation of Eurocentric culture, to be discussed in more detail in Chapter 10 (see Horton, 1993), the future becomes a commodity for investment, and if one does not properly plan and invest, it (the future) can reek disaster and defeat the individual's effort to control and manipulate it. Ani (1994) refers to this cultural obsession to control and manipulate the future as *the ideology of progress.* A major objective of what she refers to as a uniquely Eurocentric phenomenon is to provide "order to otherwise directionless motion" (Ani, 1994, p. 495). This need to provide order to and compete against the future can induce personal stress, if indeed the person perceives that the future is getting the best of him or her. From this framework, substance abuse can be understood as a method through which the individual can compensate for his or her perceived failure to successfully compete against and overcome the future (Schiele, 1996). Thus, the crux of this explication of substance abuse maintains that the acceptance of an extreme materialist view of human relations and social reality is a contributing factor of substance abuse because it despiritualizes and commodifies all aspects of reality and compels the individual to interpret these aspects as potential sources of personal destruction. Furthermore, it is assumed that the foundation for the despiritualization and commodification of reality is the Eurocentric worldview, which pervades most of the socializing structures and institutions of U.S. society.

What is particularly deleterious about the Eurocentric worldview, as it concerns substance abuse, is that it does not encourage the kind of harmony between the individual and broader environment that some believe is important in preventing and treating substance abuse (see Grant, Martinez, and White, 1998; Jackson, 1995; Jackson, Stephens, and Smith, 1997; Morell, 1996). By undergirding institutions and socializing structures such as the family, the polity, and education, the Eurocentric worldview's elements of rugged competition, extreme individualism, and materialism can disrupt and preclude reciprocally nurturing relationships between the individual and the broader society (Ani, 1994; Asante, 1990, 1988; Kambon, 1992). The notion of alienation discussed by Emile Durkheim, Karl Marx, and others has at its core feelings of disconnection from other people, society, and nature. From an Afrocentric viewpoint, much of this alienation is culturally determined by the values that buttress the Eurocentric worldview and places many persons at risk of substance abuse because the alienation can influence a lack of purpose, sense of loneliness, and perceived personal failure, which some contend are central reasons why many persons become substance abusers (see Carroll, 1993; Chickerneo, 1993; Maton and Zimmerman, 1992; Mathew et al., 1996). So, what many Western thinkers describe as a lack of mutual reciprocation or transactions between the individual and the broader social milieu is what would be called a lack of harmony within the Afrocentric lexicon. At the core of this disharmony is a sociocultural and political economic entity that is despiritualized, a society that represses the sublime (see Haronian, 1972).

Recommendations for Substance Abuse
Prevention and Treatment

To prevent and treat substance abuse and addiction from a sociospiritual perspective, the Afrocentric paradigm recommends (1) sensitizing U.S. institutions to the role they may play in cultivating and facilitating substance abuse, (2) advocating social policies that not only provide more services to substance abusers but that also strengthen the harmony or spiritual bond between individuals and their wider and intimate social milieus, and (3) integrating counseling and therapeutic techniques that help and instruct abusers to achieve greater spiritual wellness and development.

It is extremely important, from an Afrocentric perspective, that institutions in U.S. society become more sensitive and aware of the role they may play in placing many people at risk of substance abuse. From a sociospiritual viewpoint, the primary problem is the marginalization of the spiritual within these institutions. Instead, as Chandler and colleagues (1992) posit, the spiritual should not only be conceived as an additional component of human wellness and wholeness but rather as the entity that interpenetrates and underlies all other components. For the polity, this implies that political decisions and policymaking should always consider the implications a policy may have for spiritual wellness. For schools, this means that more classroom dialogue needs to take place about spiritual wellness, and for the family, it implies that caretakers and children should participate in rituals and practices that reinforce human interconnectedness and interdependency.

Often, opponents of the greater integration of spiritual values and dialogue in U.S. institutions maintain that this dialogue is counterproductive to a democracy because it inevitably raises issues of religious tolerance. From the left or progressive wing of the political spectrum, there is fear that too much emphasis on spirituality will enhance the power of the religious right to attack what they perceive as cultural and moral relativity related to the repudiation of Christian values. However, as Chandler, Holden, and Kolander (1992) convey, it is important to note that spirituality can be conceptualized independent of religion; "that is, spirituality can occur in or out of the context of the institution of organized religion, and not all aspects of religion are assumed to be spiritual" (p. 170). Semmes (1993) and Asante (1988) contend that religion tends to be particularistic in that it is the expression of the deification of some group's cultural values. Thus, a major step toward rendering U.S. institutions more aware of their role in fostering and facilitating substance abuse is to radically alter how these institutions conceptualize spirituality by promoting the view that spirituality is, in essence, the affirmation and practice of *interconnectedness*.

If substance abuse is going to be more effectively prevented and treated, there is a critical need for more social policies in which the elimination or reduction of spiritual alienation is a primary objective. Many social policy advocates have validated and embraced the concept of interconnectedness in their policy advocacy efforts, but greater attention still needs to be given to spirituality, especially discussions that offset concerns about cost-effectiveness, efficiency, and reduction—which are important—with deeper discussions about the moral good and principles of a policy. To be discussed in more detail in Chapter 8, an Afrocentric viewpoint would assert that a policy must be examined for the degree to which it (1) promotes the union of the spiritual with the material, (2) validates the subjectification, and not objectification, of human beings, (3) fosters the notion of collective failure and collective success, and (4) advances a holistic and organic view of people that includes concerns about not only the mind and body but also the soul. Social policy advocates and legislators should recognize the potential for spiritual wellness and development to interpenetrate and underlie all other human needs and all human interactions.

Several writers have discussed techniques that can help abusers and recovering abusers achieve greater spiritual wellness and development in their lives. Jackson, Stephens, and Smith (1997) state that a critical component essential in substance abuse counseling to raise the spiritual wellness of abusers is the value of harmony. For them, harmony implies recognition of the interdependency of the spiritual, mental, and physical realms of life and that harmony begins by bringing a sense of destiny into one's consciousness. This sense of destiny, which is believed to empower the recoverer and give him or her a greater sense of life purpose, is assumed to be accomplished when people gain a better and more intuitive understanding of the self. However, to do this, the abuser must become keenly aware of the importance of both feelings and intellect and how each can facilitate more comprehension and honesty about one's self and one's feelings (Jackson, Stephens, and Smith, 1997).

The previous techniques help to assist the abuser to regain harmony internally, but the concept of harmony also can be extended to human relationships. Jackson, Stephens, and Smith (1997) contend that abusers must be taught that drugs and substance abuse disrupt harmonious relationships in a way that upsets the natural and divine order of the universe. If this is true, then substance abusers may gain a more in-depth appreciation of harmonious human relationships that place these relationships in a broader context of a universal order sanctioned by the Creator. In this way, and consonant with the concept of harmony, substance abusers can be taught that the Creator exists in all elements, both animate and inanimate (Jackson, 1995), and this teaching could influence abusers to take on a subjectified view of God. God subjectification has been found to be helpful for recovering alcoholics. Chickerneo (1993), in her study of recovering alcoholics who used art therapy to overcome their addiction, found that each of her subjects "indicated that as they got to know God, they also got to know themselves, and/or as they got to know themselves they got to know God" (p. 210). She goes on to intimate that this close identification with a higher power helps recovering alcoholics to acquire greater peace and unity with self and to fill the void of emptiness and lack of purpose that frequently contributes to their drinking.

A primary technique used by those who advocate the integration of spirituality in treatment is meditation (see Chandler, Holden, and Kolander, 1992; Jackson, 1995; Jackson, Stephens, and Smith, 1997; Novak, 1989; Phillips, 1990; Tart, 1990). Chandler and colleagues (1992) suggest that the fundamental purpose of meditation and other techniques of spiritual development is to sacrilize or resacrilize the client or client system. Sacrilization is "sensitizing to the spiritual those who have no conscious experience of the spiritual" (Chandler, Holden, and Kolander, 1992, p. 172), and resacrilization is the process that "resensitize[s] those who have been spiritually well but have moved, consciously or unconsciously, toward repression" (Chandler, Holden, and Kolander, 1992, p. 172) of the spiritual. Meditation is said to facilitate these processes by encouraging (1) feelings of personal balance and harmony, (2) relaxation, and (3) an enhanced recognition of one's self and one's environment that "replaces feelings of isolation, provides greater personal security, and creates a sensation of being in communion with the universe" (Chandler, Holden, and Kolander, 1992, p. 173).

One caveat about using meditation strategies, from an Afrocentric perspective, is that the attention to feelings not be marginalized. Much of the focus in meditation techniques is on enhancing or bringing one into "pure consciousness" (see Assagioli, 1965; Novak, 1989). Although pure consciousness is fine, the Afrocentric paradigm would hold that pure consciousness, which tends to imply use of the cognitive domain only, must be balanced by pure (i.e., authentic) affect or feeling. The Afrocentric paradigm maintains that a deeper understanding of one's self and one's problem must be accompanied and cultivated by a willingness to express (both behaviorally and verbally) genuine emotions (Brisbane and Womble, 1991; Myers, 1988; Phillips, 1990; Schiele, 1996). Feeling the problem is thought to be the best way to gain knowledge of the problem and can ultimately lead to human transformation that is sustained and authentic (Akbar, 1984; Brisbane and Womble, 1991; Phillips, 1990). The acknowledgment and expression of one's emotions have been shown to increase the likelihood that the substance abuser will have a successful recovery (Brisbane and Womble, 1985; Chickerneo, 1993).

CULTURAL MISORIENTATION AND SUBSTANCE ABUSE

As with the previous chapter, the discussion on the effects of political economic oppression and spiritual alienation on substance abuse can be applied to a broad number of persons and groups in U.S. society. However, the effects of cultural misorientation on substance abuse, although potentially relevant to a broad grouping of people, is especially applicable to groups who have been victimized by cultural oppression. Though several groups have experienced cultural oppression, the Afrocentric paradigm is particularly interested in the effects cultural oppression has had on people of African descent. This section offers some ideas that may help to illuminate the relationship between cultural misorientation and substance abuse among African Americans. Also, since the age of onset of drug usage and experimentation for many people who have used or still use drugs is during adolescence (Chen and Kandel, 1995; Labouvie, Bates, and Pandina, 1997), this section focuses mainly on this potential relationship among African-American youths.

One of the areas that should be clarified regarding the prevalence of drug usage among African-American youths is that although the prominent view is that young African Americans use and abuse drugs more excessively than young European Americans, recent data indicate that this is not so. Data from the Monitoring the Future study indicate that from 1991 to 1998, the percentage of African-American eighth, tenth, and twelfth graders who had used alcohol, marijuana, and cocaine was consistently lower than the percentage of same-age European-American youths who had used the same drugs (Johnston, O'Malley, and Bachman, 1998). Findings from Prendergast and colleagues (1989) and from Bachman and colleagues (1991) report similar racial disparities and indicate that this trend is not new.

Although it is important to note that African-American youths use and abuse drugs less than European-American youths, those who advocate an Afrocentric point of view are usually more concerned with the effects of African-American youth drug abuse on the survival, advancement, and prosperity of the African-American community and culture. The significance of cultural survival, and culture generally, is quite prevalent among Afrocentric writers, and several social scientists and mental health professionals who write from an Afrocentric viewpoint increasingly have suggested that the paucity of proactive ethnic and cultural socialization is an important factor to address when explaining the social problems of African-American youths (see Akbar, 1991; Grant, Martinez, and White, 1998; Harvey and Rauch, 1997; Jeff, 1994; Lemelle, 1995; Oliver, 1989; Rowe and Grills, 1993; Ward, 1995). More specifically, these writers maintain that the problems of African-American youths, including substance abuse, are partly results of cultural alienation, that is, alienation from traditional African and African-American cultural values that underscore race consciousness, social responsibility and collectivity, and spirituality (Ani, 1994; Kambon, 1992; Mbiti, 1970; Schiele, 1996). These writers further recommend that to prevent and reduce the inimical psychosocial and economic effects of problems such as substance abuse on African-American youths, it is necessary to enhance these youths' exposure to, and internalization of, Afrocentric cultural values.

From the previous ideas, it can be assumed that African-American youths who abuse drugs need to be culturally aligned to gain a more positive ethnic/racial identity. This identity is assumed to not only enhance one's commitment to the survival, advancement, and prosperity of the group but also one's racial and cultural self-esteem. Both the commitment to group and positive racial and cultural self-esteem are important because a lack of commitment to one's racial/cultural group (what some refer to as racial consciousness) and low ethnic/racial cultural self-esteem have been found to place youths at greater risk of substance abuse and usage and to render them more tolerant of drugs (Belgrave et al., 1994; Foulks and Pena, 1995; Fudge, 1996; Grant, Martinez, and White, 1998; Kasee, 1995; Westermeyer, 1995). The effects of a lack of commitment to one's racial/cultural group and an unfavorable racial/cultural self-esteem—both considered outcomes of cultural misorientation—on substance abuse are elaborated in the following material by presenting a conceptual framework that relies on theoretical ideas of the author and on the existing literature. It should be stated at the outset that although group commitment and racial/cultural self-esteem are presented as separate effects, they can be seen as interrelated: as one's level of group commitment increases, one's level of racial/cultural self-esteem increases, and vice versa. In addition, the relationship can be conceptualized holistically in that both factors can be conceived as temporally occurring simultaneously, as if to form a circle as opposed to a straight line.

Group Commitment and Substance Abuse

The African self-consciousness (ASC) construct, discussed in the last chapter, can be employed as an indicator of an African American's level of group commitment to other people of African descent when one examines the four dimensions of the construct presented by Kambon (1992, p. 56):

1. Awareness of one's African identity (a collective consciousness) and African cultural heritage, and sees value in the pursuit of knowledge of self
2. Recognition of African survival and positive development as one's number one priority
3. Respect for and active perpetuation of things African: African life and African cultural institutions
4. Maintaining a standard of conduct of resolute and uncompromising resistance to all things anti-African

Together, the dimensions of ASC echo a common theme: ethnic consciousness engenders group commitment.

Regarding drug abuse, it is assumed that as a youth's ASC decreases, his or her level of substance abuse is likely to increase. It is further assumed that when an African-American youth does not internalize high ASC, he or she will probably not be as concerned with eliminating the oppression that black people face and, thus, would have little desire to advance black people politically, culturally, and economically. To the extent that a youth is not conscious of the oppression of people of African descent, one may be unaware of the manifold subtle and insidious ways the system of oppression maintains control over African Americans. The over availability of illicit drugs and liquor stores in many African-American communities probably would not be recognized by persons with low ASC as a possible strategy to dominate and manipulate African Americans. Therefore, youths with this mind-set may be at a greater risk of abusing substances because they lack understanding of the political and economic function of substance abuse within the context of oppression, as discussed earlier in this chapter. Moreover, persons with low ASC, as opposed to those with high ASC, may be less likely to participate in black liberation struggles and, therefore, may fail to acknowledge that substance abuse significantly inhibits their ability to optimally contribute to these struggles.

Some evidence suggests that the ASC construct may help to explicate self-destructive behaviors among African-American drug abusers. In the only study uncovered that has examined the effects of ASC on African-American drug abusers, Dixon and Azibo (1998) found that African-American male crack-cocaine users who had ASC scores that represented a higher level of group commitment tended to participate less in exploitative means to earn a living than those who had ASC scores that demonstrated lower levels of African-American group commitment. Earning a living via exploitative means was defined by the authors as participation in thefts, robberies, selling stolen goods, and hustling people in licit and illicit ways. Although Dixon and Azibo did not examine whether lower ASC places one at greater risk of using or abusing drugs, their findings are important in that ASC may help to explain the variance in criminal behavior among African-American crack cocaine users and abusers. Future research needs to explore the effects of ASC orientation on African Americans who become drug abusers and those who do not. In the Dixon and Azibo study, all of the subjects were drug abusers.

Although not using the ASC construct, Gary and Berry (1985) found a significant relationship between awareness of racial oppression and attitudes about substance abuse among 411 randomly sampled African Americans. Awareness that racial oppression was a reality in the United States was a major dimension of what the researchers referred to as a racial consciousness scale. When racial consciousness was correlated with their measure of "attitudes toward substance abuse," respondents who had higher racial consciousness were significantly less likely to tolerate substance abuse than those who had lower racial consciousness. Indeed, in this study, racial consciousness was more important in explaining substance abuse attitudes than were gender, age, church involvement, education level, marital status, and community involvement.

When commitment to one's ethnic group has been conceived as an outcome of drug abuse, adverse consequences also have been reported. Westermeyer (1995) demonstrates how substance abuse can be pernicious to one's ethnic affiliation and cultural participation. The abuse is adverse because it can cause what he refers to as *cultural disruption,* a disruption not only in one's participation with the group but also in one's internalization of the group's values, norms, and customs. In other words, the person becomes less committed to the ethos and interests of his or her cultural group. Westermeyer also suggests that the relationship between cultural disruption and substance abuse is reciprocal in that the disruption can increase the severity of the abuse. This is indicated by his statement that "The longer that these [cultural disruptive effects] have been present, the longer the substance abuse is likely to have been present. If the cultural disruption is extensive, the substance abuse is likely to be severe" (1995, p. 596). Applying Westermeyer's ideas to this discussion could imply that lower levels of ASC for African-American youths are tantamount to cultural disruption and could place them in jeopardy of drug abuse and addiction.

Since spirituality has been offered in this book to be an essential aspect of the Afrocentric worldview and Afrocentric cultural values, it may be an important factor in enhancing an African-American youth's ASC and thus lessening that youth's chances of becoming hooked on drugs. This could be because of spirituality's core themes of interconnectedness and God consciousness. The interconnectedness theme could enhance and support ASC in that African-American youths can become conscious of the spiritual bond that connect people of African descent, despite their geographical locations and economic and educational levels. This consciousness could reinforce in African-American youths the belief that despite the differences among people of African descent, there is a common origin and perhaps a common destiny for all these people. This may help youths become more in tune to their personal destiny, which might help them become more concerned with identifying and achieving personal goals, such as going to and completing college, forming and sustaining substantive interpersonal relationships, or just gaining greater insight into who and what they are. The relationship between consciousness of their cultural group destiny and their personal or individual destiny is viewed as a central factor in substance abuse recovery among African Americans (Jackson, Stephens, and Smith, 1997; Rowe and Grills, 1993). It could be suggested that the less an African-American youth affirms the interconnectedness of people of African descent, and thereby decreases the understanding of how his or her personal destiny is related to and can shape the collective destiny of people of African descent, the more likely she or he might become prone to abuse drugs.

The degree to which an African-American youth adopts the God consciousness aspect of spirituality also may have some bearing on one's level of ASC and, inevitably, on one's level of substance abuse. Gary and Berry (1985) and Maton and Zimmerman (1992) have found religiosity, which can be construed as an indicator of God consciousness, to be an important correlate of substance abuse among African Americans. Gary and Berry (1985) found that church involvement, their measure of religiosity, was positively and significantly correlated with attitudes toward substance abuse. Respondents who were not active members of a church tended to have significantly more tolerant attitudes toward substance abuse than those who were active members of a church. Similarly, in their investigation of the frequency of drug use among African-American male adolescents, Maton and Zimmerman (1992) found that spirituality significantly explained marijuana and hard-drug usage among the respondents. The more spiritual the male adolescent, the less frequently he used drugs. In fact, as a correlate of marijuana and hard-drug usage, spirituality was more important in some of their statistical analyses than were social support, stress, and internal well-being. Maton and Zimmerman measured spirituality using three items, two of which, "I experience a personal, close relationship with God" and "I experience God's love and caring on a regular basis" (1992, p. 84), can be interpreted as dimensions of what I refer to as God consciousness.

These findings suggest that the internalization of a God consciousness, whether cognitively or behaviorally manifested, helps to reduce the risk of substance abuse among African Americans, generally, and African-American youths, specifically. Although the authors of the latter studies do not provide an elaborate explanation of why a God consciousness could reduce this risk, it may be that when one acknowledges the Creator, or God, and the presence of this spirit in one's self, one may become concerned about whether one's life reflects the highest of moral principles and standards of excellence. One may attempt to think and do the "right" thing and also seek to execute one's activities in the best and most competent way possible. Such persons may endeavor to behave in a manner that legitimates the greatness and wisdom of the Creator, perhaps because they acknowledge that God is inside of them (i.e., God subjectification). Therefore, acts of mediocrity and malice may be reduced, avoided, or disdained. To the extent that the abuse of drugs, which can not only weaken but kill, is considered a malicious act that places one at risk of committing mediocre acts, young African-Americans with this orientation may be less likely to abuse drugs than those who have lower levels of God consciousness.

Racial/Cultural Self-Esteem and Substance Abuse

In the literature, what is construed as racial/cultural self-esteem is what some writers refer to as racial or ethnic identity (see Brookins, 1996; Jacobs and Bowles, 1988; Reese, Vera, and Paikoff, 1998). Generally, racial/cultural self-esteem is the degree to which the person is not only conscious of his or her group identity and cultural values but also feels good or proud about being a member of the group. It is this "feel good" or "feel proud" aspect of racial/ethnic identity that I am referring to as racial/cultural self-esteem. Some researchers have found this form of self-esteem to be important in explaining substance abuse among African Americans (Belgrave et al., 1994; Foulks and Pena, 1995; Gary and Berry, 1985; Grant, Martinez, and White, 1998). In their study, for example, of African-American cocaine abusers, Foulks and Pena (1995) found that low self-esteem and negative self-concept were important factors that contributed to the cocaine abuse of their subjects. The investigators stated that this may be a significant factor for African Americans because of the "color prejudice in white America" (p. 630) that too often serves to demoralize and stigmatize African Americans. Foulks and Pena further contend that because of this demoralization and stigmatization, African Americans may abuse drugs as a means to "self medicate for inner-personal problems" (1995, p. 611) and may participate in the drug culture as a self-affirming strategy to offset the effects of psychic pain engendered by low self-esteem.

This same rationale has been used by the Nation of Islam (NOI) to explain drug abuse in the African-American community. Having a successful track record in helping African Americans to recover from drug abuse (Lusane, 1991), the NOI advances the idea that the system of white supremacy and the relics of slavery have debilitated the self-concept of African Americans in a manner that places many of them at risk of self-hatred and of acquiescing to a slave mentality (Muhammad, 1965). Drug abuse, from this perspective, is an avenue to compensate for feelings of negative self-pride toward people of African descent, generally, and themselves, specifically.

Belgrave and colleagues' (1994) examination of African-American fifth graders' attitudes toward drugs also demonstrates the importance of racial/cultural self-esteem. For their measure of racial/cultural self-esteem, they used the Children's Black Identity Scale, which was developed by the authors. A few items on the scale were, for example, "I feel that being black is a good experience" and "I feel good about being an African American." Belgrave and colleagues' (1994) analysis revealed that African-American children who had a higher and/or a more positive black identity felt significantly more than those who did not that drug use and abuse were pernicious. Furthermore, a significant dimension of Gary and Berry's (1985) measure of racial consciousness, which was used to explain substance use attitudes among African Americans, was the degree to which respondents "had a positive view of black people" (p. 46). Although there was a second dimension to their racial consciousness measure, they found higher racial consciousness to be significantly associated with lower tolerance of substance use.

What these latter findings and observations suggest are that when African Americans, generally, and African-American youths, specifically, feel ashamed about being black, they are at risk of abusing drugs and/or tolerating substance abuse. This implies that the system of Eurocentric cultural hegemony, of which white supremacy is a component, might contribute directly or indirectly, via informal institutions such as the family and friendship ties, to the substance abuse of African-American youths. These youths may be internalizing the negative messages and images of black people projected by and within Eurocentric culture. What may be needed, then, are programs that seek to address and eliminate cultural misorientation and other consequences of racial oppression among African-American substance abusers.

AFROCENTRIC DRUG TREATMENT PROGRAMS

Recently, some programs have been designed to infuse and integrate Afrocentric assumptions into substance abuse treatment interventions aimed at transforming African Americans. One of these programs has been described by Longshore and colleagues (1998). The project they present, known as the Engagement Project, is undergirded by the philosophy of *cultural congruent* treatment, which, for the authors, implies providing interventions that are consistent with the heritage, styles, symbols, and values of African and African-American culture. To achieve cultural congruence, the project is based upon six core principles that guide the counseling process. These principles are as follows:

1. Substance abuse dependence is conceived as an individual affliction and as a community disorder rooted in cultural and power disparities between African Americans and dominant white institutions.
2. The route of recovery is understood as a process that involves the acquisition of power in the forms of knowledge, spiritual insight, and community health.
3. Discussion of clients' drug use is framed in a context that recognizes the totality of life experiences faced by the client as an African American in an unfriendly social/political environment.
4. An emphasis is placed on the importance of changing one's environment not only for the good of the individual client but also for the greater good of the community.
5. A focus is placed on drug use alternatives that underscore personal rituals, cultural traditions, and spiritual well-being.
6. Equality is sought in the therapeutic relationship between counselor and client; there is a deemphasis on counselors being socially distant and nondisclosing.

The intervention techniques used in the Engagement Project are threefold: (1) brief intervention, (2) focused dyadic counseling, and (3) motivational interviewing. In the project, brief intervention is manifested as the process in which the client undergoes minimal counseling, is shown an educational video, and is provided referrals for continual assistance, if needed. The educational videos in the Engagement Project combine voiceovers with photos, documentary footage, and excerpts from commercial films on African Americans. The videos, which are shown before counseling sessions and which can serve as springboards of these sessions, mainly focus on ethnic relations, self-esteem, community conditions, the etiology of drug abuse, and pathways to recovery. Affirming the critical elements of brief interventions, counselors in the Engagement Project offer feedback to clients in ways that (1) encourage clients to assume responsibility for decisions about their recovery process; (2) provide clients with a range of alternative treatment interventions rather than just one intervention, (3) convey empathy via both verbal and nonverbal cues, and (4) identify and communicate to clients evidence of their strengths and competence that can be used in recovery.

The purpose of focused dyadic counseling is to assist African-American clients to draw into and on the collective and communal themes of African-American culture. To facilitate collectivity in the treatment process, the Engagement Project relies on the African oral tradition, "a tradition based on the presence of others who affirm the reality of the thought, feeling, circumstance, or experience called into being by a speaker" (Longshore et al., 1998, p. 325). This is achieved in the project by including a second client in the counseling session (i.e., a client dyad), and the counselor seeks participation from both clients by probing more important issues as they arise. This strategy is also believed to help both clients feel less isolated as they share their pain and experiences. Sometimes, however, the second client is a counseling peer. These are persons who are former drug users who can (1) empathize and validate the client's feelings and (2) reinforce the ideas and comments of the counselor. To more appropriately integrate the African oral tradition in treatment, the counselor also is encouraged to rely on Ebonics, a dialect of English that infuses African vestiges of syntax and communication style (Williams, 1973, 1997). Longshore and colleagues (1998) state that the use of Ebonics is important in assisting clients to gain greater comfort that can lead to more authentic participation in the counseling sessions.

The last technique used, motivational interviewing, strives to enhance a person's motivation to seek and remain in counseling and is most appropriate for the screening and intake phases of treatment. Longshore and colleagues (1998) identity five fundamental principles of motivational interviewing, which are as follows:

1. Expressing empathy: the counselor accepts clients' feelings without judging, criticizing, or blaming.
2. Developing discrepancy: clients are led to recognize discrepancies between their present behavior and broader goals.

3. Avoiding argument: the counselor does not directly confront clients on any aspect of their lifestyle or behavior.
4. Rolling with resistance: the counselor gently moves clients toward appropriate insights and decisions by using their own words and thoughts to guide them.
5. Supporting self-efficacy: clients are encouraged to view the counselor as someone who will help them do what they already know they can do. (pp. 325-326)

Two significant strategies employed in the Engagement Project are the integration of music and food into the therapeutic process. Music has been shown to be a primary aesthetic feature of African and African-American culture and was thoroughly integrated into many aspects of social life in traditional African societies (Asante, 1988, 1990; Martin and Martin, 1985; Mbiti, 1970; Walker, 1995). In the Engagement Project, background music of jazz and rhythm and blues permeates the community center in which the project is housed. Also, after the intake interview, clients are fed a traditional African-American meal, and during the meal, counselors and peers (i.e., former drug users) involve the client in informal conversation. For Longshore and colleagues (1998), the food, music, and informal talk help elicit feelings of "home" and positive attributes of clients' families and communities.

A second program described by Jackson (1995) and Jackson, Stephens, and Smith (1997) also validates the need for Afrocentric drug treatment. Their treatment program, known as Iwo San (House of Healing), serves African-American women and their dependent children. It is based on the assumption that noncompliance among African-American women in drug treatment can be diminished if treatment programs would incorporate Afrocentric concepts and practices into the drug recovery process. These concepts and practices are applied in a number of ways. First, and congruent with the Afrocentric paradigm, discussions of spirituality are interwoven throughout the treatment program. One's drug recovery is not separated from one's spiritual development in Iwo San. In addition, the twelve-step program is an integral component of drug treatment for Iwo San participants.

Second, African-American history and traditional African and African-American ceremonial practices are drawn upon in Iwo San. All residents, including the children, are exposed to African and African-American history at the global and local levels. To support this endeavor, field trips to local African-American exhibits, art museums, and cultural events are sponsored. Some of the ceremonial practices are those which commemorate certain holidays, such as Kwanza, which celebrate rites of passage and which affirm the preparation of traditional African foods. The Iwo San program includes diverse rites-of-passage ceremonies to facilitate the achievement of several program goals. Some of these are (1) to foster client internalization of Afrocentric thought and philosophy, (2) to alleviate and eliminate egocentricism so that it can be substituted with a sense of commonality and community, and (3) to reduce and extinguish negative defenses.

One way in which the notion of shared responsibility for treatment is reinforced in Iwo San, which stems from the value of conceiving everyone in treatment as a community, is to have what is called a council of elders (COE). In traditional African societies, the COE was a group of older persons who served as the cabinet to the chief or head administrator of the village or town. Its role was to provide guidance and recommendations to the administrator from the general public. In the Iwo San program, members of COE are selected democratically, and they must be held in high esteem among and by fellow residents, staff, and the local residential community. The COE consists of representatives from the community, the staff, residents, and consultants, and the role of the COE in Iwo San is fourfold: "(1) express wisdom, (2) offer guidance and leadership, (3) facilitate moral, cognitive, and spiritual development, and (4) infuse Afrocentric philosophy in the treatment process" (Jackson, Stephens, and Smith, 1997, p. 90). One of the most important functions of the COE is to determine if a client should be discharged. This not only occurs when the client has completed the program but also when she has violated program taboos. By having clients participate on the COE, they have an opportunity to feel ownership of the program in which they are a part and, thus, can feel that they are essential and relevant in the lives of others, perhaps for the first time ever.

A third manner in which Afrocentric concepts and practices are incorporated in the Iwo San program is the way drug abuse is conceptualized. The program embraces the view that the critical question regarding African-American female drug abusers is, what cultural factors place African-American women at risk of abusing drugs (Jackson, Stephens, and Smith, 1997)? The Iwo San program embraces the idea that poverty and racial oppression often have confined the social roles of African-American women and that their participation in the drug-using lifestyle is a mode through which they adopt a meaningful self-concept. The emphasis on increasing cultural awareness and on collectivism in Iwo San is believed to provide the African-American female with greater options from which to define herself and from which she can maximize her full positive potentiality as a human being, generally, and an African-American woman, specifically. Last, to further foster this process, the program encourages what can be referred to as a strengths perspective. Jackson, Stephens, and Smith (1997) maintain that clients should be encouraged to identify and draw upon their individual and community strengths to address their problems.

A discussion by Rowe and Grills (1993) also is relevant and corroborates the ideas of the latter programs. In their article, Rowe and Grills contend that a primary shortcoming of conventional drug treatment programs for African Americans is that they are predicated on the cultural ideas of Western society. Reliance on these cultural ideas is problematic because (1) they are inconsistent with the cultural values and traditions of people of African descent, (2) they reinforce the values of Eurocentric culture and therefore preclude a systematic critique of these values, and (3) the individualistic focus of Eurocentric culture is "inadequate for resolving issues affecting complex interrelationships, and implicitly serve[s] to maintain existing positions of power and privilege" (Rowe and Grills, 1993, p. 25). To correct and reverse the adverse consequences of Eurocentric treatment values on African-American substance abusers, Rowe and Grills offer seven alternative assumptions they believe should shape and guide substance abuse treatment with African Americans:

1. The conceptualization of the problem of substance abuse and its recovery must go beyond individual affliction and view the cultural and political environment of the United States as "diseased" and as the basis through which European-American hegemony over African Americans can be maintained.
2. Effective substance abuse treatment must acknowledge the power that stems from awareness of the interconnectedness between human beings and God.
3. Effective substance abuse treatment should be predicated on African-centered precepts and values.
4. Effective drug abuse treatment and recovery must underscore the positive potentiality inherent in human beings and should be predicated on a value system dedicated to the greater good of humankind.
5. Effective substance abuse treatment and recovery must be protracted and multidimensional, addressing all aspects of African-American development and transformation.
6. The conceptualization of substance abuse treatment must be based on reciprocity, equality, and respect between the healer and the client.
7. African Americans must be aware of how their recovery is related to the overall healing and advancement of the African-American community.

This examination of various ideas on substance abuse treatment and recovery for African Americans presented here reveals several common denominators of Afrocentric drug abuse treatment. The most conspicuous themes are (1) strong emphasis on spirituality, which is interwoven throughout the programs; (2) focus on the psychosocial effects (i.e., cultural misorientation) of racial oppression for African Americans; (3) considerable attention devoted to viewing treatment as a collective process through which the clients and staff are closely related and in which clients play major and active roles in their recovery and in the recovery of their peers; (4) the belief that exposure to traditional African and African-American cultural rituals and the enhancement of African and African-American cultural awareness is critical to the recovery process; and (5) the value placed on the nexus between the healing of an individual African-American substance abuser and the collective healing of the African-American community.

Chapter 7

The Afrocentric Paradigm and Social Welfare Philosophy, Ideology, and Policy

AN AFROCENTRIC CRITIQUE OF AMERICAN SOCIAL WELFARE PHILOSOPHY

The Need for an Afrocentric Critique

Despite those who suggest that American social welfare philosophy and policy include some benevolent and well-intended features, social welfare policy throughout the history of the United States can be generally characterized as callous, reluctant, and residual (Ehrenreich, 1985; Feagin, 1975; Jansson, 1997, Piven and Cloward, 1971, 1982). The callousness revealed in these policies toward the poor is often attributed to values endemic to the American landscape, such as individualism and the Protestant work ethic (Jansson, 1997; Trattner, 1994), or to the political economy of capitalism (Blau, 1999; Piven and Cloward, 1971, 1982). A relationship between individualism, the Protestant work ethic, and capitalism also has been observed (Weber, 1958), and there is considerable debate as to which is the chicken and which is the egg. However, substantial evidence suggests that the Protestant work ethic, along with American frontierism, rendered the United States especially conducive for the acceleration of capitalism (Jansson, 1997; Kohl, 1989; Novak, 1982; Weber, 1958).

Although analyses of the effects and dynamics of capitalism, Protestantism, and frontierism are important in understanding the values inherent

Portions of this chapter originally appeared in "An Afrocentric Perspective on Social Welfare Philosophy and Policy," *Journal of Sociology and Social Welfare,* 1997, 24(2), pp. 21-39. Reprinted with permission from Western Michigan University School of Social Work.

137

in American social welfare policies, more factors need to be explored to broaden our comprehension of the emergence of these values. The Afrocentric paradigm can be applied to help better understand the dynamics of these values. Its contribution to grasping the character of American social welfare philosophy and policy is that it underscores the important role of the Eurocentric worldview and contends that by acknowledging and examining this role, a more in-depth understanding of the values that undergird social welfare policy in the United States can be gained. In this regard, a comprehensive critique of the Eurocentric worldview—its attributes and its effects on social welfare philosophy and debate—has been downplayed, if not neglected.

Too often in discussions on social welfare philosophy and policy, culture is separated from, and viewed as an epiphenomenon of, the political economy. From an Afrocentric viewpoint, the underlying cultural attributes of a society are assumed to be the springboard from which political and economic institutions emerge, albeit a dynamic relationship is acknowledged. The Afrocentric paradigm can offer an additional avenue through which American social welfare philosophy can be critiqued and understood. Although some of its commentary may parallel some existing criticisms of American social welfare philosophy, the application of the Afrocentric paradigm to the analysis of American social welfare philosophy facilitates a more expanded and inclusive dialogue on American social welfare philosophy, one that validates the cultural interpretations and ideas of people of African descent.

An Afrocentric critique of American social welfare philosophy also views the political labels of conservative, moderate, liberal, and radical as insufficient to capture the major philosophical and political themes of the Afrocentric paradigm. Each of these political ideologies stems from the political and cultural ethos of European/European-American culture and history. Although each can be adopted by the Afrocentric paradigm, they do not fully legitimate the themes and ideas of the Afrocentric paradigm. Moreover, each political ideology deemphasizes racial oppression in its conceptualization of power, the state, resource distribution, societal relationships, and social problems, generally. Of the four, the radical political ideology comes the closest to approximating the perspective of the Afrocentric paradigm. Its focus on unraveling and critiquing the adverse consequences of a capitalist economy are consistent with the social justice values found in the Afrocentric paradigm. However, because many of its proponents embrace a Marxist or neo-Marxist analysis of social problems, the radical ideology tends to view racial oppression as an epiphenomenon incapable of being conceived independently of capitalist ideology (Asante,

1990; Dove, 1995). The Afrocentric paradigm, though unequivocally recognizing that capitalism exacerbates and inflames racial tensions, conceives racism as not exclusively emanating from a particular economic mode but rather as emerging from the character of a much broader and overarching entity known as the worldview.

The Eurocentric Worldview and Its Relation to Capitalism, Racism, and Sexism

Probably the most fundamental reason for the character of social welfare philosophy in the United States is the mode through which members of American society, especially those in power, conceive reality. The underlying assumptions about conceptions and interpretations of reality form what some call *worldview,* which was defined in Chapter 1. From an Afrocentric framework, the Eurocentric worldview is assumed to primarily shape the underlying philosophical assumptions prominent in the United States. This is because the majority of people in the United States—particularly the power elite—are European American, proclaiming Europe as their ancestral and cultural homeland.

For many of the reasons identified in Chapter 4, several writers (Akbar, 1994; Baldwin and Hopkins, 1990; Burgest, 1981; Kambon, 1992; Schiele, 1994) believe that the Eurocentric worldview inherently fosters oppression and inequality, mainly because of its attributes, which are individualism, rationalism, and materialism (Akbar, 1984; Ani, 1994; Asante, 1988; Schiele, 1994). Together, these attributes are assumed to nurture political economic structures and social institutions that allow human degradation and spiritual alienation to flourish (Ani, 1994; Kambon, 1992; Karenga, 1993; Leonard, 1995; Schiele, 1994), and they served to undergird explanations of poverty that imbue the character of American social welfare philosophy and policy.

A major reason why some contend that the Eurocentric worldview inherently engenders oppression and inequality is its association with the political economic system of capitalism. From an Afrocentric perspective, capitalism is assumed to be an outgrowth of the Eurocentric worldview. Some maintain that the Eurocentric worldview emerged because of the geological evolution and physical environment of Europe, which produced shortages in natural resources and which created aggressive and competitive behavioral adaptations to a harsh and barren physical milieu (Bradley, 1991; Diop, 1978). Others contend that the worldview stems from the philosophical traditions of Plato and Aristotle that emphasized objectification of the universe and dichotomous logic (Ani, 1994; Burgest, 1981; Rashad, 1991). It is believed that these factors eventually generated more concern in Europe for material and technological development than for spiritual and human development (Ani, 1994; Akbar, 1994; Bradley, 1991). This concern over material and technological advancement is believed to have prompted the overemphasis on values such as individualism, competition, material accumulation and comfort, and the rationality (i.e., efficiency) of production, all of which are associated with capitalist societies, especially what is generally referred to as bourgeois society (see Horkheimer, 1972). Although the structural origins of modern capitalism can be found in the collapse of feudalism in Europe (Hobson, 1949), the precipitous growth of capitalism occurred when European nations began to colonize, enslave, and exploit nations and people of color during the sixteenth through nineteenth centuries (Blaut, 1993; Hobson, 1949; Williams, 1944). Thus, capitalism expanded in the world because of the greater emphasis placed on exploiting natural resources and human labor for profit, which, from an Afrocentric viewpoint, is a function of the Eurocentric worldview.

It is important to acknowledge that although some writers maintain that there were capitalist forms of economy in Africa prior to European colonization and world domination (Blaut, 1993), others maintain that *traditional Africa* (i.e., Africa prior to Arab and European influences) relied more on a communal mode of economy (Asante, 1990; Clarke, 1991; Nyerere, 1968). If the practice of using private property to disadvantage another person or group is a significant indicator of capitalism's existence, then there is little evidence that traditional Africa was capitalistic. In traditional Africa, everyone had the right to use and live on the land (Biebuyck, 1964; Nyerere, 1968), and, more important, the aspiration of personal wealth, via land ownership, to dominate and disadvantage others was almost nonexistent (Asante, 1990; Diop, 1987; Nyerere, 1968).

Further, it can be argued that societies with similar economic modes may not have similar sociocultural and economic characteristics. This is because cultural values of a society can significantly mediate the effects of an economic mode on a people's living standard and conditions (Asante, 1990; Nkrumah, 1970; Williams, 1993). Thus, even if capitalist forms of economy were found in traditional Africa, their manifestation would have been different from European capitalism because of divergent sociocultural environments.

From an Afrocentric viewpoint, both racism and sexism, critical attributes of American social welfare philosophy and policy, also are consequences of the Eurocentric worldview. This is primarily because of the Eurocentric worldview's attribute of rationalism, which undergirds a fragmented and dichotomous logic and conception of human beings (Burgest,

1981; Kambon, 1992; Schiele, 1994). This fragmented and dichotomous view leads to a focus on difference and exclusion (Baldwin and Hopkins, 1990; Schiele, 1994) rather than on similarity and inclusion. Although difference can be seen as positive and can be celebrated, the fragmented and dichotomous view of human beings found in the Eurocentric world-view debases difference and uses it to justify the exclusion and oppression of people with "different" material (i.e., outer) characteristics. The debasement of difference does not complete the process. Rather, the process is furthered by hierarchical thinking used to rank order people into categories of, say, good to bad, high to low, superior to inferior (Ani, 1994; Burgest, 1981; Schiele, 1994). Thus, outer human characteristics (i.e., Eurocentricity's materialism) are viewed as negatively different and then are used to create categories (e.g., race and sex) within which people are hierarchically and normatively ranked.

The Eurocentric Worldview and Assumptions About Poverty

To demonstrate how American social welfare philosophy is undergirded by the Eurocentric worldview, three basic assumptions about poverty are examined. These assumptions tap into the core of American social welfare philosophy on poverty. The assumptions are as follows:

1. Poverty is a function of individual deficits and behavior.
2. Despite economic hardships and societal inequalities, people should be able to maintain self-sufficiency and economic independence.
3. The poor should be punished, not helped, because they lack the initiative and perseverance to be financially self-sufficient.

At a glance, the attribute of the Eurocentric worldview that appears to reflect these assumptions the most is that of individualism. The first assumption affirms the notion that all success and failure (in this case poverty) is attributed to something the individual lacks, such as initiative or perseverance, or to something the individual is (e.g., being a teenager and/or a single parent). It accentuates the individual and holds him or her exclusively accountable for failure. This assumption negates the role of the social, political, and economic milieu in poverty and neglects to acknowledge that milieu's connection to an oppressive worldview that can cultivate human misery. By viewing poverty as solely an individual matter, the existence of poverty is thought not to be an indication of an oppressive worldview but as evidence of individual failure at internalizing and manifesting core values such as the work ethic, fortitude, and individual initiative.

The second assumption reinforces the idea of the first, with the addition of two more notions. First, it supports the view that people should be strong enough to deal with life's adversities, and, second, the assumption advances the idea that human misery (i.e., poverty) and societal inequalities are independent of each other. As it concerns the idea of individual fortitude, the Eurocentric worldview fosters a belief in the "survival of the fittest." Although this slogan is usually associated with nineteenth-century social Darwinism, it permeates the essence of the Eurocentric worldview because, within it, conflict and antagonism are viewed as natural outcomes of human and social behavior (Ani, 1994; Asante, 1990; Bell, Bouie, and Baldwin, 1990). The Eurocentric worldview assumes that if phenomena (including people) are in continuous conflict, then there will be those which survive and those which do not (Baldwin, 1985; Baldwin and Hopkins, 1990). Poverty, therefore, is viewed as a natural outcome and as an indication of one's failure to survive and adapt to societal demands of living.

The assumption that human misery and societal inequalities are unrelated, separate entities is supported by the Eurocentric worldview's linear and dichotomous logic (i.e., its rationalistic focus). Within this logical system, individual misery is thought to be extraneous to societal circumstances. It is as if the individual were in a social vacuum or cocoon, completely impervious to the influences and effects of the broader society. Further, even if a reciprocal relationship between the individual and broader society is conceded, it usually is believed that the individual wields more influence over the broader society than the broader society has on the individual, with the exception of some macrosociological theories and paradigms. This false dichotomy between what Mills (1959) called *personal problems* and *public issues* is sustained by the Eurocentric notion of the inner-directed, autonomous person who is influenced only, or at least primarily, by his or her independent and distinctive will; thus, one's destiny is of one's own making.

The third assumption merely echoes themes of the former, with more emphasis on punishment. This punishment is justified by the view that the poor have failed at surviving and at adapting to the demands of the social environment. It is as if the social environment naturally expels people who it sees as undesirable, and, since the poor are deemed natural and intractable undesirables, they are considered a threat to the free-flowing progress and survival of the social system. Within this framework, the social system has no alternative but to punish, or even eliminate, the poor. This is because of the Eurocentric worldview's materialistic character that causes the poor to be viewed as "objects" who cannot be emotionally and spiritually connected to those who are not poor, or who think they are not poor. More-over, to the extent that objectification facilitates epistemological frag-mentation and emotional distance, it nurtures the emergence of ideas that justify the exploitation and elimination of people.

The Eurocentric worldview's attribute of materialism also influences the assumptions about poverty. As aforementioned, the materialism found in Eurocentricity establishes conditions for the rise and maintenance of capitalism. This is because a materialistic focus underscores a "person to object" axiology (Nichols, 1987) in which the highest social value lies in the acquisition and accumulation of material objects. Attention to spiritual development and to the collective welfare of people are marginalized and superseded by the personal and corporate profit motive. This can be most saliently detected in the federal budgetary imbalance between funding for socioeducational development and funding for military buildup and corpo-rate gains. Moreover, the controversy in Congress that led to the passing of the Personal Responsibility Act of 1996 should be placed within the con-text that the old AFDC program only constituted about 1 percent of the overall federal budget before it was abolished (see U.S. House of Repre-sentatives, House Committee on Ways and Means, 1993). A program that was only 1 percent of the federal budget is severely scrutinized, while other federally sponsored initiatives, which are aimed, for example, at providing tax credits to businesses or bailing out the savings and loan scandal of the 1980s, are given cursory attention. This unequal attention is attributed to the focus on materialism within the Eurocentric worldview that fosters a sociopolitical and socioeconomic climate conducive for es-tablishing social welfare philosophy and policies that sustain power and wealth among an uncompassionate ruling elite (Schiele, 1997a).

FOUNDATIONS OF AN AFROCENTRIC POLITICAL IDEOLOGY

Because the political ideologies of conservatism, liberalism, and radi-calism emerge from the history, cultural themes, and interpretations of Europeans and European Americans collectively, the Afrocentric para-digm maintains that traditional African values and practices, examined in Chapter 2, concerning power, governmental responsibility, morality, re-source distribution, and societal relationships be used as a backdrop to develop and promote an Afrocentric political ideology. This ideology should not only reflect the historical themes of the way people of African descent conceived and managed societal relationships and resource dis-tribution but also should embrace the collective political and economic interests of people of African descent. Last, because the Afrocentric paradigm is concerned with eliminating spiritual alienation, an Afrocentric political ideology should promote positive human transformation for all. Keeping with the dual themes of particularism and universalism, an Afrocentric political ideology is equally interested in the specific liberation needs of people of African ancestry as in the spiritual and moral development of the world (Asante, 1997; Karenga, 1993; Kershaw, 1992).

However, many Afrocentrists contend that before people of African ancestry can begin to help other people and groups advance spiritually and morally, special and particularistic efforts need to be targeted to assist people of African descent in overcoming the pernicious psychological consequences of years of Eurocentric cultural oppression. These efforts are aimed at overcoming the shackles of cultural misorientation and low cultural self-esteem, and often calls for black self-help solutions are championed by Afrocentrists. These self-help strategies are conceptualized as opportunities for people of African descent to gain a greater sense of self-confidence and self-mastery, which have been undermined by oppression (Akbar, 1996; Davis, 1980; Kunjufu, 1991). For African Americans, the institution of slavery and its vestiges have immensely damaged their desire and willingness to take the risks to establish organizations, businesses, and other institutions that are managed and financed by them (Akbar, 1996; Kunjufu, 1991; Muhammad, 1965). Although this call for black self-help is frequently criticized for encouraging cross-racial-group hostility, an emphasis on within-racial-group solidarity and self-help is not inherently associated with animosity and resentment (Asante, 1992). Even so, the Afrocentric paradigm contends that it is better for the hostility held by many oppressed groups to be channeled into more positive activities such as self-help initiatives rather than in acts of random and heinous violence, often perpetrated against other persons who share the same burden of oppression.

Further, the self-help component of an Afrocentric political ideology suggests that group autonomy for the oppressed not only enhances collective self-confidence and self-mastery but also enables an oppressed group to institutionalize its culture and history beyond the scope of friendships and family relations (Cabral, 1973; Karenga, 1996; Martin, 1986; Schiele, 1997b). Perhaps cultural oppression's most injurious and insidious consequence for the oppressed may not be political and economic disempowerment but, as Martin and Martin (1995) argue, cultural amnesia. Martin and Martin (1995) define cultural amnesia as the process through which a cultural/ethnic group's memory of its history and cultural traditions has been loss or suppressed, and this void frequently precludes the desire of the oppressed to seek and accept information about their past and traditions. The establishment of black self-help institutions can provide expansive avenues for people of African descent to resurrect, restore, and promote their historic cultural themes and practices (Karenga, 1996; Stuckey, 1987).

Indeed, a more conscious and fervent validation by African Americans of their historic cultural themes and practices can help them to contribute more substantively to the development of a multicultural society and world. As Mahubuti (1998) states, "How can an individual be multicultural when she or he is not knowledgeable of her or his own group's cultural history and traditions?" If respect for the dignity and worth of each group's culture is a desired societal goal, authentic multiculturalism would require the ability of members of a cultural/ethnic group to have easy access to the values and ideas that characterize their heritage so that they may be culturally competent enough to teach others about their history and traditions. Thus, an Afrocentric political ideology, out of which an Afrocentric social welfare philosophy grows, should be grounded in the cultural values and traditions of people of African descent, should legitimate and promote positive human transformation for all, and should advocate for the establishment and maintenance of self-help institutions among people of African descent.

Before proceeding to the particulars of social welfare policy recommendations from an Afrocentric viewpoint, it is important to distinguish between the Afrocentric and black conservative political ideologies because they both advocate self-help solutions for African Americans. The self-help solutions advocated by black political conservatives, such as radio talk show hosts Larry Elder and Armstrong Williams, Supreme Court Justice Clarence Thomas, and former U.S. Congressman Gary Franks, are predicated on the belief that African Americans have developed a victim's mentality that produces considerable and unnecessary indulgence in government assistance (see Faryna, Stetson, and Conti, 1997; Franks, 1996; Watson, 1998). This indulgence, they argue, plays unjustly on the culpability of European Americans, making contemporary European Americans liable for the wrongdoings of the past. It also creates in the mind-set of African Americans the insidious notion that white assistance, through governmental handouts, is indispensable for the advancement of African Americans, which causes African Americans to become incarcerated in a mentality of white dependence and paternalism (Faryna, Stetson, and Conti, 1997; Franks, 1996; Watson, 1998).

Black conservatives also maintain that governmental assistance is perilous because it stigmatizes African Americans and causes whites and other Americans to view them as a drain on society, as a ball and chain hindering the progress and full fruition of the values of a free-market economy, in which black conservatives believe everyone has an equal chance at success. African Americans who receive benefits from certain forms of the "wrong kind" of affirmative action policy, such as predetermined quotas, are interpreted as undeserving of their success and achievements. So, based on this logic, the university graduate or professional student suffers because peers and many professors might question his or her capabilities, causing self-doubt that could lead to lower academic performance and even perhaps academic attrition. Further, the black corporate manager who receives a promotion because of the "wrong kind" of affirmative action can experience superfluous ridicule and insubordination from co-workers and subordinates. This ridicule and disrespect, the logic continues, can not only have deleterious implications for how the new black manager perceives himself or herself but also can impede workplace comradery, eventually reducing worker production and efficiency.

Last, African-American conservatives assert that able-bodied African Americans who receive income or welfare assistance without seeking employment or who just receive governmental relief even while exploring employment options are stigmatized because they are seen as indolent and shiftless. Though most African-American conservatives are opposed to able-bodied persons receiving welfare assistance—regardless of race, arguing that it compromises the work ethic, they nonetheless contend that even well-intended welfare recipients, who may need temporary assistance, are viewed negatively and thus may internalize these pejorative labels and behave accordingly (Faryna, Stetson, and Conti, 1997; Franks, 1996). Ultimately, they argue, the convergence of stigmatization and paucity of enthusiasm for the work ethic has created a black underclass that tolerates immoral acts and rejects moral certitude. The primary source of this moral and economic wretchedness, African-American conservatives suggest, is the failed governmental policies of the Kennedy-Johnson years, in other words, governmental dole. From an African-American conservative perspective, the only salvation for African Americans is for them to disavow governmental handouts, work fervently to embrace the values of a free-market economy, and purge from their minds that they are victims of racism (Faryna, Stetson, and Conti, 1997; Franks, 1996; Watson, 1998).

Although the Afrocentric political ideology agrees with the black conservative ideology that many African Americans have been circumscribed into a mentality of white economic dependency—justifying the necessity of black self-help—the Afrocentric political ideology disagrees with the sources of this mentality and advocates for a more expansive notion of self-help. From an Afrocentric viewpoint, the origin of the mind-set of black dependency is not the injudicious governmental spending of the 1960s but rather the system of Eurocentric domination, of which governmental programs are just *one* component. Years of intergenerational Eurocentric domination have caused undue psychosocial crises for African Americans and has placed them at an economic and political disadvantage. To completely understand the African-American predicament, the Afrocentric political ideology would suggest that the interplay between the domination and psychosocial development of African Americans be acknowledged and examined. In this way, the factors that have influenced the psychological evolution of African Americans are not historically decontextualized and politically fragmented to only accuse one segment of Eurocentric domination (e.g., the Kennedy-Johnson Democrats) for the harm that has been done to African Americans.

In addition, because the Afrocentric political ideology recognizes the historic and intergenerational effects of Eurocentric domination on African Americans, it does not fall prey, as does black conservatism, to a binary analysis that views advocating for governmental assistance as antithetical to calls for black self-help. The Afrocentric political ideology simultaneously argues for governmental assistance and black self-help. One does not oppose the other because, as Karenga (1986) notes, "while the oppressor is responsible for our oppression, we [blacks] are responsible for our liberation" (p. 52). Since intergenerational oppression, in which U.S. government policies have played a major role, is responsible for the current adverse predicament of many African Americans, it is logical and deemed just, from an Afrocentric viewpoint, that U.S. governmental assistance of any kind be provided to help African Americans catch up from historical, economic, and political deficits produced by intergenerational oppression. Likewise, albeit this government assistance is considered justifiable and morally correct, Afrocentric political ideology suggests that African Americans should not passively wait on the enactment of governmental programs. Rather, they should draw on their internal resources and establish organizations, schools, and businesses that are managed and financed primarily by them.

The Afrocentric political ideology, unlike the black conservative ideology, also includes a more comprehensive notion of black self-help. Black conservatives only view black self-help from a microeconomic perspective, with the goal being that African Americans should enthusiastically embrace the work ethic and reject their racial victim mentality so that they can provide for their families with little, if any, governmental assistance. Although the Afrocentric paradigm supports the value of productive work, its conception of self-help validates the belief that African Americans should collectively advance themselves through the affirmation of a collective cultural consciousness. Termed African self-consciousness earlier, the Afrocentric political ideology views African Americans as not just a group of citizens, as does the black conservative ideology, but also as a cultural/ethnic group with a distinct history, set of cultural traditions, and worldview. To this end, the development of self-help institutions among African Americans is a mode through which African-American cultural traditions and values can be preserved and promoted, and it is a strategy through which African Americans can overcome the effects of cultural amnesia discussed earlier. In addition, since the U.S. government, in many instances, has forfeited the interests of African Americans collectively, black self-help from an Afrocentric perspective is politically and economically necessary to guard African Americans against both the planned and capricious forces of continued racism and Eurocentric oppression (Karenga, 1993; Shujaa, 1994; Wilson, 1993).

Although many black conservatives, and even some black liberals (see Wilson, 1987, 1996), declare that white racism is declining in significance, the Afrocentric paradigm suggests that Eurocentric domination is not diminishing; rather, it is mutating from domination by terror to domination by seduction (Schiele, 1998, in press). In many ways, domination by seduction is deemed more effective than domination by terror because its methods of oppression cloak and conceal underlying intentions of exploitation and oppression, thereby placing greater numbers of dominated groups and persons at risk of being deceived into believing that the social system is working on their behalf (Bauman, 1992; Marcuse, 1964; Schiele, 1998, in press). If the latter is true, then the Afrocentric political ideology would contend that black self-help is perhaps more essential today than in the past.

AFROCENTRIC SOCIAL WELFARE POLICY RECOMMENDATIONS

Universalistic Policies

The focus on the ideological themes of universalism and particularism in the Afrocentric paradigm shapes the foundation for Afrocentric social welfare policy recommendations. Universalistic Afrocentric policy recommendations that could benefit all persons within the United States would encourage (1) enhanced educational opportunities, (2) guaranteed minimum incomes to working and poor families, (3) universal health care coverage, and (4) friendly and cooperative workplace atmospheres.

Enhanced Educational Opportunities

To enhance educational opportunities, the Afrocentric paradigm would advocate (1) collective responsibility for the costs of higher education, (2) making high school training more akin to college training, and (3) inclusion and affirmation of multicultural curricula. The escalating costs of higher education in the United States are increasingly rendering higher education a privilege for the affluent rather than a civil right for all. Since the Afrocentric paradigm adopts a communitarian perspective on human relations, it would possibly recommend that the costs of higher education be defrayed by citizens of the entire society through not only personal income and sales taxes but also through corporate taxes. These taxes should not be flat or universally proportional but rather reflect the actual amount of money held by a person, household, or corporation. The higher the actual income or assets, the greater the tax. Corporations should bear a significant share of this revenue generation since they are among the most frequent beneficiaries of the skills that education and training afford people.

Making high school training more akin to college or post-high school training is a way to not only enhance educational and training opportunities for citizens but also to reduce the cost of training. Afrocentric social welfare policy would advocate the need to make secondary school education more time efficient by rendering the training more specialized. Instead of requiring one to defer a career choice until college or even graduate school, Afrocentric social welfare policy would encourage students to make that decision around the ninth to eleventh grades, if possible. The rationale behind this is that (1) the current secondary school training in the United States can be characterized as too redundant and generalist; (2) to require youths to attend twelve years of school and then require that they attend four (college) or even six to ten years more (graduate or professional school) can be too much of a burden for some; (3) by the time students are in their teens, they have the capacity for formal operational thought (Newman and Newman, 1991), which enables them to intelligently ponder a career choice; and (4) if secondary school training was more specialized, the amount of money needed for higher education would be minimized and reduced. Of course, for this to work, employment and career standards across professions and employment settings would have to be radically altered.

Last, there is a need to make educational curricula more inclusive of the contributions and paradigms of cultural groups whose perspectives and traditions historically have been suppressed and absent in public education. Inasmuch as social welfare policies seek to affirm the dignity and worth of all members and groups within a society, social welfare policies should endeavor to dismantle cultural oppression by insisting on cultural pluralism. Schools are often one of the first institutions in society that formally and repetitiously expose one to views and images of self and others. When views and images of self and one's cultural group are absent or disparaged in the educational process, significant psychological damage, such as low cultural self-esteem, inappropriate labeling, and behavioral resistance can occur (Asante, 1991; Hale-Benson, 1982; Hilliard, 1987). Further, those whose views and positive images are dominant can develop low disregard for the disparaged or *curriculum absent* cultural group and assume an exaggerated sense of their cultural self (Asante, 1991). The importance of this inequality is that, too often, absent or disparaging views of one's cultural self can turn one off early to learning and achievement, thus contributing to future problems in emotional and career development for that person (Boykin, 1983; Kunjufu, 1985).

Guaranteed Minimum Income

An Afrocentric welfare policy would also support a guaranteed minimum income for working and indigent families. The guaranteed minimum income was proposed in 1969 by the Nixon administration under the Family Assistance Plan (FAP) but was never implemented. The problem with FAP, and most other income maintenance programs and proposals in the United States, from an Afrocentric viewpoint, is (1) the conservative and restrictive strategies by which eligibility is determined, (2) the reliance on the practice of "less eligibility," and (3) the use of workfare as a form of punishment.

An Afrocentric welfare policy would not rely on conservative and restrictive methods to determine eligibility for assistance; instead, more relaxed strategies would be proposed, based on calculations of cost-of-living and poverty levels that relied on both the assumptions of relative and absolute poverty. Relative poverty estimates are those which assume deprivation to be "relative" to the standard of living experienced by others in a society (Karger and Stoesz, 1998). Relative poverty does not compromise on meeting basic needs of people, but it focuses attention more on equality of income and resource distribution than does absolute poverty estimates that rely on precise and quantifiable standards for survival (Karger and Stoesz, 1998). Although it is noble for any society to establish absolute criteria of poverty, the problem with current U.S. welfare policy, from an Afrocentric perspective, is that criteria used to determine absolute deprivation have been too conservative. In determining criteria for absolute deprivation from an Afrocentric perspective, one would not have to exhaust all or most of their resources, and the remaining citizenry, especially those with copious resources, would be responsible for sustaining the needy. However, if educational and training opportunities are increased early in life, there would be less need for income assistance because people would have stable work that pays them sufficiently.

The reliance on the concept and practice of less eligibility would also be unnecessary in Afrocentric social welfare policy. Less eligibility, which contends that welfare payments should be less than the lowest societal wage, is useless in Afrocentric social welfare policy because wage labor would not be placed in competition with welfare assistance, especially when the wages for labor are excessively low, and it would not be presumed that people are loath to work or would intrinsically seek to exploit welfare benefits or others. However, given a society such as the United States, which endeavors to suppress the power and positive potentiality of many, it is not surprising that people feel cheated and, in turn, seek to exploit the system that has exploited them.

Afrocentric social welfare policy would not use workfare as a means to punish people. There would be no need because Afrocentric social welfare policy would focus more on enhancing the wages of people, their opportunities to find stable employment, and their opportunities, early in their educational experience, to identify and locate a career that would bring them high job satisfaction. When people can find employment that is stable, that remunerates them fairly for the labor they produce, and that brings them considerable intrinsic satisfaction, work becomes an enjoyable activity.

Universal Health Care Coverage

Another critical feature of Afrocentric social welfare policy would be universal health care coverage. From an Afrocentric viewpoint, no one should have to be concerned whether, if they become sick, they will be treated or whether they will be able to visit a physician or other health care professional regularly. Afrocentric social welfare policy would preclude health care, and human misery in general, from being used as a means for excessive profit. A fee-for-service system would not be considered inherently unjust in Afrocentric social welfare. However, when profit is deemed a central feature of service delivery, considerable emphasis is placed on efficiency of services as opposed to quality of services. Although efficiency is important and is said to increase quality, quality of care in the U.S. health system is usually given less attention than is cost of and access to health care (Starr, 1994). The Afrocentric perspective would regard cost containment and access to health care as important but would give equal attention to quality, especially to a more holistic conception of quality of care, such as the relationship between care provider and care receiver, perceived satisfaction of consumer, prevention, and long-term rather than short-term effects of treatment. To achieve greater balance among cost containment, access, and quality of care, an Afrocentric health care policy would approximate the National Health Service proposed by Congressman Ron Dellums in the late 1970s. It is based on the belief that health care is a right of citizenship, a fundamental, moral obligation of society, and that the profit motive in health care compromises quality of care and unnecessarily elevates service costs.

The concept "universal" in health care policy, from an Afrocentric viewpoint, also would imply diversification of the theoretical models and practitioners of health care so that a "complete oneness" in the delivery of health care services can be achieved. Just as there is Eurocentric hegemony in the social sciences, there is also hegemony in the analysis and treatment of human health. This dominant health care model highlights treatment, not prevention, and a materialistic view of human health. The spiritual or unseen and the social/psychological aspects of human health have traditionally been ignored in the United States and are only recently beginning to receive attention. From an Afrocentric perspective, a more holistic and spiritual view of human beings should be integrated in health care policies and practices. In traditional Africa, significant authority in the area of health care is given to spiritualists or mediums whose primary objectives are to use spirits, energy sources, and prayer in treatment (Brisbane and Womble, 1991). Further, since many health problems are associated with life stress, particularly concerning financial insecurity, it is imperative from an Afrocentric viewpoint to never separate the political economy from problems of physical and mental health.

Friendly and Cooperative Workplace Atmospheres

Afrocentric social welfare policy also would accentuate the need for friendly and cooperative workplace atmospheres. From an Afrocentric viewpoint, such an atmosphere would provide workers with (1) more autonomy, decision making, and less-rigid supervision, (2) ample family leave and vacation time, and (3) child care services at the workplace. Studies have shown that when the autonomy and decision-making ability of workers increases, job satisfaction increases (Kadushin and Kulys, 1995; Knoop, 1995). This finding is often explained by the assumption that people feel more comfortable at work when they feel they can be trusted and when they believe what they do is important to the organization. Afrocentric welfare policy supports this belief and significantly rejects the validity and dominance of McGregor's (1960) theory X, which views humans as inherently recalcitrant, lacking in self-regulation, and in need of constant and rigid supervision and monitoring.

Sufficient family leave and vacation time is also essential. With the overemphasis on production and efficiency in Eurocentric organizational theories (Schiele, 1990), it is no wonder that one of the most inimical issues between workers and employers is family leave and vacation time. The overemphasis on production and efficiency, which maximizes profits or conserves costs, can undermine worker health, leisure, and rest. From an Afrocentric perspective, there is a critical need to offset this focus on production and efficiency in the workplace by shortening the workweek and by restructuring workplaces—such as staggering work hours—to accommodate the family and vacation needs of workers rather than the avarice of a ruling, corporate elite.

Last, an Afrocentric workplace policy would advocate the provision of child care at the workplace. With the increase in single-parent families, two-working-parent families, and the erosion of traditional systems of child care brought on by an ever-increasing, geographically mobile workforce, child care has become more problematic for families. The primary problems are the high costs of child care and trusting child care providers. Providing child care at the workplace can take care of both these concerns. First, if child care was provided at the workplace, the cost could be absorbed by the organization. The worker should not have to pay because the worker is already selling his or her labor for, and contributing to, the survival of the organization. Thus, a reciprocal relationship of "service" between worker and company would exist. Second, companies providing child care on site might reduce the level of distrust workers may have of child care providers and the amount of family leave necessary because the child/children and worker would be located at the same site during work hours.

Particularistic Policies

Particularistic or race-specific policies that advance people of color, generally, but African Americans, specifically, also are critical from an Afrocentric perspective. In the context of the United States, race-specific policies can be defined as social policies that offer specific political, economic, and employment opportunities to racial groups for whom consistent and historical patterns of abuse, mistreatment, and discrimination by local, state, and federal governmental entities, as well as private agencies, have been carefully observed and documented. Many social policy analysts have discouraged race-specific policies in the United States (see, for example, Glazer, 1975; Sowell, 1989; Steele, 1990; Wilson, 1987). Some of the criticism regarding these policies centers on them being impractical because the majority of American citizens are European American and do not support race-specific policies, on the interracial conflict that the policies generate, and on the observation that remedies for racism can be sufficiently dealt with if significant structural changes would occur in the American economy of capitalism. Although each of these criticisms has credible aspects, the Afrocentric paradigm advocates for race-specific policies on the grounds that (1) they are morally sound; (2) when they are explained using terms like "enhanced opportunities" rather than "preferential treatment," more European Americans agree with their utility; and (3) the range of possible race-specific polices has not been exhausted, fully explored, and publicly debated. With this in mind, the Afrocentric paradigm would advocate for three race-specific policies to enhance the political and economic status of African Americans: (1) some form of financial reparations for the pain and injustice of slavery and its relics; (2) affirmative-action policies, especially in regard to higher education, and (3) the Racial Preference Licensing Act, examined fictionally by Bell (1992).

Reparations for African Americans

Since the Afrocentric paradigm underscores the tragedy of American slavery and assumes its vestiges to continue, it would support some form of financial reparations to the descendants of slaves here in the United States. Proponents of reparations to African Americans have argued that since the institution of slavery was promoted by the U.S. government, state and local governments in the United States, and the thirteen colonies out of which the U.S. government was formed, the descendants of U.S. slavery should be awarded reparations for the damage engendered by the institution of slavery (see, for example, Allen, 1998; Baraka, 1998; Lumumba, Obadele, and Taifa, 1993; Robinson, 1997).

Proponents maintain these damages have taken on sundry forms, from political and economic to social and psychological. Politically, proponents of reparations argue that although the Thirteenth, Fourteenth, and Fifteenth Amendments to the U.S. Constitution were important in this country's acknowledgment of both the human and civil rights of African Americans, these amendments do not sufficiently compensate for the 205 years during which African Americans were treated as animals and property with no rights at all (Allen, 1998; Baraka, 1998; Lumumba, Obadele, and Taifa, 1993; Robinson, 1997). Also, after these amendments were passed, they were soon nullified by many state and local mandates, which came to be known as Jim Crow laws. Although many of these laws emanated from state and local jurisdictions, their validity was solidified and given the ultimate stamp of approval by the U.S. Supreme Court in the 1896 *Plessy v. Ferguson* ruling that authorized the doctrine "separate but equal" as constitutional. Because of this ruling, proponents of reparations contend that the political rights of African Americans were denied, and this disavowal fostered another sixty-nine years of political disenfranchisement and disempowerment that did not end legislatively until the 1965 Voting Rights Act.

Economically, reparations are recommended because of (1) the free labor provided by enslaved Africans for over two centuries and (2) the wretched material conditions of African Americans spawned by the injustices of slavery. Proponents of reparations argue that because the free labor of enslaved Africans was the foundation for both initiating and advancing capitalism in America (for a discussion, see Bailey, 1992), descendants of enslaved Africans deserve not only compensation for their ancestors' unpaid labor but also for their ancestors' critical role in building a strong economic base for the United States that has benefited many, including those whose ancestors were major investors in the transatlantic slave trade (Allen, 1998; Baraka, 1998; Lumumba, Obadele, and Taifa, 1993; Robinson, 1997). Second, since the abolition of slavery, African-American families historically have had lower family and household incomes and net worth than European-American families, and African Americans have held some of the lowest-paid, lowest-status jobs in the United States (Bennett, 1966; Franklin, 1980). Proponents of reparations suggest that although racial discrimination has explained much of why African Americans have held such positions, racial discrimination must not be understood separately from its origins in American slavery (Allen, 1998; Baraka, 1998; Lumumba, Obadele, and Taifa, 1993; Robinson, 1997). The institution of American slavery, they argue, laid the foundation for questioning the intelligence, competence, and worth of African Americans that is at the heart of hiring and promotion decisions.

Socially, proponents of reparations contend that many of the social problems found in the African-American community can be attributed significantly to the culture of slavery. The family, as several authors suggest, was one of the social institutions adversely impacted by slavery. For example, Frazier (1927) suggested that one of the most devastating consequences of slavery for the African-American family was that it severed the cultural continuity from Africa. Frazier asserted that this cultural disconnect had demoralizing consequences for sex mores and for family control among enslaved Africans and many African-American families after slavery. One of the most appalling effects of slavery on the African-American family was, as Frazier believed, that its members had not internalized sexual monogamy as a cultural norm and that this factor was prominent in creating considerable marital instability and disruption. This lack of internalization of sexual monogamy caused by slavery, according to Frazier, had particularly adverse consequences for many African-American men, whom Frazier (1939) referred to as "tribeless." One of the primary characteristics of these men was their tenuous and emotionally ephemeral relationships with women, rendering them as perpetual deserters of their women and often the children they bore together.

Moreover, Akbar (1996) maintains that because enslaved Africans were valued exclusively for their physical skills and abilities, and because enslaved African families frequently were displaced and separated, the concepts of motherhood and fatherhood were significantly compromised. Enslaved Africans, although developing creative strategies to cope with the atrocities, challenges, and pressures placed on their family lives (Gutman, 1976; Nobles, 1974) were confined in their ability to optimally protect, nurture, and exercise responsibility for their offspring (Akbar, 1996). More fundamentally, enslaved African women frequently had little or no control over birthing offspring because they were viewed and used as breeders, constantly subjected to the capricious and pernicious sexual desires and fantasies of slave holders (Abramovitz, 1996; Akbar, 1996; Stampp, 1956). The paucity of control over their bodies, lives, and destinies engendered by slavery, Akbar states, substantially compromised many enslaved Africans' ability to assume and internalize the roles necessary to be responsible, caring, and nurturing mothers and fathers. Although considerable research demonstrates that many African-American parents are responsible, loving, and caring (McAdoo, 1997; McAdoo and McAdoo, 1985; Staples, 1994), this documentation does not rule out the possible latent burden of the intergenerational effects of slavery on African-American families' ability to optimally function and prosper.

Last, proponents of reparations assert that the relics of slavery have damaged and distorted how African Americans view themselves culturally and ethnically. Earlier, in Chapters 5 and 6, Kambon's (1992) concept of cultural misorientation was employed to suggest that many African Americans lack knowledge and appreciation of their history and their traditions as descendants of Africa. Conceptualized as low cultural self-esteem or low ethnic/racial identity, the origins of cultural misorientation, according to Kambon, were the institution of American slavery and its cultural depreciation, marginalization, and vilification of all artifacts and people associated with Africa. Proponents of this view contend that the psychological damage of slavery had precluded African Americans from having the level of confidence, self-assurance, and cultural pride necessary to establish viable and long-standing institutions, organizations, and businesses that reflect traditional African cultural values and to educate and expose others to the cultural integrity and contributions of people of African descent (Asante, 1988; Kambon and Hopkins, 1993; Karenga, 1996). Reparations could be used here to help establish institutions, schools, organizations, and other facilities that can reeducate African Americans and others about the contributions of Africans and African culture.

Why not African Americans? One of the consistent questions raised by proponents of reparations for African Americans is "How and why have other victims of government-sponsored atrocities received reparations and African Americans have not?" They underscore the inconsistencies in the treatment of the African Americans' atrocity of slavery relative to other oppressed groups' calamities. Thus, questions such as the following are frequently asked: (1) Despite the horrors associated with the interment of Japanese Americans during World War II—who received financial reparations from the U.S. government—was this interment any worse than the sale and enslavement of Africans here in the United States? (2) Since the U.S. government forced Saddam Hussein to pay reparations to the Kuwaitis after his invasion of that country, did the Iraqi invasion engender any more harm than American slavery generated for Africans and their descendants in the United States? (3) Since the United States was a critical player in the war crime trials that demanded Germany pay reparations to Jews and others victimized by Hitler's Third Reich, why does not the U.S. government view the injustices inherent in slavery as sufficient evidence to offer reparations to African Americans? Proponents of reparations maintain that the U.S. government's denial of the gravity of pain caused by slavery, while simultaneously openly acknowledging and atoning for the injustices imposed on others, is hypocritical and may demonstrate a yearning to repress and expunge memories of slavery from the annals of U.S. history and the American psyche (Allen, 1998; Baraka, 1998; Lumumba, Obadele, and Taifa, 1993).

Current initiatives. Recently, two initiatives have increased the likelihood of reparations being granted to African Americans: (1) a U.S. House of Representatives Reparations Bill and (2) legal settlements in the Rosewood, Florida, case. In November 1989, Representative John Conyers (D-Mich) introduced bill HR 3745, known as The Commission to Study Reparation Proposals for African Americans Act. Its purpose, as stated in the bill, is as follows:

To acknowledge the fundamental injustice, cruelty, brutality, and inhumanity of slavery in the United States and the 13 American colonies between 1619 and 1865 and to establish a commission to examine the institution of slavery, subsequent de jure and de facto racial and economic discrimination against African Americans, and the impact of these forces on living African Americans, to make recommendations to the Congress on appropriate remedies, and for other purposes. (U.S. House of Representatives, 1989)

The Conyers Bill is the first of its kind ever introduced in the U.S. Congress, and the primary objectives of the commission it proposes to establish are as follows:

1. Examine the institution of slavery which existed within the United States and the colonies that became the United States from 1619 through 1865 . . .
2. Examine the extent to which the Federal and State governments of the United States supported the institution of slavery in constitutional and statutory provisions, including the extent to which such governments prevented, opposed, or restricted efforts of freed African slaves to repatriate to their home land.
3. Examine Federal and State laws that discriminated against freed African slaves and their descendants during the period between the end of the civil war and the present.
4. Examine the lingering negative effects of the institution of slavery . . . on living African Americans and on society in the United States.
5. Recommend appropriate ways to educate the American public of the Commission's findings.
6. Recommend appropriate remedies in consideration of the Commission's findings . . . (U.S. House of Representatives, 1989)

The commission is to be composed of seven members, with three members being appointed by the president of the United States, three appointed by the speaker of the House of Representatives, and one member appointed by the president pro tempore of the U.S. Senate. The Reparations Study Bill has been introduced every year in Congress by Representative Conyers since 1989. Currently referred to as HR 40, the bill was most recently introduced on January 6, 1999. As of yet, the bill has never been subjected to a floor vote, nor a committee or subcommittee vote. Since its introduction, the bill has died in house committee deliberations and currently has been referred to the House Judiciary Committee.

Second, in May 1994, nine African Americans collectively were awarded $2.1 million by the Florida State Legislature to compensate for loss and damages suffered in the Rosewood, Florida, massacre (see Anonymous, 1994, 1995; Florida House of Representatives, 1994; Jerome and Sider, 1995). In this massacre, which occurred in 1923, a mob of white men burned every resident of and home in Rosewood, an all-black town, in an attempt to locate a black man who allegedly had raped a white woman. However, before the complete destruction of the town, a few adults were able to escape with children to nearby woods where they hid in a swamp until they were rescued several days later. The children who escaped and who were rescued are now elderly and were the claimants and recipients of the reparations in the Rosewood case. The Rosewood Reparations Case is the first time a state legislature, or any other governmental entity in the United States, has financially compensated African Americans for the negligence of law enforcement officials in protecting the personal safety and property of African Americans from acts of racial aggression. In 1997, film director John Singleton directed and released a movie on the calamity titled *Rosewood* (see Anonymous, 1997).

Affirmative-Action Policies

The Afrocentric paradigm also supports affirmative-action policies for African Americans, other groups of color, and women in the workplace, in the awarding of governmental contracts and in educational admissions policies. Affirmative-action policies seek to correct for past discrimination practices against people of color and women who have experienced political and economic injustices via institutionalized racism and sexism (Cahn, 1995; Karger and Stoesz, 1998). The basic premise of affirmative-action policies is that since the U.S. government actively participated in discriminatory practices against people of color and women or did not actively protect the rights of these persons for many years, it should correct its past wrongdoings by taking "affirmative action" to ensure that people of color and women are provided fair and ample opportunities in the workplace and in the pursuit of higher education (Cahn, 1995; Karger and Stoesz, 1998). Multiple viewpoints both oppose and promote affirmative action as a legal and governmental remedy. The viewpoints focus on central issues, some of which are as follows: (1) Is not affirmative action reverse discrimination? (2) Is preferential treatment a proper strategy when nondiscriminatory policies such as the Civil Rights Act of 1964 exist? (3) Should compensation for historic injustices only be provided to individuals who have suffered them or to entire groups? (4) Can and should equality of outcome be ensured and protected by the state, or is variance in performance outcome a natural component of human talents and abilities?

(5) Do affirmative-action policies harm the intended beneficiaries by implanting in their minds a sense of inferiority?

Reverse discrimination. Implied in the first question regarding reverse discrimination is another question: Is it fair to punish those who have not imposed injustices or unfair treatment against others? To address the question, the Afrocentric paradigm would contend that although many contemporary persons of historically privileged groups do not practice racial or gender discrimination and may be exemplary in demonstrating kindness and fairness toward others, their physical and phenotypical attributes continue to place them at an advantage. This observation is supported by the assumption that in a social system wherein privileges, resources, and opportunities significantly vary by physical or phenotypical attributes, advantages are automatically provided to all members of the physically or phenotypically privileged group relative to the physically or phenotypically unprivileged group. This is because, in a society such as the United States, certain physical characteristics, such as gender and race, have become politicized; that is, official policies and, more important, institutional practices, have intentionally sought to suppress the power and positive potentiality of groups whose physical attributes have been associated with additional uncomplimentary characteristics, such as mental inferiority, indolence, or cultural inadequacy. This type of institutional oppression or suppression of power, and its pervasiveness and consistency, provides an inherent edge to all members of the physically privileged group, even though this advantage is not evenly distributed and is based on a host of other factors, such as economic class.

However, the Afrocentric paradigm agrees with Dubois (1935) and Amott and Matthaei (1991) that even when economic class and other common factors that occur across both historically privileged and unprivileged groups are controlled for or taken into consideration, the power and pervasiveness of institutional oppression continues to support members of the historically privileged group in ways that can provide what Dubois (1935) called a *psychological wage.* What Dubois meant is that the status and privileges afforded by race in the United States could compensate for exploitative class relationships between and among whites. Thus, there was a wage for being white in the United States that transcended economic class. Though the Afrocentric paradigm would prefer that all persons and groups who share a similar sociopolitical and geographical space be provided opportunities to enhance their positive potentiality, it does recognize that the inequality in privileges, opportunities, and resources created by institutional oppression is historic and its vestiges continue to this day. Any strategy aimed at remedying this inequality should place contemporary social relations within this unfortunate historic context. In this regard, perhaps an unkind reality inherent in a nefarious social system such as institutional oppression is that the sins of the fathers and mothers might have to be paid by the burdens of the sons and daughters.

Preferential treatment and nondiscriminatory policies. Concerning the second question of whether preferential treatment is necessary when state policies support nondiscrimination practices, the Afrocentric paradigm reinforces the ideas of President Lyndon B. Johnson in his 1965 speech at Howard University, in Washington, DC, in which he stated:

> You do not take a person who for years has been hobbled by chains and liberate him, bring him up to the starting line of race and then say, "you're free to compete with all the others," and still justly believe that you have been completely fair. Thus it is not enough just to open the gates of opportunity. All our citizens must have the ability to walk through those gates. . . . We seek not . . . just equality as a right and a theory but equality as a fact and equality as a result. (quoted in Cahn, 1995, p. xii)

A major theme in the passage from Johnson's speech, as Cahn (1995) observes, is "that fairness required more than a commitment to impartial treatment" (p. xii). Johnson understood that years of historic oppression would require not only nondiscriminatory policies but also an "extra push" or helping hand from the government and the private sector that fostered historically oppressive relationships. In this way, the enactment and enforcement of nondiscriminatory policies is just the first step in correcting historic injustices; it only prevents further injustices from occurring, but it does not compensate for previous years of historic maltreatment. For justice to be complete, from an Afrocentric viewpoint, a second step of compensation should be combined with the first step of terminating legal racial and gender discrimination.

In addition, another problem with the nondiscrimination laws enacted by the U.S. government is that they generally employ language that decontextualizes the discrimination by not identifying the group or groups that have legally perpetuated the discrimination. This is a critical flaw of these policies, from an Afrocentric perspective, because without contextualizing the discrimination, that is, identifying who the discriminators were, nondiscrimination policies can be used, as they are today, by some descendants of historic legal discriminators and others to contend that any assistance by the government or a private firm to advance members of historically oppressed groups constitutes reverse discrimination and thus violates nondiscrimination laws. Whether written to intentionally or unintentionally produce this effect, the wording of U.S. nondiscrimination laws allows descendants of the perpetrators of legal discrimination and others a loophole to sustain their dominance and to further ensnare the descendants of the victims of legal discrimination.

Compensation to individuals or groups? The third question raises the issue of whether compensation should be given to entire groups or just individuals who have been victimized by unjust practices. Those who oppose compensation to entire groups suggest two points: (1) group membership per se is not the primary reason for discrimination but rather the attributes, such as inferiority or indolence, that are ascribed to *individuals who just happen to be members of a specific group* (Cowan, 1995), and (2) under U.S. jurisprudence and based on the values found in the U.S. Constitution, rights are believed to be the exclusive domain of individuals, not groups (Glazer, 1975; Novak, 1982; Sowell, 1989). From an Afrocentric perspective, the problem with both these arguments is that they are predicated primarily on a circumscribed understanding of human behavior that accentuates the value of individualism found in Eurocentric political thought (see Jansson, 1997; Kohl, 1989). Within this understanding, human behavior is too often reduced to individual thoughts, attitudes, strengths, and deficits. Though group attachment is acknowledged, it is believed that the individual has the power to be independent of group influence and that the individual is solely or primarily responsible for both favorable and unfavorable actions toward others (Jansson, 1997; Kohl, 1989). Therefore, the degree to which individual pleasure and individual pain are associated with broader, collective patterns of human beings is either denied or downplayed. Within this line of reasoning, affirmative action is not only imprudent because it tends to indict all persons who are believed to be beneficiaries of injustice but also because it provides misguided compensation to all "individuals" in so-called "victimized groups" who may not have been victimized at all.

Congruent with the characteristics of the Afrocentric worldview discussed in Chapter 2, the Afrocentric paradigm recognizes and underscores the tenacious and persistent effect of collective identity on individual thought and behavior. Although, clearly, injustice against people of color and women was, and is, committed by individuals, these individuals are not disconnected from broader themes and values found in both their primary and secondary groups. Likewise, though harm against members of historically oppressed groups is most poignantly felt and seen by narratives told and the pain experienced by individuals, these individuals were not random targets of aggression and injustice; rather, their physical characteristics placed all the members of that group at risk of being victimized, albeit perhaps differentially. Even if one accepts the argument that the physical attributes were (are) less important than the characteristics ascribed to them, it is still the physical attributes that trigger emotions of hatred, fear, and anxiety, all believed to be cornerstones of racism and oppression (Baldwin, 1980; Hacker, 1992; Thomas and Sillen, 1972; Turner, Singleton, and Musick, 1984; Wright, 1984).

Can equality of outcome be ensured and protected? The fourth question spoke to concerns of whether the state should or can ensure equality of outcome in such areas as workplace diversity and performance or academic enrollment and achievement. Opponents of affirmative action and other state-sponsored programs aimed at helping specific, disadvantaged groups suggest that although the state should affirm equality of opportunity, it cannot guarantee equality of outcome (Glazer, 1975; Murray, 1984; Novak, 1982). Novak (1982) contends that equality of outcome is impossible if one accepts as true the notion that human performance will inevitably vary, that some will always do better than others, despite conditions or circumstances. However, although the Afrocentric paradigm embraces the idea of inherent variance in human skills and abilities, it does not accept that this variance should be understood outside a societal context that promotes oppression of all sorts. Again, opponents of affirmative action and other such programs rely heavily on a circumscribed interpretation of human behavior that perhaps not only reflects their philosophical orientation but also helps to advance their political agenda of continued domination. From an Afrocentric standpoint, the conspicuous group differences observed between members of historically privileged and oppressed groups on a host of outcomes suggest that there has been an institutional pattern of discrimination that is wrong. Woodruff (1995) asserts that "A pattern of discrimination is wrong when it makes membership in a group burdensome by unfairly reducing the *respect* [italics mine] in which the group is held" (p. 40). Both people of color, especially African Americans, and women have been regarded by the U.S. power elite as being less competent and less valued (Abramovitz, 1996; Gilligan, 1989; Hacker, 1992; Pinderhughes, 1989; Solomon, 1976), and this devaluation undergirds practices of discrimination and oppression (Pinderhughes, 1989; Rothenberg, 1990; Solomon, 1976; Young, 1990). Because of the Afrocentric paradigm's affirmation of the latter analysis, it favors the practice of state-sponsored efforts to even out the variance in outcome. Much of the discussion, however, emanating from opponents of affirmative-action about equality of opportunity versus equality of outcome commits a fallacy about the United States being a beacon for equality of opportunity. By promoting the belief that there is equal opportunity for all, opponents of affirmative action are better able to market their objection to affirmative-action policies by disseminating a seductive argument about the impossibility of equality of human outcome.

A sense of inferiority? The last question addressed whether affirmative-action policies generate feelings of personal inferiority among the beneficiaries. This concern over psychological harm has been expressed mostly by opponents of racial preferences in university admissions and hiring practices. Opponents of these policies argue that beneficiaries of affirmative action are harmed by these policies because they place them in competition with others who are exceedingly more qualified than they (Connerly, 1996; Gingrich and Connerly, 1997; Steele, 1990; Thernstrom and Thernstrom, 1999). These commentators note correctly the significantly lower standardized test scores of African Americans compared to European and Asian Americans. From these data, it is concluded that African Americans are handicapped when they are placed in educational settings with others who score higher, and that racial preferences only reinforce in the minds of African-American students—whether consciously or not—that they are intellectually inferior. Indeed, in their critique of Bowen and Bok's (1998) *The Shape of the River,* in which affirmative-action policies in higher education admissions are shown to be effective and beneficial for African Americans and others as well, Thernstrom and Thernstrom (1999) subtly imply that because Martin Luther King Jr. scored in the bottom half of all test takers on the GRE, he probably was better off and more comfortable at Morehouse College, his alma mater and a school that admitted weaker test performers, than at a more "selective" school such as Princeton, where the majority of students would have scored significantly higher. Hence, King would have been harmed by race-sensitive policies and perhaps may not have become the illustrious orator and leader he became. Last, the critics of university race-sensitive policies contend that the continued reliance on racial preferences obfuscates the real problem: poor primary and secondary schools that African-American students mostly attend. Gingrich and Connerly (1997) suggest further that racial preferences are malicious to children in these schools because they detract attention away from the substantive change that needs to occur in these "uncaring educational bureaucracies" (p. 15).

Problems with the inferiority assumption. From an Afrocentric perspective, there are at least three problems with the analysis regarding the psychological adversity of affirmative-action policies for beneficiaries: (1) the validity of standardized tests are never questioned; (2) the possible political function of the tests are never identified; and (3) the harm the relics of slavery and institutional racism may have on many African Americans' willingness and desire to achieve is not explored.

First, opponents of affirmative action in higher education never challenge the validity of standardized tests used in admissions decisions. As one of the criteria employed to evaluate the quality of a test or measure, validity can be defined as the degree to which a test or measure elicits the kind of information it purports to measure (Rubin and Babbie, 1993). In this sense, the crucial validity question for standardized tests such as the SAT and GRE is, do they elicit the full range of information needed to sufficiently evaluate the readiness of a student for undergraduate or graduate training? Also, are the items on these tests valid predictors of one's future success as a student and as an effective and influential professional? Considerable research has examined these questions, and the evidence suggests that although these tests are fairly good indicators of the quality of a student's previous education, their ability to predict a person's future performance as a student or professional is dubious (Chenoweth, 1997; Keller, 1994; Linn, 1990). In addition, since the United States is composed of culturally diverse groups who not only have distinct cultural values but also many different learning and epistemological styles, some recommend that standardized tests should be more reflective of the diverse sociocultural panorama of the American people (Bell, 1994; Gonzalez, 1996; Hale-Benson, 1982; Wilson, 1980; Wyche and Novick, 1985).

Critics of affirmative action are right when they recommend that more attention be given to ensuring a quality education for all at the primary and secondary levels. Attention to quality education at the lower grades, however, is not contradictory to a critique of the validity of standardized tests adopted in higher education. If standardized tests are acknowledged as "culture tests" (see Wilson, 1980), then their ability to tap more diverse ways in which people obtain, process, and share knowledge can be expanded. Moreover, their limitations in identifying the readiness and potential of students to do good work also can be more thoroughly recognized and investigated.

Second, opponents of affirmative-action policies in higher education also never entertain, at least publicly, the political function of standardized tests. The Afrocentric paradigm maintains that, similar to the political and economic institutions of U.S. society, science and its creations also can be interpreted as instruments of oppression (Akbar, 1984; Asante, 1988, 1990; Kershaw, 1992; Nobles, 1978). The rationale for this observation is found in the fact that many of the earlier developers of standardized tests, such as Lewis Terman, were eugenicists who were motivated to design such tests to provide scientific evidence that persons of non-northern European and non-western European background, particularly people of color, were mentally inferior to those with northern European or western European ancestry (Gould, 1981; Hilliard, 1987; MacKenzie, 1981). Though opponents of affirmative action would argue that America has significantly transformed since the days of the eugenics movement, contemporary ideas advanced by such authors as Herrnstein and Murray (1994) indicate that the motivation to prove certain groups inferior has not been extinguished. More important for this discussion, and consistent with the assumptions of the Afrocentric paradigm, these ideas should not be construed as anomalies from eccentric and provocative scholars but rather as cornerstones of the American ethos and vision.

Last, critics of university affirmative-action policies who identify the negative psychological effects of these policies rarely consider the pernicious consequences of institutional racism and the relics of slavery on many African-American students' willingness to achieve. These opponents assume that since many Asian-American students perform well on standardized tests, even better than many European-American students, the argument about the abominations of institutional racism and discrimination is bogus. However, as Ogbu (1978, 1988) observes, it is erroneous to lump all minority groups in one homogeneous category and assume that their experiences with the dominant Eurocentric society have been uniform. Ogbu (1978) asserts that minority groups must be distinguished by their incorporation into, or arrival in, a country and their unique experiences with the members of the dominant group. He particularly admonishes that a distinction be made between two types of minorities: (1) caste minorities and (2) immigrant minorities. Compared to immigrant minorities such as most of the Asian-American groups, for example, Chinese, Koreans, and Japanese, caste minorities, which would include African Americans, differ in the following ways: (1) Unlike immigrant minorities, caste minorities entered the United States involuntarily; African Americans are the prime example in that they were imported to this country as slaves. (2) Membership in a caste minority is obtained permanently at birth; thus, their place in society is more or less well defined. (3) Because of their castelike status, caste minorities have restricted access to resources that remains impervious to educational level and skill expertise. (4) Caste minorities, while not always endorsing the ideology of the dominant group, are generally more affected by the ideology of superiority and inferiority. (5) Since they have been incorporated into U.S. society involuntarily and then relegated to subservient status, caste minorities tend to attribute much of their social and economic problems to institutional racism and discrimination, which they believe to be permanent (Ogbu, 1978, 1988).

The differences between caste and immigrant minorities suggest that cast minorities have more unfavorable experiences with the dominant group and its institutions than do immigrant minorities. These unfavorable experiences, Ogbu (1978, 1988) maintains, adversely affect caste minorities' optimism about succeeding in society, which may stymie their motivation to achieve academically. On the other hand, since immigrant minorities' entry into the United States was voluntary, and because they are less affected by the ideology of superiority and inferiority, Ogbu (1978, 1988) concludes that these minorities have more favorable experiences with, and perceptions of, U.S. society and, therefore, are more likely to be inspired to learn and achieve in school. In short, the experiences of slaves significantly diverge from the experiences of the immigrants.

Akbar (1996) expands more on the specific effects of slavery on the aspirations of African Americans. He claims that the lack of aspiration to achieve academically for many contemporary African Americans can be ascribed to the social and psychological circumstances of slavery. In slavery, Akbar contends that the conception and treatment of African Americans as chattel and as servants to please and entertain slave owners was not conducive for nurturing higher expectations of human possibility. This plantation milieu helped to foster a self-concept among the enslaved that they were at their best when they demonstrated physical prowess and capabilities. With these social circumstances and expectations, coupled with the prohibition against reading and writing among enslaved Africans, Akbar concludes that it is no wonder that many African Americans find academic work boring and a waste of time. Because the sociopolitical conditions and societal expectations of African Americans did not change after the official abolition of slavery by the Thirteenth Amendment to the U.S. Constitution, but rather continue even to this day, Akbar posits that the "plantation ghost" of slavery has haunted African Americans intergenerationally. From an Afrocentric lens, for opponents and others interested in race-sensitive policies to disavow the inimical effects of institutional racism, discrimination, slavery, and its relics on African Americans psychologically is to confine and decontextualize understanding of the aspiration of many African-American students.

The Racial Preference Licensing Act

The last race-specific or particularistic policy that the Afrocentric paradigm would offer consideration is the Racial Preference Licensing Act, which is presented fictionally by Bell (1992). Bell's (1992) *Faces at the Bottom of the Well* is a set of fictional short stories in which the consistent theme is the intractability of racism in America. In the third story, titled

"The Racial Preference Licensing Act," Bell's fictitious president of the United States offers the fictional policy as an alternative to traditional race-sensitive policies. The fictional act mandates the following:

> all employers, proprietors of public facilities, and owners and managers of dwelling places, homes, and apartments could, on application to the federal government, obtain a license authorizing the holders, their managers, agents, and employees to exclude or separate persons on the basis of race and color. . . . Once obtained, it require[s] payment to a government commission of a tax of 3 percent of the income derived from whites employed, whites served, or products sold to whites during each quarter in which a policy of "racial preference" was in effect. (Bell, 1992, p. 48)

Essentially, as the previous quote suggests, the license allows those who would purchase it to openly acknowledge their racial preferences at a fee. To compensate African Americans for years of racial injustice, the fees and commissions paid by those who purchase a license would be placed in an equality fund. This fund would underwrite the establishment of black businesses, would be used to provide no-interest mortgage loans for black home buyers, and would offer scholarships for black students seeking college and vocational education. Thus, the costs of overt racial preference would be a license used to provide educational and financial incentives to African Americans.

A closer examination of Bell's chapter on the Racial Preference Licensing Act reveals five fundamental assumptions on which the act is predicated:

1. Racial nepotism rather than racial animus has been the primary obstacle for the advancement of whites and the discrimination experienced by blacks. In this sense, racial groups in the United States are akin to families, with all of the emotions of attachment, comfort, and familiarity.
2. White group self-interest has been more of a factor in the enactment of civil rights legislation than has white altruism or concerns about racial injustice.
3. People should have the right of nonassociation.
4. The law enforcement model, upon which civil rights legislation is based, is ineffective because though many whites may not be discriminatory themselves, many may identify more readily with the discriminators than with the victims of discrimination.

5. Civil rights laws have done nothing to reduce the black crime rate, drug abuse, and other social problems that disproportionately affect African Americans.

A major problem with the Racial Preference Licensing Act, from an Afrocentric perspective, is that it appears to accentuate a one-way-street approach to human biases and preferences. The act appears to be more concerned with validating the preferences and rights of free association among European Americans than among African Americans. This focus is based on the logic that it has been the preferences of European Americans that have yielded adverse consequences for African Americans, instead of the reverse. Although the Afrocentric paradigm would agree with this logic, it would suggest that if open racial preferences are to be sanctioned by the government, then the "right to prefer" needs to be extended to all who would purchase the license. What the logic of the Racial Preference Licensing Act tends to omit is that not only do many European Americans have racial-association preferences but so do many African Americans and perhaps other racial and ethnic groups as well. For example, many African-American professionals who can afford to move into predominately European-American suburban neighborhoods choose instead to reside in the growing number of predominately African-American suburbs, with the best example being Maryland's Prince Georges County (see McCall, 1997; Meyer, 1991).

What the Racial Preference Licensing Act addresses is the power of race in the United States in shaping people's preferences and associations. Ironically, though many Americans' preferences and associations are influenced significantly by race, many Americans oppose what they view as government-sponsored race preferences, especially when those preferences are perceived to benefit some at the expense of others. From an Afrocentric interpretation, a few critical questions concerning this issue of racial preferences are as follows: (1) If preferences and associations continue to be heavily influenced by race and ethnicity, should America continue to advance race neutrality as an ostensible value? (2) Does an emphasis on racial preferences in human associations automatically lead to racial anger and hatred? (3) If the latter two questions are answered in the affirmative, and if the values and ideology associated with race in America completely dissipate, would group preferences develop around different distinctions and characteristics? (4) If the latter is so, is the emergence of an ideology that accentuates some characteristics to the vilification of others a natural human outcome? The Afrocentric paradigm contends that the answer to the last question is found in, and relative to, the overarching worldview that pervades a society. The central problem of the ideology of race—which mandates attention to race-specific policies—is a problem of the worldview that dominates a society. In the United States, that worldview, from an Afrocentric interpretation, is the Eurocentric worldview that, ultimately, if human relationships are to be transformed to achieve greater respect and appreciation of human diversity, should be the target for change.

Chapter 8

The Afrocentric Framework
of Social Welfare Policy Analysis

OVERVIEW OF THE AFROCENTRIC POLICY
ANALYTIC FRAMEWORK

The Afrocentric paradigm also can be employed as a foundation for an Afrocentric policy framework to examine and evaluate various social welfare policies. Karger and Stoesz (1998) define a policy framework as "a systematic means for examining a specific social welfare policy or series of policies" (p. 39). At the core of this systematic method are questions that emerge from a set of philosophical assumptions that both describe and prescribe how social welfare policies are and should be analyzed, formulated, and implemented. Most frameworks used to analyze social welfare policies focus more on how a policy is formulated and on examining its content than with the policy's implementation (Copeland and Wexler, 1995). To date, most of the formal social welfare policy analytic frameworks have emanated from not only a Eurocentric framework but also almost exclusively from European-American social welfare scholars. Some of the predominant policy analytic frameworks have stemmed from persons such as Gill (1992), Dobelstein (1996), Gilbert and Specht (1986), Karger and Stoesz (1998), and Prigmore and Atherton (1986). Although these models have their unique, progressive attributes and contributions, many of these frameworks collectively share some common characteristics: (1) They present their frameworks as if they can be applied universally to all social policy situations, social problems, and targeted populations, with little, if any, alterations. (2) They accept the notion that social welfare policy formation, though having nonrational features, is mostly a rational and linear process. (3) Although they acknowledge the influence of cultural factors in the policy formulation, implementation, and analytic process, they often neglect to recognize and underscore how their policy frameworks reinforce core themes of the Eurocentric worldview. (4) They tend to omit or minimize Eurocentric domination as a chief attribute of the policy formulation, implementation, and analytic process, opting instead to highlight the importance of social class and universal concerns dealing with economic stratification or inequality.

The Afrocentric framework of social welfare policy analysis, though having a similar goal of examining and evaluating the development and implementation of a social welfare policy, and affirming the social justice values found in many existing frameworks, does not claim universalism, that it can be widely applied to fit all social policy situations and social problems. It states up front and unequivocally that its features are based heavily on traditional African/African-American philosophical assumptions. In addition, although it is concerned with the impact of social welfare policy on all vulnerable populations in the United States and throughout the world, the Afrocentric policy analytic framework is particularly concerned with the consequences for people of African descent.

Another point about the Afrocentric framework of policy analysis relates to the concept of analysis itself. The concept "analysis" can take on multiple meanings but generally is referred to as the fragmentation of a whole (e.g., an idea) into constituent parts and then comprehending the parts in a linear, straight-line fashion. Although the Afrocentric paradigm recognizes the necessity for such an interpretation of social phenomena, especially when attempting to gage the historical evolution of events, it also accepts that social phenomena, such as policy analysis, should be understood more holistically and circularly in a manner that synthesizes seemingly contradictory and unrelated components. The Afrocentric framework of policy analysis is not opposed to linear causation but rather the idea that linear causation, particularly in its more mechanistic form, is the best method of knowing.

One of the problems, however, with communicating the themes of Afrocentric epistemology and using it as a basis to evaluate social welfare policies that predominately emerged within the cultural context of Eurocentric domination is the English language. Emerging from a combination of languages from three closely related European groups—the Jutes, the Angles, and the Saxons—English reflects the cultural and epistemological themes and preferences of these early Europeans who populated the region of northern Europe about 1,500 years ago (Bloomfield, 1976). An authentic communication of the ideas and preferences of the Afrocentric policy analytic framework would best be achieved through one of the indigenous languages of West African ethnic groups, such as the Ibo, Akan, Dogon, or Ashanti. Thus, my communication of the tenets and attributes of the Afrocentric policy analytic framework, as with my description of the Afrocentric paradigm generally, is hampered and even distorted somewhat by the medium of the English language. With this in mind, the following is a presentation of some beginning ideas that may characterize an Afrocentric framework of social welfare policy analysis.

FEATURES OF THE AFROCENTRIC FRAMEWORK OF POLICY ANALYSIS

Implications of Policy for Vulnerable Groups

This first feature of the Afrocentric policy analytic framework is to examine the extent to which the policy has both pernicious and helpful implications for vulnerable groups in a society, but particularly people of African descent. Vulnerable groups of a society can be defined as groups whose physical characteristics, value orientations, behavioral patterns, and/or economic circumstances are stigmatized by those in power and are used as a justification to suppress the positive potentiality of the group and to prevent it from gaining power in society. In the United States, some of these groups are women, gays and lesbians, the differently abled, political critics, people of color, and low-income groups, especially those who receive governmental assistance. Among these groups, however, there is considerable diversity in vulnerability status and level. To this extent, the Afrocentric framework openly acknowledges, unlike many other social welfare policy frameworks, the phenomenon of what Titterton (1992) refers to as "differential vulnerability." To determine how much at-risk groups in a society differ in their vulnerability status, the Afrocentric framework of social policy analysis draws on the work of Young (1990). In her book, *Justice and the Politics of Difference,* Young includes a chapter titled "The Five Faces of Oppression." In the chapter, Young identifies five faces or attributes of oppression. The faces are (1) exploitation, (2) marginalization, (3) powerlessness, (4) cultural imperialism, and (5) violence. Young contends that they can be used as criteria to ascertain the degree of oppression or vulnerability a group may experience. She asserts that "these criteria can plausibly claim that one group is more oppressed than another without reducing all oppression to a single scale" (1990, p. 65).

The first criterion, *exploitation,* refers to "a steady process of the transfer of the results of the labor of one social group to benefit another" (Young, 1990, p. 49). Here, Young uses a Marxist concept of exploitation to imply the manner in which class divisions in a society engender structural relations that define the rules of work, that is, how people are compensated and by whom. Those who have little control over these definitions, and thereby have less of a society's cumulative wealth, are placed at a greater risk of not being remunerated fairly for the value of their work. Whereas exploitation may affect all employed persons who have little control over the rules of work, *marginalization* refers to those persons in society whom "the system of labor cannot or will not use" (Young, 1990, p. 53). Referred to by Young as *marginals,* these persons lack the skills needed to find and maintain gainful employment and could be considered, as Willhelm (1970) notes, as "economically irrelevant." The most conspicuous examples of marginals, Young claims, are the growing number of persons known as the underclass of the inner cities as well as persons, due to illness, stigmatization, and disabilities, who cannot secure or are blocked from obtaining essential skills for meaningful work participation.

Though anyone who lacks substantive control over the rules of work can experience exploitation, Young (1990) uses the term *powerlessness,* the third face of oppression, to describe the extra burdens endured by persons who are not professionals. Professionals, as opposed to nonprofessionals, are privileged in ways that nonprofessionals are not. Professionals generally can exercise more power in the workplace, can work with considerably more autonomy, can make more money, and can elicit more societal respect because of their educational level and the higher value placed on their work. Nonprofessionals—those with little or no advanced, specialized training—have very few of these privileges, if any. Relative to professionals, they are powerless and often are the victims in the workplace of the rules and decisions rendered by professionals.

The latter forms of oppression for Young reflect the social division of labor. The fourth face of oppression, *cultural imperialism,* deals more with the control a group has over determining the cultural history, meanings, and values of a society and influencing which meanings and values will be excluded or marginalized. In cultural imperialism or oppression, there is " the universalization of a dominant group's experience and culture, and its establishment as the norm" (Young, 1990, p. 59). In this way, the extent to which the cultural values and interpretations of a group are deemed marginal and/or nonexistent by the dominant group is the measure of that group's cultural oppression. Conversely, when the cultural values and interpretations of a group are analogous to the dominant group, that group is not likely to experience cultural vilification. The last feature of oppression for Young is *violence.* Young's primary meaning of violence is that of physical abuse and victimization. Groups who are targets of various "hate" crimes and who live in constant trepidation of being physically attacked are included in this form of victimization. Young also, however, includes in this category groups who are disproportionately targets of lesser forms of aggression, such as harassment, intimidation, and ridicule.

Using Young's five faces framework, we can see how groups, even vulnerable ones, can vary in their level of vulnerability and oppression. Although Young admits that the existence of any one of the five faces is sufficient to consider a group oppressed, and thereby vulnerable, not all conditions are applicable to all social groups in society. As Young (1990) states:

> Working class people are exploited and powerless, . . . but if employed and white do not experience marginalization and violence. Gay men, on the other hand, are not qua gay exploited or powerless, but they experience severe cultural imperialism and violence. . . . Racism in the United States condemns many Blacks and Latinos to marginalization and . . . members of these groups often suffer all five forms of oppression. (p. 64)

If what Young maintains is correct, and using her five criteria, or faces, then people of African descent, at least in the United States, can be considered one of the most vulnerable groups in society. Nonetheless, Young's (1990) model also can be employed to frame questions about the implications of the policy for various vulnerable groups, despite their degree of vulnerability. The critical questions that need to be asked regarding the policy as it concerns vulnerable groups are as follows:

1. To what extent does the policy exacerbate the exploitation of the labor of working people, both professionals and nonprofessionals? Does the policy attempt to generate more wealth for exploited persons and enhance the value of their labor, or does it attempt to extrapolate more labor at the expense of less remuneration, or both?
2. To what extent does the policy facilitate or hinder the conditions of persons whom Young calls the marginals? Since the urban underclass is a substantial component of this group, what provisions of the policy block or create opportunities for the underclass to gain skills, to become important contributors to the economy and the world of work? What about the policy's provisions for the elderly and the mentally and physically disabled, two more categories of marginals? If job training is provided in the policy, to what extent is the training commensurate with, and appropriate for, the changes occurring in technology?
3. To what extent does the policy enhance or hamper opportunities for nonprofessionals (i.e., the powerless) to obtain further academic/

professional training? Does the policy include provisions that increase workplace power and influence for nonprofessionals, and does it include workplace friendly provisions that provide ample family leave and vacation time, flexible/staggered work hours, and child care services, which are especially needed by nonprofessionals who have less disposable income?

4. To what degree does the policy exclude or include interpretations and cultural values from the group or groups targeted by the policy? In this regard, to what extent does the policy acknowledge or deny the strengths, contributions, and cultural integrity of the group or groups for which the policy was developed?

5. To what degree does the policy include provisions that protect the target group from physical harm, hate crimes, and other forms of harassment, intimidation, and stigmatization?

These latter questions are quite appropriate to determine the policy's impact on people of African ancestry, but since the Afrocentric framework of policy analysis is particularly concerned with the policy's implications for this group, a few additional questions also are applicable:

1. To what extent does the policy include provisions and themes that reinforce and promote continued Eurocentric domination? This not only includes an analysis of whether the policy reinforces Eurocentric political and economic dominance but also the degree to which the policy is imbued with values and philosophical themes that stem from and validate Eurocentric interpretations of social problems, human needs, and policy formulation and implementation.

2. Since the descendants of African Americans gave 205 (1660-1865)* years of free labor to the economic development of the United States and suffered another 100 years of political disenfranchisement and economic exploitation, totaling 305 years of marginalization, to what degree does the policy include provisions that offer additional opportunities for African Americans to advance themselves educationally and professionally? Also, because the U.S. government participated willingly and prominently in the political disenfranchisement and economic exploitation of African Americans, to what extent does the policy include provisions to transfer wealth to African-American

---

*The date 1660 is used because it was then when Virginia introduced the first slave codes into the newly formed English colonies. It was these codes that committed Africans into servitude for life (see Bennett, 1966; Day, 1997).

families in an effort to redress the injustices it perpetrated in the past?

3. To what extent does the policy acknowledge the strengths and resources within African-American communities and families and include African Americans in its formulation and implementation? In this regard, does the policy acknowledge the self-help traditions in African-American communities and families and does it support the continuation of these traditions? Also, does the policy include interpretations of social problems, human needs, and policy formulation and implementation that are grounded in traditional African/African-American philosophical assumptions and cultural practices?

Historical Antecedents of Policy

Similar to the policy frameworks of Gill (1992) and Karger and Stoesz (1998), the Afrocentric framework of social welfare policy analysis contends that an analysis of both the long-term and immediate historical antecedents and policy precedents is necessary to grasp a holistic understanding of a policy. These historical factors can be specific policy precedents and/or can entail political, economic, social, and cultural factors that help to usher the policy into law.

Policy Precedents

Specific policy precedents are those policies which precede the current policy in time, are related to the current policy by the social or economic problem it attempts to address, and contain provisions on which the rationale for the current policy is based. Alternatively, the precedent policy may lack some important provisions that the current policy may include, partly because of a critique of the precedent policy. For example, the passage of the 1965 Voting Rights Act in part came about because of a critique of the 1964 Civil Rights Act for not including within the realm of civil rights the domain of voting rights (Quadagno, 1994; Watson, 1990). The passage of the Supplemental Security Income legislation of the early 1970s can be attributed partly to criticism of the previous legislation for being too fragmented and uncoordinated regarding the indigent aged and the disabled (Jansson, 1997; Trattner, 1994). These examples demonstrate how current policies often address the provisional or programmatic "gaps" of precedent policies.

However, to assume that policies progressively build on each other in succession, as is assumed in much of the scholarly writing, is to deny the reality of much of policy development in the United States and to validate the notion that policy formation is inherently progressivistic, that is, that policy formulation is a process of successive improvement in addressing social problems and enhancing human relationships. Although the meaning of a progressive (i.e., good) policy can vary significantly by such factors as political ideology, definition of human need, conceptualization of a social problem, and ideas about effective intervention, precedent policies can be, and often are, interpreted as more progressive and morally affirming than the contemporary policies upon which they may be based. For example, many social welfare analysts are predicting that the Personal Responsibility Act of 1996 is a moral and social devolution in social welfare policy thinking because of its significant absolution and removal of the federal government from the administration of income maintenance and job-training programs (Children's Defense Fund and National Coalition for the Homeless, 1998; Leven-Epstein, 1996; Schiele, 1998). Conversely, because of its federal devolution and workfare thrust, others view the act as an extremely necessary, progressive, and effective social welfare policy change (Casse, 1997; Haskins, 1999).

In addition, though the interpretation of progressivistic is important to consider, the Afrocentric framework of policy analysis holds that social welfare policy development in the United States must be conceived as a series of strategies that has little to do with advancing the positive potentiality of ordinary persons, but more to do with furthering oppressive social relationships. In this way, if the character of "progressivism" is in American social welfare policy, it is progressivism toward more effective and efficient containment and monitoring of the aspirations, critical consciousness, and power of a host of groups, but especially the vulnerable groups delineated earlier. Although many social welfare policy scholars admit this "social control" function of the welfare state and social policies, generally, many of them also acknowledge an equally important "treatment" or humanitarian function, suggesting that American social welfare policy development has an equally affable side (see Day, 1997; Dinitto, 1995; Dobelstein, 1996; Gilbert and Specht, 1986; Jansson, 1997). To be fair, many of these writers argue that this humanitarian side frequently emerges from power and protest movements that leverage concessions from the government. Although this is true, many of these scholars—some more explicit than others—contend that certain American values, such as democratic equalitarianism, seek good intentions via social welfare policy development, though they admit the values have been applied differentially to various groups in society (see Day, 1997; Jansson, 1997; Richan, 1988). Also, the tendency is to view the values of treatment and control as competing and contradictory when, in fact, they may be conceived as different components of an overall unified agenda of oppression and domination, the kind often referred to in Marxist perspectives found in Marcuse (1964) and Piven and Cloward (1971).

The Afrocentric framework of policy analysis maintains that if a society practices gross divergence in the treatment and protection of groups, as expressed through social welfare policies, with some groups receiving far more historical preferential treatment than others, then that society cannot be depicted as having "good" or benevolent intentions, no matter how benign. It can be argued that the United States has clearly and consistently applied social welfare policy differentially in ways that place many groups, especially people of color and women, at risk of vulnerability. The Afrocentric framework maintains that American social welfare policy, while being good to some, has not been beneficial to many, and, thus, whatever treatment, benevolent, or social betterment features it may have do not outweigh the tremendous harm it has caused significant numbers of persons, often intergenerationally. In this sense, the Afrocentric framework embraces perhaps a more critical view of the intentions of American social welfare than many other perspectives. This is because it is grounded in, and informed by, the experiences of pain, disappointment, and oppression African Americans have endured since their importation to the United States in 1619.

Political Factors

Although precedent policies can be encompassed under political factors affecting a policy, additional political factors should be considered when attempting to understand the influence of antecedents on the emergence of a policy. Some of these factors are the results of political elections, judiciary decisions, voting patterns of the electorate, corporate influence, and protest politics.

Political elections. Since social welfare policy formulation occurs through the activities of legislators and political administrators, the consequences of political elections can significantly shape the policy agenda and the passing of one piece of legislation over another. Throughout the history of the United States, the dominance of one political party over another, in both the legislative and executive branches or both, is often a harbinger of upcoming social welfare policies. The limitation of the American two-party, winner-take-all system renders the Democrats and the Republicans dominant over social welfare debates and in shaping social welfare legislation. This results in the suppression of ideas about social welfare policy that arise from persons and groups with divergent political affiliations. Thus, in examining the influence of election outcomes on the development of a policy, the Afrocentric framework encourages recognition of the manner in which the values, parameters, and provisions of a policy have been significantly confined by the dominance of the two-party, American political system.

Though social welfare policy dialogue has been circumscribed by the American two-party system, differences exist between Democrats and Republicans. Although these differences may be ever more arduous to discern today, as increasingly more liberals and moderates accept the market as the preferred locus and deliverer of social welfare policies and programs (Blau, 1989; Karger, 1994; Karger and Stoesz, 1993), a continued difference is that Democrats still tend to rely more on state-sponsored remedies to address social problems than do Republicans. Republicans tend to yield more to market trends and solutions found in local, privately sponsored charity and community-based organizations. Given this reality, then, election outcomes can produce political forces that either place greater emphasis on state-sponsored solutions or market-driven, privately sponsored ones. The dialectic between these two forces has characterized the development of American social welfare policy at least since the 1930s, but, from an Afrocentric framework, this tension is being assuaged by the increasing eclipse of market-driven and private charity advocates over state-sponsored ones. This implies that, in the near future, if indeed the dominance of the two-party system remains, election outcomes may have little to do with explaining the variance in policy dialogues and social welfare policy proposals that emerge in Congress, the White House, and the various state legislatures throughout the country.

Judiciary decisions. Decisions that emanate from case law and judicial pronouncements also heavily influence the development and implementation of social welfare policy. Though the courts themselves do not sponsor or advocate legislation, they often decide on the constitutionality of legislation, and the interpretation rendered can substantially impact the survival and implementation of policy. This was demonstrated in the 1950s with the "man in house" rule and "night raids" that were established as appropriate social welfare procedures in many localities. The "man in house" rule stated that if an AFDC caseworker found an able-bodied man living in or frequently visiting the home of an AFDC recipient, the money allocated to the recipient could be reduced. The rule was predicated on the assumption that if the mother of children receiving AFDC benefits is intimately involved with a man who either lived with or frequently visited her, she may receive unreported income from the man that would enhance her family income and thereby warrant a reduction in her benefits or render her ineligible for AFDC (Axinn and Levin, 1982; Trattner, 1994). Night raids were unannounced visits by AFDC caseworkers to the homes of AFDC recipients with the aim of monitoring recipients' homes and determining if men were indeed living in the homes or visiting frequently. Both the "man in house" rule and night raids were extant for some time, especially in the 1950s and early to mid-1960s, but each was found unconstitutional by the U.S. Supreme Court on the grounds that they violated recipients' right to privacy (Axinn and Levin, 1982; Trattner, 1994). In this sense, courts have been used to nullify existing social welfare practices and policies that are interpreted as constitutional violations.

However, nullification of social welfare policies oftentimes contributes to the advent of new social welfare ideas and sometimes new policies. The legal death of one policy can effectuate the legislative birth of another. An excellent example of this was the 1954 *Brown v. Board of Education of Topeka, Kansas* Supreme Court ruling that found separate but equal schools unconstitutional. This ruling legally nullified the fifty-eight-year-old *Plessy v. Ferguson* Supreme Court ruling that legalized the separate but equal doctrine. The legal death of the *Plessy* case brought on by the 1954 ruling served as a legal foundation for the legislative birth of the 1960s civil rights policies that challenged and further eroded state-sponsored racial segregation and discrimination.

Although many policy pundits maintain that the judiciary is more detached from the legislative process and exerts a more objective force in shaping social welfare policy, the Afrocentric paradigm suggests that this may not be true. First, the views of judges who are appointed by executives, such as the president or a governor, rarely diverge significantly from the politicians who appoint them (Louthan, 1979; Lyles, 1996). Second, and perhaps more important, the U.S Constitution, which many judges interpret, can be conceived as a document imbued with the political and sociocultural values of the American descendants of Europe who lived during the eighteenth century, particularly white men who owned considerable property. A major component of the U.S. Constitution is Jeffersonian philosophy, which is the notion that government should exert very little control over the lives of citizens (Jansson, 1997; Licht, 1992; Quadagno, 1994). According to this philosophy, citizens should have the freedom to conduct their social and business affairs without the potentially harmful intrusion of the state. This viewpoint has led to a strong emphasis in the Constitution on suspicion of governmental authority and on individual liberty as opposed to social and economic equality (Jansson, 1997; Quadagno, 1994). Although some social welfare writers, such as Jansson (1997), acknowledge the effects of American frontierism on the emergence and popularity of Jeffersonian philosophy, it also can be reasoned that this restricted concept of liberty derives from broader historical factors and a more prolonged cultural tradition that validated the need to be cynical of governmental authority (see Ani, 1994; Diop, 1978; MacPherson, 1962). Nonetheless, the tradition of governmental cynicism has strongly hindered the development of progressive social welfare policies and government-sponsored social programs in the United States and has led Jansson (1997) to refer to the United States as a "reluctant" welfare state. Thus, the U.S. Constitution, which the judiciary is responsible for interpreting, can be understood as a particular document that has much to subjectively say about issues of social welfare and social relations.

Third, because judges are seen as more analytical, and thus less subjective, the subjectivity they apply to interpret the Constitution is frequently overshadowed and downplayed in media discussions. The views and opinions of judges can be influenced by factors such as personal experiences, gender, race/ethnicity, and social class background (Louthan, 1979; Wice, 1992). Another important factor that can shape the opinions and decisions of judges is professional or legal socialization (Louthan, 1979; Wice, 1992). Legal socialization can include the law school attended, key preceptors, legal practicums and clerkships, prior work experience, and professional organizations with which the judge is associated (Kennedy, 1982; Wice, 1992). The experiences from this socialization provide a conceptual guide that, among other things, delineates philosophical assumptions about how social relations and events should be explained and interpreted legally (Kennedy, 1982; Wice, 1992). The influence of the legal paradigm on legal interpretations of social welfare policy should not be underestimated because it, perhaps more so than other personal factors, is the one a judge may be more willing to acknowledge as affecting his or her legal decisions. In this way, although the other factors may be important, a judge may be more conscious of his or her legal paradigm and view it as a more legitimate influence over his or her legal deliberations. From an Afrocentric framework, therefore, knowing the political and ideological viewpoints of the politician who appoints the judge, conceding the Constitution as a cultural document that reflects the cultural traditions and beliefs of an elite cadre of eighteenth-century European-American leaders, and recognizing the significance of the legal paradigm that can affect a judge's legal values and decisions all are pivotal factors that can hinder or facilitate the continuation of social welfare policies.

Voting patterns of the electorate. The frequency and method through which citizens vote in elections and their attitudes about social issues can significantly influence the kind of social welfare policy supported by legislatures, administrators, and the judiciary. In a democracy, wherein all the citizens have the right to elect their political leaders, and wherein each vote counts equally, the voters become essential players in the policy process. Voting patterns can play a critical role in the type of social welfare policy that ends up becoming the law of the land.

Attitudes about social issues and those regarding the value of voting are crucial in determining voting patterns. Attitudes about social issues can be influenced by several factors, such as personal experiences, views about the appropriate role of government, race/ethnicity, social class, geographical region of residence, gender, age, and a host of other characteristics. The multiplicity of these factors would suggest then a wide range of diverse attitudes about social issues. Although these factors can and should produce this kind of diversity, there is a common denominator through which this diversity is filtered and reduced into confined philosophical and ideological dimensions: the visual and print media.

The power the media have on shaping ordinary citizens' attitudes is well documented (Jhalley and Lewis, 1992; Kellner, 1990; MacDonald, 1983). Since ordinary citizens have little control over what airs on television and radio or is printed in newspapers and magazines, they are subjected to informational decisions made by a few. There is considerable debate, however, over the degree to which the media respond to the preferences of the public or whether the public's preferences are influenced by the media elite. Although the Afrocentric policy framework acknowledges some degree of reciprocity between the two forces, it assumes that the influence of the media elite is greater, primarily because of the corporate interests involved. Corporations own the major media outlets in the United States, and fewer numbers of corporations increasingly control greater numbers of media outlets (Alger, 1998). This constant expansion of media power by fewer corporations allows these corporations, and their media employees, to wield substantial control over what the public sees and hears and the interpretations (spins) offered to explicate these events (Alger, 1998).

Coverage of social welfare issues and social problems is not exempt from the media spin and, as with many other issues, is filtered through the two dominant political ideologies of the conservatives and the liberals (Blau, 1999; Karger and Stoesz, 1998; Quadagno, 1994). These dominant political ideologies are used to frame the strengths and shortcomings of issues in a way that invariably and exclusively presents only these two sides or shades of an issue. Indeed, from an Afrocentric perspective, the media's repetitious and effective presentation of only these two sides of a social issue places the public at risk of conceiving social issues exclusively from these vantage points. Even the media entity C-SPAN, though allowing much more diversity of social and political viewpoints than perhaps visual media outlets owned by big corporations, reinforces the dominance of the conservative/liberal political debate. Thus, citizens' attitudes, although having some degree of media autonomy, are shaped significantly by the informational hegemony of the media elite, which further reinforces the voting public's reliance on the two-party political system to define and offer solutions to social problems. This informational hegemony can ultimately affect voting patterns, causing the public to either side with the popular conservative spin or the popular liberal one.

Public attitudes about voting, whether the public views it as a worthwhile activity, also are important in shaping voting patterns. Data from recent presidential and other elections reveal that generally about half or slightly less than half of eligible voters vote (U.S. Bureau of the Census, 1998). For example, in the 1996 congressional elections, only about 46 percent of the eligible voting-age population voted, and in the 1996 presidential election, only about 49 percent of eligible persons cast their ballots (U.S. Bureau of the Census, 1998). Many factors can influence voter turnout, but some political analysts believe that voter apathy is a central reason (see Amy, 1993; Guinier, 1994). Many reasons can be called upon to explain voter apathy, but the Afrocentric policy framework assumes that much of it may be attributed to the effects of oppression.

One of the major outcomes of oppression is a feeling of despair and powerlessness. These feelings can render the oppressed apathetic about voting because they realize, at a very conscious level, that the American political system is heavily influenced by the corporate and power elite. Although many of them would not desire to relinquish their right to vote, some would perhaps argue that there is an equally tenacious right that protects their choice not to vote. Further, since many politicians in the United States are still older European-American males of affluent economic status and family background, many who do not fit these demographic attributes may conclude that their interests and viewpoint will not be adequately represented and advanced. This observation about the potential influence of oppression is confirmed by evidence that shows that those who possess personal and demographic characteristics distinct from many politicians—younger, poor, and nonwhite—tend to be less likely to vote. For example, younger persons tend to vote less than older persons; lower-income persons tend to vote less than higher-income persons; and African and Hispanic Americans tend to vote less than European Americans (U.S. Bureau of the Census, 1998). Although, clearly, additional factors may explain these voting patterns, the Afrocentric policy framework suggests that oppression, and its corollaries, is a primary factor that may cause many to devalue the practice and significance of voting.

Voting patterns also can be affected by the influence major national or world events can have on individuals' standard of living or on their emotions and feelings. Major national or world events are those social, political, or economic phenomena which have either wider personal impact or broad personal appeal to a prodigious and varied range of persons. Also, since the media elite exercise considerable control over the informational dissemination process, the events they decide to cover and place substantial emphasis on can significantly influence how individuals vote. Two examples are illustrative of this point: the Iran hostage crisis of 1979-1980, and the Clinton congressional impeachment hearings of 1998-1999. Both of these events had a significant influence on many Americans who tuned in to media outlets; many Americans were emotionally charged by both events, causing them to form strong opinions.

In regard to the Iran hostage crisis, some political pundits today maintain that if President Jimmy Carter's failed hostage rescue attempt of American prisoners in Iran had been successful, he probably would have won reelection to the presidency—in spite of the double-digit inflation and other perceived deleterious consequences associated with Carter Administration policies, events that perhaps were more personally relevant to American citizens than the Iran hostage situation. Furthermore, the event's broad emotional appeal was so monumental that, in the 1980s, allegations emerged that then-presidential candidate Ronald Reagan and his campaign supporters worked out a deal with the Iranian hostage holders not to release the hostages until after the 1980 presidential elections. It was further alleged that, if elected, President Reagan promised the Iran hostage takers valued and state-of-the-art military armament. In 1980, Reagan was elected and, if the allegations are true, was able to manipulate the emotions of the electorate by exploiting a big political event.

The overwhelming media coverage of President Bill Clinton's 1998 impeachment hearings may have affected voting patterns in the 1998 congressional elections. In January 1998, allegations were brought by Independent Counsel Kenneth Starr that President Bill Clinton had committed perjury before the grand jury in the Paula Jones sexual harassment case brought against President Clinton in which Jones alleged that the president had sexually harassed her while he was governor of Arkansas. Also, Kenneth Starr alleged that President Clinton had obstructed justice by directing a former white house intern and witness in the Paula Jones case, Monica Lewinsky, to not reveal all she may have known about her own sexual affair with the president, which at first was denied by the president, although later he publicly acknowledged it. Many felt that the overwhelming coverage of the story in the media, which elicited strong emotions of support for, and opposition against, the president, would hurt the Democrats in the 1998 congressional elections because the President himself was a Democrat. However, some pundits predicted that the story would hurt the Republicans more since many polls showed that although the majority of the public felt that Bill Clinton probably did perjure himself to conceal his extramarital affair with Lewinsky, they also believed that it was not an impeachable offense. Many Americans, according to the polls, believed that the Republicans and their ally, Kenneth Starr, were overstepping their authority by attempting to impeach the president.

On the morning after the congressional elections of 1998, which occurred during the time in which the U.S. House of Representatives Judiciary Committee was holding impeachment hearings, House Republicans, who before the election were in the majority by twenty-two seats and who were widely predicted to gain seats, lost six seats. In addition, the Republican-controlled Senate failed to increase its majority. Although other factors could have influenced how voters voted in 1998, many believed that reactions to the impeachment hearings were a critical factor. Although other major events were occurring in 1998, the media elite's decision to make the impeachment hearings and President Clinton's scandal the major news story of the year restricted the range of issues on which voters could have made decisions, and this may have caused Republicans to lose seats in the House of Representatives.

The corporate influence. A fourth political factor to be considered when evaluating a policy from an Afrocentric framework is the corporate sector. The impact of corporations on the political content and analysis presented in the media, and how this content can restrict political debates and choices for voters was examined previously. However, there are additional important methods that corporations use to exert influence over the policy formulation and implementation process: (1) establishing and maintaining several well-paid lobbyists whose purpose is to influence politicians' decisions through the use of a host of financial incentives and fringe benefit strategies, (2) the financing of political campaigns either through direct contributions or through the formation of Political Action Committees (PACs), and (3) the financing of think tanks or policy institutes that conduct formal policy research and analysis.

Of the three methods, perhaps the financing of think tanks is less known and publicized. In their book, *No Mercy: How Conservative Think Tanks and Foundations Changed America's Social Agenda*, Stefancic and Delgado (1996) offer explicit data on corporations that fund conservative think tanks and describe how this funding helped to foster the ascendency of the conservative political mood popular today and such conservative social policies as those which emanated from the Republicans' infamous Contract with America. The authors show how conservative think tanks such as the Heritage Foundation, the Cato Institute, the American Enterprise Institute, and the Hudson Institute are heavily financed by major corporations, which often contribute the largest proportion of these institutes' annual budget. The strategy often used by corporations to fund these think tanks is to establish corporate foundations. For example, the Joseph Coors Foundation, of the renowned Coors Beer Company, played a primary role in establishing the Heritage Foundation in 1973 and remains one of its largest contributors (Stefancic and Delgado, 1996). The John M. Olin Foundation, which was established in 1953 by inventor and industrialist John Merrill Olin is another major contributor to conservative think tanks. For example, according to Stefancic and Delgado (1996), in 1992 and 1993, the Olin Foundation gave $740,910 to just one conservative think tank, the American Enterprise Institute. Much of the money was used to fund research activities of well-known conservative policy analysts such as Judge Bork, Irving Kristol, and Dinish D'Souza (Stefancic and Delgado, 1996). Thus, the policy analyst working from an Afrocentric framework is well advised to discern how corporate dollars directly and indirectly can influence social policy debates, formulation, and implementation.

Protest politics. A last political factor that should be examined when analyzing a policy from an Afrocentric framework is the role of protest politics. Protest politics can be defined as the pressure disenfranchised or other disgruntled groups in society place on politicians through public demonstrations and additional public displays of defiance that involve massive numbers of people. These protests, if well organized and consistently placed in action, or if they pose a substantive threat to social and economic stability, can have a significant impact on policy debates and development. Protest politics emerging from the poor and oppressed frequently have caused politicians to make certain concessions (Morris, 1984; Piven and Cloward, 1971, 1982). The social protests of the 1930s and the 1960s are viewed consistently by scholars as being the chief impetus behind social reform legislation that came about in both decades (Abramovitz, 1996; Day, 1997; Ehrenreich, 1985; Quadagno, 1994; Weir, Orloff, and Skocpol, 1988). The labor movements of the 1930s and the civil rights movement of the 1960s compelled politicians in both eras to offer concessions, perhaps more out of the motivation to maintain social order than out of a sense of promoting equality and justice. This cynical understanding of American politics, which is clearly consistent with the Afrocentric framework, was expressed poignantly by Piven and Cloward (1971) in their book *Regulating the Poor*. Drawing on a neo-Marxist analysis, Piven and Cloward suggest that social welfare relief serves two functions relative to labor: (1) relief augments a shrunken labor market, and (2) relief helps overcome the poor fit between labor market requirements and the characteristics of the labor force. The primary point in the Piven and Cloward analysis is that since the free-market system of capitalism does not and cannot ensure that all persons will work—thus reducing control over those persons' civil behavior—the system of social welfare serves to compensate for the market's weakness in controlling behavior. Since much of protest politics aims to secure greater economic and employment opportunities for oppressed groups, and because protest politics often is viewed as civil disorder by the power elite, social welfare programs can function to (1) provide employment and training opportunities for the oppressed that then (2) help quell their need to protest and to continue a strident critique of the existing social structure. The influence of protest politics on social welfare policy development indicates that even ordinary persons, when organized and committed, can affect social and economic legislation, oftentimes in a more powerful and sweeping manner than the aforementioned political forces. Though the legislation created may not go far enough to completely resolve a social problem, the protest that fostered it can help change policy debates and justify the need for additional legislative amendments.

Part of the emphasis on protest politics in the Afrocentric framework is predicated on the historic role African Americans have played in protest movements. The gains that have ensued from these movements, although still lacking in critical areas, often elevated not only the political and economic status of many African Americans but also helped shape current and future policy debates. A policy analyst applying Afrocentric principles to the policy analysis process would be remiss in overlooking the role of protest politics in formulating a social policy and in influencing the debate in the area that the policy addresses.

Economic Factors

Economic factors also can influence the formulation and content of a social welfare policy. Some economic factors that can shape social welfare policy formulation and content are (1) unemployment rates, (2) inflation, (3) the gross national product, (4) job creation, (5) wages, (6) labor shortages, (7) interests rates, and (8) taxes. The significance of these factors, collectively and individually, was most dramatically demonstrated in U.S. history by the effects of the 1929 stock market crash on the Depression and on the New Deal legislation of the early 1930s. Unemployment nationally in the early 1930s was about 25 percent, and in some cities, such as Norfolk, Virginia, the unemployment rate was over 40 percent (Day, 1997; Jansson, 1997). The injudicious economic and production practices of U.S. corporations in the late 1920s, which helped cause the crash (Day, 1997; Trattner, 1994; Wenocur and Reisch, 1989), and the corollary of massive numbers of people out of work forced politicians and the business community to devise a series of government-sponsored programs to relieve the unemployed or, acknowledging the more critical view discussed earlier, to socially control the poor by suppressing their spirit of insurgency and protest. The problem of unemployment led the U.S. government to enact an array of economic policies and relief agencies in the early 1930s that culminated in the 1935 Social Security Act. The significance of the crash of 1929 in generating the federal economic policies and relief agencies to address the massive social problems of the early 1930s is seen in the observation that, up to that point in U.S. history, the U.S. government had only supported two other social welfare initiatives, namely, the Freedmen's Bureau of the 1860s and the Sheppard-Towner Act of 1921 (Day, 1997; Trattner, 1994).

Although presented separately from the political factors, it is important, from an Afrocentric viewpoint, to conceive the economic and the political as inseparable. The injudicious production and pricing practices of many U.S. corporations in the late 1920s, which led to the 1929 crash, were supported by many politicians of that day, including then-President Herbert Hoover (Day, 1997; Jansson, 1997; Trattner, 1994). Moreover, workfare policies supported by many politicians throughout U.S. history have received their thrust from corporate concerns that there be a continued adequate supply of low-wage labor (Blau, 1994; Rose, 1989). Last, the role of corporations in affecting the decisions of politicians through their financing of lobbyists, PACs, and think tanks is, Afrocentrically, no accident either. Consistent with Marx's analysis of capitalism, the Afrocentric framework of policy analysis contends that capitalism must be understood organically. To isolate the parts that drive capitalism is not only to fall victim to an incomplete analysis but also obviates comprehension of how capitalist ideology is employed to advance the interests of the power elite (Horkheimer, 1972). It is this understanding that is assumed to be a chief foundation of social welfare policy debates and decisions in the United States.

Social Factors

Social factors, as with economic factors, also are important in examining a policy from an Afrocentric framework. Since all human behavior occurs within a social context or has social implications and meaning, social factors could include a broad range of phenomena. However, for this discussion's purpose, social factors are conceived as those factors which generate considerable shifts and changes in the demographic picture or landscape of a nation. These factors could be birthrates, marital and divorce rates, migration and immigration patterns, and morbidity and mortality rates. Perhaps birthrates and mortality rates and migration and immigration patterns have been some of the major social factors influencing social policy debates and formulation. Take, for example, the impact of birthrates and mortality rates on the 1990s debate regarding Social Security. Conventional wisdom suggests that the current Social Security funding strategy will have to be altered drastically in the future if the policy is to survive. Currently, the program is funded through a compulsory tax on the wages of most employed persons to contribute to the financial needs of primarily retired elderly persons over the age of sixty-five in perpetuity. Both birthrates and mortality rates have placed significant strain on the viability of this funding strategy. On the one hand, elderly persons are living longer today and life expectancy is projected to increase in the future (U.S. Bureau of the Census, 1998). On the other hand, the birthrates of the generation that followed the famed "baby boomers," who were born between 1946 and 1963, were significantly lower than the baby boomer generation, the older of whom will be at retirement age (sixty-five) beginning in the year 2011. The confluence of an aging baby boomer generation with an ever-increasing and longer-living elderly population is generating an ever-shrinking dependency ratio (i.e., the ratio of contributors supporting beneficiaries), with the number of beneficiaries steadily increasing relative to the number of contributors on whom the involuntary Social Security tax is levied. These social events are likely to radically change Social Security policy in the very near future, as can be gleaned from current congressional debates and proposals.

Migration and immigration patterns also have affected, and can affect, social welfare policy legislation. An excellent example of this was the effects of massive Chinese, Japanese, and eastern and southern European immigration on the passing of the 1924 Immigration Act. This act restricted the immigration of most ethnic groups, with the exception of those from northern and western Europe. Persons from other ethnic groups were deemed undesirable because of the political conservatism that followed World War I, a critical component of which being the protection of the racial purity of "true" Americans whose descendants rained from western and northern Europe (Jansson, 1997; Trattner, 1994). Recently, a similar fear about the effects of massive numbers of Hispanic immigrants, who frequently end up on public assistance, has been suggested as a primary reason why new welfare reform measures increasingly make it difficult for legal immigrants to receive public assistance in the United States (Yang, 1996). The latter concerns about population control should especially be attended to by the policy analyst relying on the Afrocentric framework because the Afrocentric model assumes that the growing birth and immigration rates of groups of color in the United States poses a significant challenge for continued dominance of European-American cultural values, language, and general lifestyles.

Cultural Factors

The Afrocentric paradigm supports the notion that culture embraces and informs all other social phenomena in a specific society (Ani, 1994; Asante, 1988, 1997; Henderson, 1995). From this organic view of culture, cultural factors could be everything that characterizes a society—politics, economics, religion, education, military institutions, and so on. If we rely on the definition of culture as a fundamental worldview statement about social reality, the major cultural factors that can affect social welfare policy debates, development, and implementation are values or value orientations. Similar to most other social welfare policy frameworks, the Afrocentric framework of policy analysis contends that value orientations constantly inform and pervade social policy debates, dilemmas, and development. From this vantage point, the Afrocentric policy analyst seeks to examine how the value orientations that characterize the Eurocentric worldview shape and influence the provisions of a policy and the manner in which it is implemented. Eurocentric value orientations from the public, the corporate sector, politicians, political think tanks, and political lobbyists should be examined to determine (1) which cadre exerted the most impact on the formation of the policy and (2) the degree of variance among the previous groups on their acceptance of core Eurocentric cultural values.

Some of the core Eurocentric value orientations that should be identified are as follows: (1) insular or possessive individualism, (2) the association of one's economic status with one's moral and personal worth, (3) the Protestant work ethic, (4) white supremacy, (5) exclusive conception of a materialist social reality, (6) deemphasis on a collective understanding of the social problem for which the policy was designed, (7) overemphasis on protecting individual liberties at the expense of protecting the interests of the public and, more specifically, the entire group for which the policy has been developed, (8) extreme focus on economic competition, (9) separation of federal, state, and local government; community; and individual responsibility in resolving the problem that is the focus of the policy, (10) protecting the economic and political interests of the corporate elite, and (11) nonparticipation of corporations in funding and providing the services mandated by the policy. These values, from an Afrocentric perspective, are believed to be some of the primary philosophical underpinnings of social welfare policy development in the United States.

In addition, the Afrocentric policy analyst is encouraged to examine the degree to which the policy includes interpretations and cultural values that stem from the group or groups for which the policy was established. Consistent with the strengths perspective of social policy analysis and development offered by Chapin (1995), the Afrocentric framework of policy analysis asserts that the group for which the policy is designed should have substantive influence over the character and content of the policy and whether a policy should be formulated in the first place. This participation should fundamentally elicit the target group's definition and interpretation of the problem or whether it considers the phenomenon a "problem" at all. Although the targeted group's views about the problem or event are essential, the Afrocentric framework admonishes that these views should be weighed against the views of others who are directly or indirectly affected by the problem or event. This should be the case because, though the problem might be relatively isolated within a certain segment of society, the reality of shared social space by manifold groups in society suggests that problems can affect the lives of others for whom the policy may not be intended. An example of this would be a policy designed to prevent street crime within certain residential communities. Although the bulk of the policy might focus on providing services and educational opportunities for those at risk of perpetrating a crime, the policy would also have implications for anyone who happens to travel or spend any time in the targeted communities. Thus, ideas and interpretations should be elicited not only from those who are at risk of committing the crimes but also from those who frequent the targeted communities, which enhances their chances of being potential crime victims. The role of the Afrocentric policy analyst in this case is to identify whether this kind of elicitation figured into the design of the policy and to identify what group's interpretation of the problem most heavily influenced the provisions, content, and implementation of the policy. The important point here is that the Afrocentric policy analyst is encouraged to unearth not only the value orientations that shape the policy but also the sources or groups to whom the value orientations belong.

Collective Emphasis of Policy

Another component of an Afrocentric policy analysis framework is determining the degree to which the policy promotes a collective emphasis. A collective emphasis comprises at least three aspects: (1) the degree to which the policy promotes the union of the material and spiritual aspects of human need, (2) the degree to which the policy validates concern for the collective interests and welfare of all in the society, especially those most vulnerable to human suffering and despair, and (3) the extent to which the policy promotes values of collective success and collective failure.

Union of Material and Spiritual

A critical role of the Afrocentric policy analyst is to examine the degree to which spiritual aspects and needs of human beings are addressed. Much of the content in most, if not all, social policies in the United States focuses exclusively on meeting the material needs of humans. These needs are those of food, clothing, shelter, and money to consume goods and to maintain a minimal standard of living. Rarely are issues of the spiritual needs of humans, such as self-worth, securing meaning in life, nurturing internal peace and tranquility with oneself and others, and addressing issues and ideas regarding transcendental forces, examined in social policies or policy analysis, and when they are, these issues are considered secondary to concerns of material sustenance (Canda and Chambers, 1994). Perhaps two reasons for the reluctance to incorporate spiritual needs in social policy formation are, as Sullivan (1994) contends, that "common definitions of spirituality are broad and vague . . . [and] spirituality becomes indistinct from religious doctrine, which often has a built-in status quo bias" (p. 71). First, and as has been discussed, spirituality is viewed as both separate from and a part of religious dogma in the Afrocentric paradigm (Asante, 1988; Schiele, 1997; Semmes, 1993). The central idea that spirituality communicates, from an Afrocentric perspective, is interconnectedness, both within the material and unseen domains as well as between them. This interconnectedness implies wholeness or a feeling of completeness and meaning for the individual, feelings that lead one to desire to participate in life constructively, not destructively, and to contribute positively to the advancement of the human family.

With this definition as a foundation, Sullivan's (1994) second point about spirituality being too broad and vague is irrelevant. If one prefers quantitative measurement as a way to gauge human feelings and behavior, then feelings or attitudes that lead one to want to participate in life constructively and to contribute positively to the advancement of the human family can be measured and even further fractionalized and reduced. Scales can be designed—and have been (see, for example, Jagers and Owens-Mock, 1993; Montgomery, Fine, and Myers, 1990)—to tap these feelings. However, although the Afrocentric paradigm does not discourage measurement, it concomitantly does not disparage broad and seemingly vague constructs. Indeed, broadness and vagueness can help to promote a collective emphasis among humanity for at least three reasons. First, broadness can help expand human perspectives and rescue these viewpoints from reductionistic thinking that can bring about provincialism. Provincialism, or isolated thinking, some say influences the practice of domination because it fails to consider or integrate the ideas and concerns of others (Mosse, 1978; Myers, 1988). Second, vagueness can promote a collective emphasis by blurring seemingly important differences between and among people, between humans and the environment, and between humans and the metaphysical world. Last, if a critical goal of spirituality is to better tap into the wisdom and vastness of the Creator (i.e., God subjectification), as is true in the Afrocentric framework, it appears that an orientation which encourages broad and vague definitions or interpretations of phenomena might be appropriate, and even essential.

Another possible reason why spirituality principles are devalued in policy content and analysis is the false dichotomy between relationships between people and relationships between people and a higher power. The Afrocentric paradigm suggests that the higher power can be manifested in human relationships and that these relationships can benefit considerably from this acknowledgment. Sullivan (1994) argues that the main concern about incorporating spiritual principles is "the diversity of beliefs and practices" among Americans and the ability "to create a universal code of ethics" (p. 71). However, the problem with his analysis is that he does not conceive spirituality as inseparable from religious dogma, as does the Afrocentric paradigm. If the notion of interconnectedness can be agreed upon as a synonym of spirituality—a notion that validates and recognizes that all people stem from a common source and that it is mutually beneficial for all to accept this interconnectedness if only to preclude global annihilation—then social policies would be emancipated to integrate spirituality, to facilitate a more complete vision of human needs, and to more effectively foster honest, harmonious, and mutually satisfying human relationships. The role of the Afrocentric policy analyst, therefore, is to identify the extent to which a policy encourages this kind of interconnectedness.

The Collective Interests and Welfare of All

A policy analytic framework based on Afrocentric principles also is concerned about the degree to which the policy protects the collective interests and welfare of all. This concern should be particularly examined to identify the policy's capacity to protect and advance those who are most vulnerable. One of the methods through which the interests of the most vulnerable can be advanced and protected is to provide greater specificity and a goodness of fit between the policy and the group for which the policy is designed. In this way, and consistent with the postmodernist notion of rejecting a unified subject (see Bauman, 1992; Leonard, 1995; Penna and O'Brien, 1996; Seidman, 1994), the Afrocentric paradigm encourages social policy development that emerges from, and speaks to, the specific needs and ethos of a group. This should be the case in multiethnic and multicultural societies such as the United States in which a diversity of definitions of social problems and human needs exists. This does not suggest that there can be no common ground nor shared interests across diverse groups in a manner that accentuates the value of interconnectedness discussed previously. This perspective, however, does acknowledge that cultural diversity implies diversity of experience and interpretation; thus, there can be social policy unity without social policy uniformity. The balance of social policy unity with social policy diversity can be said to reflect and protect a sort of *pluriversal collectivity.* Within this collectivity, difference and solidarity are conceived as equal social realities, and to deny one is to discredit a comprehensive explication of a social space shared by distinct cultural groups. Social policy development, as with other human productions, should better reflect the need to maintain order and cooperation among diverse groups yet tailor social interventions to more closely approximate the needs, interests, and interpretations of a specific group.

Here, the Afrocentric policy analyst attempts to identify the extent to which the policy is specific to the interests and interpretations of a group without engendering substantial harm, or ideally no harm at all, to the collective welfare of others who share the same geographical space. Specifically, the Afrocentric policy analyst is looking to identify (1) whether the policy's definitions of social problems and human needs are shaped significantly by the group for which the policy is established, (2) whether the implementation aspects include members of this group as major decision makers and administrators, (3) the degree to which attention to group specificity in the policy violates shared social arrangements that are mutually beneficial to all who occupy the social space, and (4) the degree to which the policy challenges or fosters a hegemonic universalism that seeks to reinforce discourses that emanate predominantly from one group. Of course, seeking to identify these aspects of a policy ultimately raises questions about competing values of a policy and whether the methods employed to resolve the competition are fair or hegemonic. Determining whether the resolution is fair or unfair is a significant objective of the Afrocentric policy analyst. One indicator of fairness would be the extent to which the policy includes interpretations from various subsegments within the group for which the policy is designed. Although social analysts, especially of the cultural-competence genre, often advocate for inclusion of different interpretations across and between groups, attention also must be given to diversity within cultural/ethnic groups and whether this diversity is fostered or suppressed in social policy development and implementation.

What this discussion suggests is that the dialectic between honoring diversity and specificity and maintaining some sense of social commonality through the policy development process is a formidable task. The point here, from an Afrocentric perspective, is that the current process is far too hegemonic, excluding and suppressing multiple narratives about definitions of human need. The Afrocentric policy analyst, therefore, evaluates the policy from the vantage point of whether the policy's content and its development conform to the value of *pluriversal* collectivity.

Collective Success and Failure

A last dimension of determining whether a policy validates a collective focus is the extent to which it embraces themes of collective success and collective failure. Themes of collective success and failure are ideas that conceive individual success and failure, to a considerable extent, as outcomes of collective social actions of both the wider and more intimate social environments (Gyekye, 1992; Karenga, 1996; Williams, 1993). Failure and success are shared phenomena, not events that are the exclusive products of isolated, intrapsychic attributes (Gyekye, 1992; Karenga, 1996; Williams, 1993). Since most social welfare policies are designed to address some failure, whether real or perceived, hegemonic or agreed upon, the primary goal of the Afrocentric policy analyst is to ascertain if ideas of collective failure have been incorporated into the policy's provisions and procedures. Some questions the policy analyst can ask that might help to achieve this end are as follows:

1. Does the policy consistently adhere to individualism as a chief explanation of the problem?

2. Does the policy include sociopolitical and sociohistorical factors as major explanations of the problem?
3. If oppression and domination are central attributes of the social system in which the policy emerges, does the policy acknowledge oppression as contributing to the problem?
4. Does the policy allow for collective solutions to the problem that place responsibility not only on individuals thought to have the problem but also on those in the individuals' intimate and broader social environments?
5. Does the policy's funding mechanism include contributions from multiple factions in society, factions that may have helped to create the problem as well as those which can benefit psychologically, politically, and economically from the problem's resolution?

In the latter question, the analyst should observe if financial contributions from the corporate, government, volunteer, and local community segments of society are present. If so, what is the distributional pattern of the contributions? That is, who is contributing the most and the least?

Chapter 9

The Afrocentric Paradigm
and Human Service Organizations

Since most human service work occurs within a formal organizational context, the applicability of the Afrocentric paradigm to both explain and provide prescriptions for human service organizations is critical. Human service organizations process, sustain, or change individuals (Hasenfeld, 1983, 1992; Hasenfeld and English, 1974). Within these organizations, human beings are considered the "raw material" (Hasenfeld, 1983, 1992). Some examples of human service organizations are social service departments, hospitals, health maintenance organizations, schools, mental health agencies, and churches. This chapter applies the Afrocentric paradigm (1) to critique existing, Eurocentrically oriented organizational theories by identifying some differences in the way organizations are conceptualized from a Eurocentric and an Afrocentric viewpoint, (2) to help human service organizations become more effective in enhancing positive organizational potentiality, and (3) to examine the need for people of color to establish human service organizations that reflect their cultural ethos and advance their political interests.

DISTINCTIONS BETWEEN AFROCENTRIC
AND EUROCENTRIC ORGANIZATIONAL THEORIES

Some fundamental distinctions in the conceptions of organizations are found between Afrocentric and Eurocentric (mainstream) organizational theories. Although similarities exist between the Afrocentric model and

This chapter consists of a reworking of three previously published articles: "Organizational Theory from an Afrocentric Perspective," *Journal of Black Studies,* 1990, 21(2), pp. 145-161; "The Afrocentric Paradigm and Workplace Diversity," *Workplace Diversity, Issues, and Perspectives,* 1998, pp. 341-353; "Malcolm X's Example for Social Work," *Black Caucus,* 1996, 2(2), pp. 8-20. Reprinted with permission from Sage Publications, the National Association of Social Workers, and the National Association of Black Social Workers, respectively.

199

some Eurocentric organizational theories, a major difference lies in what I will refer to as *organizational normality* (i.e., that which is considered the standard or accepted reality for organizations). Many mainstream or Western organizational theories—with the exception of the neo-Marxist perspective—concentrate on the factors affecting organizational productivity (i.e., how fast, how much, and how well something is produced or, in the case of human service organizations, how well and how efficiently people are processed, sustained, or changed). This focus is in the theory of bureaucracy's principle of rationality (Weber, 1946); in the scientific management's notion of maximum productivity (Hasenfeld, 1983); in the human relation's assumption that increased worker satisfaction will induce increased productivity (Kaplan and Tausky, 1977); in the decision-making theory's concepts of "satisficing" and "performance gap" (Hasenfeld, 1983); in the energy expended by Lawrence and Lorsch to identify the attributes of a "highly effective organization" (Lawrence and Lorsch, 1967); in the natural system model's emphasis on goal displacement and how this displacement causes the unattainment of formal, official goals (Scott, 1967); and in the political economy's focus on how the distribution of power and the availability of resources, both within and outside organizations, shape the choice of service technologies used for production. As Perrow (1978) astutely observes, even when such theories as the natural systems and human relations theories reject mechanical and rationalistic notions of organizations and accept informal, humanistic, and natural characteristics, these characteristics are viewed as constraints on the organization in becoming more efficient (rational) in achieving its announced goals—in other words, constraining its rate of production.

Another fundamental characteristic of mainstream or Eurocentric theories of organizations is the emphasis placed on the individual organization member. Even the human relations model, with its focus on small group processes, uses this group process to affect the individual's job satisfaction and productivity. Part of this individual focus is a function of the manner in which "individual" is conceived in the Eurocentric tradition, especially in western social science. Akbar (1984) comments on this observation in his discussion of what he calls the Eurocentric social science model. Akbar maintains that one of the salient attributes of the Eurocentric model is its individualistic character. Individualism is emphasized in the Eurocentric model, according to Akbar, because human identity is conceived insularly: it is assumed that the individual can be understood separate from others. By focusing on this conception of human identity, Akbar contends that the individual's corporate identity (e.g., significant others such as family members, community members, and friends) is of secondary importance in conceiving the individual.

The limited conception of human identity found in the Eurocentric model is reflected in the way the "client" is conceived in human service organizational theory. Throughout the human service organization literature, until very recently, "client" was usually conceived as one individual, as if he or she lived in a vacuum and was not part of a social group.

Unlike the Eurocentric model's conception of identity, and as discussed in Chapter 2, individual identity is conceived as a collective identity within the Afrocentric model. For example, Cook and Kono (1977) state that in black or African psychology, "individuality in the sense of self in opposition to the group disappears and is replaced by a common understanding and a common goal" (p. 26). Moreover, Asante's (1988) concept of the "collective cognitive imperative" (i.e., the full spiritual and intellectual commitment to a vision by a group) and Nobles' (1980) concept of "experiential communality," or the sharing of a particular experience by a particular group of people, are important in understanding a fundamental characteristic of an Afrocentric organizational model: its emphasis on discerning similarities or commonalities among organizational workers and consumers instead of underscoring individual differences. Although differences are acknowledged and appreciated, the collective thrust in the Afrocentric organizational paradigm gives preeminence to the group: the welfare of the group takes precedence over the welfare of the individual. This group orientation has also been discussed by Hunt (1974), who asserts that the black perspective on public management is a collective orientation, wherein the public demands and interests of blacks as a group supplant the needs of blacks as individuals.

Accepting that the collective orientation assumption is valid—and being mindful that the Afrocentric model is predicated on traditional African philosophical assumptions—the interests of the organization as a whole or collective would be the primary concern within an Afrocentric framework, although individual interests and concerns would be recognized. From an Afrocentric perspective, organizational and group survival replaces productivity as the overriding concern. Organizational normality would not be defined by the quantity or efficiency of production (as is the case in many Eurocentric theories of organizations), but rather by the way in which an organization preserves itself (i.e., whether the behaviors employed by organization members maintain the survival of the organization). Although this view of survival is similar to the concept of survival found in the natural systems model—in that organizational survival is given high importance—a fundamental difference is that survival in the natural systems model places considerable emphasis on goal attainment, as if goal attainment and survival were synonymous. The Afrocentric perspective conceives survival in itself as paramount. Though goal attainment would be important within an Afrocentric organization, survival in an organization based on Afrocentric principles would include more than just goal attainment. It would, for example, include the maintenance of common objectives, concerns, and sentiments among organization members.

Besides the maintenance of common objectives, concerns, and sentiments among organization members, the Afrocentric model's concept of survival also transcends the boundaries of the organization and extends into the community. This focus highlights organization-community relations perhaps more strongly than most existing human service organizational theories. Just as it is unthinkable to understand the individual separate from others in the Afrocentric paradigm so, too, would it be to understand the organization separate from the community to which it belongs and which it serves. Therefore, to a considerable extent, the organization and the community are viewed as one: the organization's purpose is a reflection of the community's purpose. To the extent that this bond exists between the organization and the community, it is assumed that the survival of the organization is significantly related to the survival of the community, and vice versa. Hence, the collective survival notion found in the Afrocentric paradigm involves the coalescence of individual, organization, and community identities. Fundamentally, the Afrocentric paradigm differs from existing organizational theories in its view of organizational normality, its concept of human identity, and its notion of organizational survival.

THE AFROCENTRIC PARADIGM
AND POSITIVE POTENTIALITY IN ORGANIZATIONS

Now that some differences in Eurocentric and Afrocentric organizational models have been identified, it is next important to draw upon the theoretical discussions in Chapter 2 to describe how an Afrocentric organization might appear and what aspects of organizational functioning it would underscore to enhance what can be called *positive organizational potentiality.* Positive organizational potentiality is defined here as an organization's vast capabilities to be inclusive in its conceptions of human worth and in its use of culturally different strategies and interventions. When concepts of human worth are expanded and culturally different strategies and interventions are employed, an organization's ability in effectively meeting the complete needs of consumers and staff is increased.

To encourage an orientation toward greater positive organizational potentiality, the Afrocentric paradigm recommends the following: (1) the worth and dignity of organization members and consumers should be equally valued; (2) the internal differentiation of work tasks should be limited, and, when possible, work tasks should be shared; (3) more emphasis should be placed on person-to-person communications than on written communications; (4) group recognition should occur more than individual recognition; (5) there should be consensus decision making; (6) efficiency should be deemphasized; and (7) diverse ideas about hiring and performance evaluations should be incorporated.

Worth and Dignity of Organization Members

In the Afrocentric organizational model, the worth and dignity of each organization member and consumer would be equally acknowledged and nurtured. For organization members, worth and dignity, Afrocentrically, imply not only the overall self-worth of the member as part of the human family connected to a common universal source but also acknowledgment of the importance of the skill the person brings to the organization and the unique way he or she performs the skill. When focus in organizations is placed on the similar origins and spiritual connection of humans, hierarchical schemes of human self-worth that rank order people by their outer (material) qualities, such as gender, skin color, and weight, are unnecessary. In this sense, the Afrocentric paradigm encourages the development of *organizational morality.* Organizational morality refers to an organizational state in which members of an organization have the highest regard for human life and dignity and consistently display behaviors that reflect this value. This respect is not assumed to be held exclusively for organization members; it is also for consumers and others who interact with the human service organization. To this end, humanistic values, such as client and worker self-worth, worker empathy, and concern for the welfare of clients and co-workers, are moved from a status of obscurity to the forefront of organizational priorities. This is especially relevant to human service organizations whose purpose is to promote the general well-being of individuals in society (Hasenfeld, 1983, 1992).

To the extent that morality implies spirituality in the Afrocentric paradigm, the development and maintenance of organization members' spirituality would be viewed as a critical factor in shaping the mental and physical performance of members. It would be assumed that without a well-nourished and developed spirit, the mental and physical performance of organization members would be at a minimum.

The value placed on the worth and dignity of both organization workers and consumers found in the Afrocentric paradigm is predicated heavily on its person-to-person axiology. As opposed to the Eurocentric viewpoint that tends to underscore a person-to-object axiology (see Ani, 1994; Nichols, 1987), the maintenance and enhancement of the interpersonal relationship is considered the most preeminent value in the Afrocentric organizational paradigm. Such an emphasis fosters a human-centered orientation to life in lieu of an object or material orientation. Accordingly, the acquisition of an object or material item would not take precedence over maintaining and strengthening interpersonal ties.

The focus on interpersonal relationships in existing organizational models is best represented in the human relations model, with its emphasis on increasing interpersonal competence (Kaplan and Tausky, 1977), warm personal ties (Litwak, 1978), and collegial relationships (Kaplan and Tausky, 1977; Litwak, 1978). The strengthening of interpersonal competence and relationships in the human relations model, however, is used as a strategy to increase workers' satisfaction, through increased participation, to affect worker performance and increase worker productivity. Thus, increased interpersonal ties are viewed as a means to achieve an end. This weakens and undermines the interpersonal character and assertion of the human relations model. Conversely, in the Afrocentric model, the strengthening of interpersonal relationships between and among organization members and consumers would be perceived as an end in itself. This logic is predicated on the assumption advanced by Brisbane and Womble (1991) that, often, in human service work, how one is treated is just as important in influencing positive human transformation than the actual practice intervention itself.

Organizations based on Afrocentric principles also would not value some worker skills over others because the Afrocentric paradigm accentuates the mutual dependency of worker skills and talents. All skills needed for the effective operation of the organization are considered equally essential. Thus, for example, housekeeping skills, which are often seen as subordinate to others, would be valued just as much as others and even more so because the execution of additional organizational activities are predicated significantly upon a sanitary and aesthetically pleasant work milieu.

Low Internal Differentiation and Shared Work Tasks

Low internal differentiation and exchange of work tasks are important in fostering organizational collectivity and effectiveness (Daly, 1994). High internal differentiation of tasks often leads to the emergence of well-defined organizational subunits that can encourage members to become more committed to the goals and interests of their subdivisions than to the collective goals of the entire organization (Daly, 1982; Selznick, 1948). The exchange of work tasks can prevent overcommitment to subunit goals and provide organizational members with the opportunity to take on the "skill identity" of another. This can nurture a collective, organizational empathy and respect for diverse tasks that otherwise would not exist.

Person-to-Person Communication

Warfield-Coppock (1995) maintains that person-to-person communications would be appropriate in Afrocentric organizations and can facilitate greater organizational harmony among workers. This is because the exchange of ideas is not filtered through a medium (e.g., a memo) that can make communications appear impersonal and perfunctory. Person-to-person communication also provides the advantage of observing gestures and facial expressions and listening to someone's voice. In the Afrocentric paradigm, not only is what people say important but also how they express their ideas via the rhythm and tone of their voices and through their body and facial gestures (Akbar, 1976; Asante, 1980). Face-to-face communications also require organization members who may be at odds with one another to communicate rather than to sustain their animosity through avoidance.

Emphasis on Group Recognition

The Afrocentric paradigm of human service organizations would encourage group recognition more than individual recognition. This is not to imply that individual accomplishments be overlooked but that when focus is placed on individual achievement alone, the collective efforts and skills of those involved in helping an individual strive are denied or downplayed. In addition, exclusive or primary attention to individual achievement may tend to engender envy among organization members when they are not equally recognized for their accomplishments.

Consensus Decision Making

Consonant with the collective thrust found in the Afrocentric paradigm is the focus on consensus decision making. Although traditional African societies maintained an elected chief and council of elders as the governing body of a village, town, or state, they also followed the practice of eliciting public opinions from any citizen, and if disagreement arose on an issue, the council of elders would listen to arguments until unanimity was obtained (Chazan, 1993; Gyekye, 1992; Williams, 1987). The goal of these debates was not for one perspective to prevail over another, but for differences to be obfuscated so that an agreement could be reached (Chazan, 1993; Gyekye, 1992). Since these discussions could sometimes be considerably extensive, there was less concern for making swift decisions by a few for the sake of efficiency (Gyekye, 1992; Williams, 1987).

The emphasis on communalism and consensus in traditional African practice and philosophy encourages organizations to form structures and procedures that elicit the opinions of all organization members when disagreement arises. This practice can foster not only inclusion but also prudent decision making because the more people working together to solve a problem, the greater the likelihood of finding a good solution and anticipating contingencies. This was confirmed by Daly (1994) who found that the use of problem-solving communication, in which ideas from manifold workers are elicited, can assist organizations in successfully meeting the challenges of a turbulent organizational milieu. In addition, the focus on consensus decision making is extended to include the opinions and suggestions of those in the organization's environment. As aforementioned, the organization and the environment/community to which it belongs and which it serves are deemed one because the concept of organizational survival in the Afrocentric paradigm transcends the boundaries of the organization to include the preservation of the surrounding environment/community.

Although some degree of hierarchy would be expected in Afrocentric organizations, superordinate/subordinate relationships would be dissuaded. Relationships wherein one person is responsible for the actions of others would be seen less as *power-imposing relationships* and more as *compassionate power relationships*. Power-imposing relationships in organizations are built upon superordinate/subordinate relations and on the belief that workers are prone to indolence and a lack self-regulation. Compassionate power relationships are based on sincere mutual respect, the belief in worker self-regulation, and the belief that power should be shared.

From an Afrocentric viewpoint, it is also important to realize that for organization members to be able to fully participate in decision-making processes, the stress related to home and child care must be minimized. To do this, and as discussed in Chapter 7, the Afrocentric paradigm encourages flexible work hours, provision of child care services at the workplace, and ample family leave and vacation time (Schiele, 1997; Warfield-Coppock, 1995). These strategies may lead to greater perceptions of organizational support among workers. Indeed, when workers perceive that organizations care about their overall well-being, job satisfaction, and job performance, commitment to the organization increases (Daly, 1994; Eisenberger, Fasdo, and Davis-LaMastro, 1990; Witt, 1994).

Deemphasis on Efficiency

From an Afrocentric perspective, the overwhelming concern given to efficiency or speed in organizations should be diminished. This does not imply that effectiveness is compromised because efficiency and effectiveness are two different organizational entities (Bloom, Fischer, and Orme, 1995). Although some degree of attention to speed is important, its overemphasis can lessen the quality time needed for successful problem solving, change, and goal achievement. In human service organizations, this means that an overemphasis on efficiency can bring about hasty solutions and procedures that might not adequately tap the needs or problems of consumers. Because of the priority given to efficiency, consumer needs and problems can be oversimplified so that they "fit" neatly into statistical categories and hasty goal statements.

The focus on efficiency in organizations also implies that humans should, and can, work mechanistically with little or no error. The Afrocentric paradigm, which recognizes the importance of affect and spontaneity in people's lives, would suggest that mechanistic and error-free assumptions or desires in several Eurocentric organizational models are not only inappropriate but also oppressive. Upholding expectations of people as machinelike creates an unrealistic standard that can be used to superfluously criticize, reprimand, demote, or fire workers. In addition, since the speed at which activities are accomplished is usually a major organizational objective, concerns and needs of workers that are external to the expectations to perform efficiently (i.e., their socioemotional needs) are generally unmet and treated as secondary. Thus, workers are dehumanized because their worth as human beings is confined to their ability to perform efficiently.

Diverse Ideas About Hiring and Performance Standards

To the degree that an organization employs persons from culturally diverse backgrounds, the Afrocentric paradigm supports the application of diverse procedures for hiring and performance appraisal. Too often, in organizations today, uniform criteria are employed to hire and evaluate workers. This practice is usually justified by the need to uphold the values of fairness and meritocracy. However, the ideals of complete fairness and meritocracy are rarely observed in organizational practice (Arvey and

Faley, 1988). From an Afrocentric viewpoint, fairness and meritocracy in the American workplace can be viewed as smoke screens to conceal the practice of white supremacy and to promote the universalism of European-American (i.e., Eurocentric) culture. White supremacy can be defined as the individual and institutional intentions and practices of some European Americans to ensure their political and economic advantage over people of color. Eurocentric cultural universalism can be defined as the belief and projection of European-American definitions of reality as historically ubiquitous and culturally global. Both white supremacy and Eurocentric cultural universalism obviate the hiring (inclusion) of people of color in the workplace; more important, they also preclude the inclusion of additional cultural ideas about hiring and performance appraisal.

From an Afrocentric perspective, inclusion of more people of color in the workplace can be significantly aided by eliminating the hegemony of Eurocentric cultural concepts that dictate the appropriate criteria for hiring and worker performance appraisal. Some possible examples of these criteria are direct eye contact in personal conversations; the pervasive integration and use of humor in conversations; the acceptance and knowledge of Eurocentric theories of human behavior, development, and service interventions, for example, in mental health and social service organizations; the suppression of affect and bodily gestures in communication; the denial of racism or racial discrimination in organizational activities; recognizing individual achievement over collective achievement; familiarity with English and specific European-American applications of English; and evaluating workers primarily on material and specific aspects of their work that tend to conform easily to reductionistic definitions of efficiency and effectiveness.

As it concerns reductionistic definitions, which are characteristic of bureaucracies (Lipsky, 1980), and which are said to reflect a Eurocentric epistemological orientation (Akbar, 1984; Ani, 1994; Asante, 1990; Kershaw, 1992), the Afrocentric paradigm encourages a more balanced approach of determining worker performance that would include both quantitative and qualitative methods of evaluation. Because of the focus on a more holistic or organic interpretation of events, a qualitative means of understanding reality is assumed to be consistent with the Afrocentric paradigm and the cultural traditions of many groups of color. One example of a qualitative means of performance evaluation is the use of field or naturalistic observations. By observing the worker while executing his or her daily work tasks, the observer can more readily discern the intricate attributes of the worker and his or her immediate work milieu. These intricacies are difficult to tap and observe when exclusively relying on quantitative measures. As Lipsky (1980) states, "actual performance is virtually impossible to measure . . . aspects of performance can be measured . . . but the most important dimensions of service performance defy calibration" (p. 168).

The Afrocentric paradigm, therefore, advocates more culturally inclusive criteria for hiring and performance appraisal that embrace the cultural values of the diverse groups that constitute an organization. This inclusiveness also extends to those who receive organizational interventions—the clients or consumers. For example, in mental health and social service organizations, rather than exclusively applying Eurocentric standards in hiring that seek to determine the degree to which one affirms and is knowledgeable of Eurocentric theories of human behavior, development, and human service interventions, standards would include knowledge of theories that emerge from different cultural traditions and worldviews. Instead of applicants of color, for instance, being expected to limit knowledge and skills to Eurocentric theories, hiring standards would be developed to tap their degree of familiarity with, and their ability to apply, theories of human behavior and human service interventions that emanate from their unique cultural traditions and worldviews. Likewise, performance appraisals for people of color would be based on familiarity with, and application of, similar kinds of knowledge. Furthermore, since performance appraisals are predicated heavily on accepting and exhibiting organizational norms of language and communication style, and since U.S. norms validate Eurocentric standards, people of color and others who possess different language and communication styles may be unfairly evaluated. The Afrocentric paradigm recommends that existing human service workplaces base part of their evaluation of people of color on their particular language or communication styles. Diversification of organizational standards of hiring and performance appraisal, in short, would encourage cultural pluralism in the workplace with complete validation and inclusion of culturally diverse ideas about the structure and activities of organizations. In this way, organizational climates can emerge that will encourage the integration of diverse skills and ideas to address the demands of a culturally diverse organizational environment.

EMPOWERMENT THROUGH ORGANIZATIONAL AUTONOMY

Although the Afrocentric paradigm urges the inclusion of diverse ideas about organizational structure and operation that emanate from culturally excluded and oppressed groups, it also realizes that there will be some opposition to complete cultural inclusion. This opposition can stem not only from practical considerations about managing diversity in the workplace but also from efforts to maintain Eurocentric cultural hegemony. To a considerable extent, concerns raised about the difficulty in managing diversity can be interpreted as subterfuge to continue Eurocentric cultural hegemony. From an Afrocentric viewpoint, maintaining this hegemony may have less to do with concerns about hiring more culturally excluded and oppressed groups and more to do with concerns about the inclusion of culturally different organizational models that challenge the assumptions of traditional Eurocentric organizational paradigms.

Because some will continue to fight against workplace diversity of this kind for the sake of continuing Eurocentric cultural dominance, thus marginalizing the legitimacy of using the cultural values of people of color as a foundation for new organizational structures, the Afrocentric paradigm encourages culturally excluded and oppressed groups, especially people of color, to establish and support organizations which are managed and financed by them and which are structured to integrate their unique cultural style and traditions (i.e., self-help). Though self-help may sound contrary to the previous discussions about inclusion, the Afrocentric paradigm maintains that the tactic of challenging Eurocentric cultural hegemony is not inconsistent with encouraging people of color to do for themselves (Asante, 1988; Karenga, 1993). This focus also is consistent with the balance between the universalistic and particularistic themes found in the Afrocentric paradigm.

Self-help is important for all groups in the United States, but especially for those whose cultural style is most distinct from the European-American cultural model. Although some similarities in experiences of oppression cut across racial/ethnic groups in the United States, there have been significant differences between the ways various European immigrant groups and people of color have been received and treated in the United States (Lieberson, 1980; Takaki, 1993). People of color, particularly those who were victims of colonization and forced into the United States, have had a more difficult time being included and accepted (Longres, 1995). In part, this was because they were seen as more culturally different (Longres, 1995), which caused them to experience maximum cultural oppression (Blauner, 1972). Since African Americans, due to slavery, arguably represent the most extreme and prolonged examples of involuntary entry into the United States, it can be maintained that they have been among the most dehumanized victims of cultural oppression.

The cultural oppression experienced by people of color whose entry into the United States was forced renders self-help an essential option for these groups for at least three reasons. First, it prevents the group from placing all of its social change eggs in one basket. Although efforts challenging the existing European-American society to be more inclusive are worthwhile, this strategy depends heavily on the hope that a significant number of European Americans, especially those in power, will radically alter their mind-sets and, more important, the institutional structures from which they benefit economically. Though transforming the mind-set of many European Americans is definitely possible, it may not be politically and economically advantageous for European Americans collectively, particularly since many European Americans today are finding it increasingly difficult to secure stable employment themselves.

Second, self-help for people of color is important because it is an avenue through which they can eliminate the adverse psychological effects of cultural oppression. Eurocentric cultural oppression has caused many to believe that Eurocentric definitions of reality are the only lenses through which reality can be conceived (Ani, 1994; Kambon, 1992). Eurocentric cultural oppression has been psychologically damaging for both people of European descent and people of color. For people of European descent, it tends to engender a false sense of cultural superiority, whereas for people of color, it tends to create a false sense of cultural inferiority (Ani, 1994; Kambon, 1992). Thus, the very act of people of color establishing and maintaining their own human service organizations can be viewed as an essential step toward repairing and enhancing their collective self-confidence and self-esteem.

Finally, self-help can be seen as a stronger strategy to bring cultural pluralism into complete fruition. Since the United States is based on a capitalist economy, the Afrocentric perspective maintains that a group's political power in the United States is significantly related to its degree of economic autonomy. Besides enhancing opportunities for advancing their material interests, the political power generated from economic autonomy would give people of color greater political leverage for promoting their cultural values and worldviews. Thus, Eurocentric cultural hegemony would be eradicated because people of color would be better able to project and imprint their cultural styles and traditions onto the American landscape. This would effectuate a more egalitarian distribution of power among diverse cultural groups.

Since the Afrocentric paradigm emanates from the history, traditions, and visions of people of African descent, the ideas about group self-help are especially relevant for African-American human service workers. In this regard, the Afrocentric paradigm would recommend that these workers take advantage of the current downsizing and governmental devolution era by writing program proposals, collaborating with colleagues, and investigating service gaps and niches to establish their own private human service organizations. A significant component of these efforts should be greater communication of African-American human service workers with

African Americans in business and African-American ministers. For African-American human service workers to establish and maintain human service organizations, they must have a strong financial base and start-up capital. African Americans who are trained in business often have skills and knowledge about finance and capital formation that human service workers lack. The collaboration between the African-American business and human service communities could help engender foundations that could finance human service organizations that primarily serve African Americans, and others, if desired.

African-American churches probably collect more money and have more black capital than any other organization owned and operated by African Americans. For example, Lincoln and Mamiya (1990) estimated that the combined income of African-American churches across the country was over $2 billion. African-American human service workers could connect with progressive African-American ministers who have a more expansive role of religion and the church, one that equally aims to transform the spiritual and the material being. Data from Billingsley and Caldwell (1994) present a somewhat optimistic viewpoint about the degree of receptivity of black churches to participating in social service outreach. They found that about two-thirds of the churches they studied provided some form of outreach and social action service. Although, historically, there has been conflict between the secular helping practices of African-American human service workers and the sacred practices of African-American clergy (Martin and Martin, 1995), the Afrocentric paradigm suggests that the social problems faced by African Americans today are too perilous to the survival of all African Americans to not forge unity between secular and sacred factions within the African-American community.

ADDITIONAL CONSIDERATIONS

Although this chapter has described several characteristics of an Afrocentric organizational paradigm, additional conceptual work needs to be explored to fully develop an Afrocentric organizational model. For example, since organizational survival is a primary concern of the Afrocentric perspective, several research questions emerge for an Afrocentric-oriented organization to function in a Eurocentric or Western-oriented society: (1) How can collectively oriented people in an Afrocentric organization maintain a collective orientation in a society that is, to a considerable extent, antithetical to a collective, communal focus? (2) How would an Afrocentric-oriented organization, with its deemphasis on efficiency, survive in a society that places substantial value on efficiency? (3) How would other external factors, such as legal and legislative mandates and insurance reimbursements, affect the deemphasis on efficiency in an Afrocentric organization? (4) How would this type of organization establish a communal bond with members of a community who are influenced by the dominant cultural value of individualism? (5) What roles would social class, gender, and race play in shaping organization-community relations? (6) What effects would such current trends as managed care and outsourcing of services have on the collective thrust of Afrocentric organizations? These are just a few research questions that speak to organization-environment relations.

Other examples of areas needing further exploration are as follows: (1) What practice interventions would be appropriate for an Afrocentric human service organization? (2) How specifically would organizational goals be formulated in an organization based on Afrocentric principles? (3) What should be the appropriate size of an Afrocentric organization? (4) How, specifically, would an Afrocentric organization manage and implement different hiring and performance standards that seek to achieve greater appreciation and validation of an increasingly diverse workforce and consumer population? Attention to these and other research questions should contribute significantly to the application of the Afrocentric paradigm to not only the study of human service organizations but also the more effective transformation of the lives of consumers.

Chapter 10

Social Work Research
and the Afrocentric Paradigm

RATIONALE FOR AFROCENTRIC
SOCIAL WORK RESEARCH

Social work research can be viewed as a form of knowledge inquiry and knowledge development that attempts to describe, explain, evaluate, predict, and interpret behaviors, thoughts, and problems experienced by those who deliver and consume social work services. For some time, the dominant model of knowledge inquiry and development used in social work research has been positivism and, more recently, postpositivism (Fraser, 1993). Although this paradigm has been the lens through which many social work researchers perform their activities, it has received some criticism within the last ten to twenty years from perspectives emanating exclusively from social work such as the heuristic approach (Heineman-Pieper, 1981, 1989; Tyson, 1995) and the empowerment perspectives (Holmes, 1992; Solomon, 1976). Critiques of positivism also have emerged from perspectives that cut across the social sciences, such as the Frankfurt School (Adorno, 1969; Harbermas, 1971; Horkheimer and Adorno, 1994), hermeneutics and antifoundationalism (Feyerabend, 1981; Gadamer, 1989), feminism (Davis, 1986; Harding, 1991; Reinharz, 1992), and postmodernism (Bauman, 1992; Lyotard, 1984; Seidman, 1994).

The latter perspectives have made considerable strides at critiquing the positivist viewpoint. However, since these critiques have originated mostly from persons of European ancestry, or from perspectives found in European-American culture and intellectual thought, they can be considered Eurocentric. Although these critiques are often viewed as marginal, reactionary, and radical by those who promote positivism and postpositivism, they nonetheless tend to dominate ideas about knowledge inquiry and development emanating from groups of color. This is because European Americans collectively wield considerable control over the knowledge validation and information dissemination processes in the United States (Asante, 1990; Kershaw, 1992; Schiele, 1996).

African Americans have suffered from the dominance of Eurocentric paradigms in social science, since many of these ideas, which arose during the European Enlightenment, were used to justify the enslavement and racial inferiority of people of African descent (Ani, 1994; Mosse, 1978). The suffering has been not only political but also psychological in that many African Americans fail to acknowledge their African cultural heritage (Baldwin, 1985). To address the political and psychological fallout of Eurocentric knowledge hegemony, some have underscored the legitimacy of the cultural traditions of people of African descent and have maintained that they are inconsistent with many of the assumptions of Eurocentric paradigms of knowledge inquiry and development (Akbar, 1994; Asante, 1987; Kambon, 1992; Myers, 1988). This inconsistency and the need to legitimize the cultural traditions of people of African descent have prompted some to explore systems of knowledge inquiry and development that validate an African or Afrocentric viewpoint (see, for example, Akbar, 1984; Asante, 1990; Dixon, 1976; Ezeabasili, 1977; Gyekye, 1995; Kambon, 1992; Kershaw, 1992; Semmes, 1981). Although their concepts have been helpful in advancing an Afrocentric paradigm of knowledge inquiry and development, they have not applied the Afrocentric idea to social work research. This chapter builds on and coalesces existing ideas of the Afrocentric view of knowledge inquiry and development and applies them to construct a foundation for an Afrocentric social work research paradigm. It does this by discussing what might be considered some fundamental attributes of Afrocentric social work research.

DEFINITION OF AFROCENTRIC SOCIAL WORK RESEARCH

Afrocentric social work research can be broadly defined, similar to many other social work research models, as a mode of knowing, inquiring, and interpreting of social events and problems that confront consumers, potential consumers, and deliverers of social work services. Afrocentric social work research, however, is predicated on traditional African philosophical assumptions, examined in Chapter 2, that emphasize a holistic, interdependent, and spiritual conception of people and their environments. These assumptions are said to be traditional in that they depict the cultural values of Africans before the invasions of both Arabs and Europeans who sought to impose their values on indigenous African traditions (Clarke, 1991; Williams, 1987). Further, despite the deleterious effects of slavery and cultural oppression on African Americans, these traditional assumptions are believed to have survived among African Americans (Akbar, 1979; Asante, 1988; Herskovits, 1941; Martin and Martin, 1985; Nobles, 1980; Sudarkasa, 1988), albeit with modifications and different manifestations. Although these assumptions are manifold and can be applied in many ways, this chapter focuses on their relationship to knowledge inquiry and development, and, based on the works of several writers (see Akbar, 1984, 1994; Asante, 1988, 1990; Dixon, 1976; Gyekye, 1995; Harris, 1992; Karenga, 1989; Kershaw, 1992; Mbiti, 1970; Myers, 1988; Nobles, 1980; Zahan, 1979), these assumptions can be succinctly expressed as follows: (1) Since knowledge is seen as a precious gift from God, it should be used in ways that elicit the most constructive, and morally affirming, capabilities of human beings. (2) Knowledge should acknowledge both the material and spiritual aspects of human beings and nature. (3) Knowledge should reflect the interconnectedness of all elements of the universe. (4) The affective and subjective approach to knowing is epistemologically valid.

Critical to many definitions of a knowledge inquiry and development paradigm is the way it conceives the relationship between explanation, prediction, and interpretation. Afrocentric social work research does not separate, or see as oppositional, explanation, prediction, and interpretation. The debate between positivists/empiricists and those of the antifoundationalist/ hermeneutics school about whether the human sciences should be about explanation, prediction or interpretation is viewed as superfluous, myopic, and excessively competitive, from an Afrocentric perspective. The Afrocentric paradigm, which incorporates a more holistic understanding of knowledge inquiry and development, maintains that science is about the business of explanation, prediction, and interpretation simultaneously. In this model, however, interpretation is considered the foundation upon which human beings describe, explain, and predict their world (Asante, 1990). It renders all science, including the natural sciences, as subjective (Akbar, 1984, 1994).

ATTRIBUTES OF AFROCENTRIC
SOCIAL WORK RESEARCH

The Importance of Particularism

Within the Afrocentric paradigm, all social and human phenomena are potential topics of study, and no one is barred from using the Afrocentric paradigm of social work research. Since, however, it emerges from the cultural traditions and experiences of people of African descent, Afrocentric social work research is especially useful in addressing concerns of social life that have implications for African Americans and other people of African ancestry. Although universalism is not rejected in the Afrocentric paradigm, it is believed that the only route to universalism is through the particular (Akbar, 1994). This particularistic feature is not considered a problem from an Afrocentric viewpoint; it is seen as natural and essential. Indeed, application of knowledge inquiry and development paradigms that address interests and validate interpretations stemming from the group or subject from which the paradigm arises is not unusual (Mannheim, 1936). Research and knowledge development paradigms deriving from European-American culture, for example, often seek and are tailored to address the interests and to validate the interpretations of people of European descent (Akbar, 1984; Asante, 1990). Thus, Afrocentric social work research can help generate information on all human behavior and social events, especially if these behaviors and events have implications for the lives, and are interpreted from the particular worldviews, of people of African descent.

Eliminating Oppression and Enhancing Human Potential

Afrocentric social work research endeavors to eliminate human oppression and enhance positive human potential. In this regard, the Afrocentric paradigm takes on an empowerment perspective similar to the one discussed by Holmes (1992). However, unlike Holmes's, the Afrocentric view of empowerment goes beyond including "subjects" in all levels of the design and execution of a research project. It delves into the need to view experiences and values of various cultural groups as not only legitimate sources of study but also legitimate sources for establishing additional knowledge inquiry and development paradigms that may or may not be compatible with the dominant ones currently used. Moreover, the Afrocentric view of empowerment aims to use knowledge inquiry and development as a means to end all forms of oppression (Kershaw, 1992), not just those found within the confines of conducting social and social work research, that is, within the confines of identifying research problems and collecting and analyzing data.

Although Afrocentric social work research is committed to abolishing all forms of oppression, it is primarily concerned with eliminating racial and cultural oppression because both pervasively affect the lives of persons of African descent. Racial oppression can be defined as the practice of subjecting a group to unfair, immoral, and belligerent treatment simply because of visible characteristics, especially skin color, that are assumed to be racial. Cultural oppression refers to the "universalization of a dominant group's experience and culture, and its establishment as the norm"

(Young, 1990, p. 59), and, for African Americans, has taken the form of the imposition and universalization of European-American culture. The results have been that knowledge claims and interpretations about reality that originate from African-American cultural traditions and experiences frequently have been deemed marginal, illegitimate, or nonexistent. This is why, from an Afrocentric perspective, it is essential to repudiate the objective and universal viewpoint of knowledge inquiry, development, and validation and replace it with one that sees knowledge inquiry, development, and validation as cultural artifacts that vary with the particular worldview of diverse groups.

To this end, the Afrocentric paradigm endeavors to foster what Foucault (1977) calls the *insurrection of subjugated knowledges*. The Afrocentric paradigm is a form of knowledge insurrection in that it challenges interpretations of people of African descent that stem from groups who benefit from the oppression of people of African ancestry and advocates that these interpretations emerge from the narratives of black people themselves. However, unlike some from the postmodernist camp (see, for example, Bauman, 1992; Lyotard, 1984; Seidman, 1994), the Afrocentric paradigm does not view the affirmation of a subjugated group's narrative as an end in itself. The Afrocentric paradigm is materialist in that it endeavors to validate the narratives of people of African descent not only for psychological (i.e., self-esteem) and scientific (i.e., knowledge validation) reasons but also to change the political and economic conditions faced by people of African descent. Knowledge insurrection within the Afrocentric perspective defies Eurocentric universalism and strives to abolish the material conditions and consequences of racial and cultural oppression.

Similar to those within the ranks of the Frankfurt School (see Habermas, 1971; Horkheimer and Adorno 1994; Marcuse, 1964), the Afrocentric view of social work research, and by extension social theory, merges social change activities with those of knowledge inquiry and development. Unlike the proponents of "Critical Theory," the Afrocentric paradigm does not limit its social change activities to the elimination of a specific economic system with its accompanying ideology, although this is important. Rather, the Afrocentric paradigm aspires to eliminate the underlying worldview that creates the need for such an exploitative system in the first place. In essence, Afrocentric social work research encourages humans to become more at one with the Creator and the universe. This "oneness with nature and God" cosmology is thought to bring about respect and appreciation for all aspects of nature—including human beings—both for the common aspects and the different ones, and is believed to preclude the exploitative behavior that accompanies oppression (Schiele, 1994). In this regard, Afrocentric social work research generates knowledge to enhance the potential of people and societies to behave morally and in ways congruent with the belief in the oneness of the universe and humanity.

Affirming Tradition and Consensus

In Afrocentric social work research, tradition and consensus are key elements. Horton (1993) maintains that knowledge development tends to be "traditionalistic" and "consensual" within the African framework. According to Horton (1993), a traditionalistic and consensual concept of knowledge development is one in which (1) the major precepts of a community's knowledge are thought to have been developed and handed down by the ancients, and (2) theorizing is carried out in a way that accentuates the commonalities, notwithstanding differences, among diverse ideas. In contrast, a progressivistic and competitive concept of knowledge development is one wherein (1) knowledge is seen as a process of gradual but steady improvement (i.e., future knowledge is thought to be better than present knowledge and present knowledge to be better than past knowledge), and (2) the generation and advancement of ideas takes on a competitive character in which various theories compete aggressively to demonstrate their superiority over rival theories in explaining and predicting social and human phenomena.

If Horton (1993) is correct about the Afrocentric paradigm's focus on tradition and consensus in the knowledge development process, then that focus might be based on at least three assumptions:

1. *Knowledge that stands the test of time is worthy of continuation* (Horton, 1993). This adage advances the belief that much of what we need to know today about human behavior can be found in the wisdom of the ancients. It asserts that for knowledge to be valid, it must endure the ultimate test of time. Time is essential because it is through the repetitious use of ideas by various groups across generations that the validity of ideas can be adequately assessed. If ideas have been useful for past generations, it is suggested that they are, and will be, relevant for present and future generations. This is in contrast to what Horton (1993) refers to as the "progressivistic" feature of knowledge development in the West (i.e., knowledge is seen as a process of gradual but steady improvement).

2. *African ancients—especially those of the Nile Valley—are thought to have possessed supreme wisdom because their objective was to generate knowledge that would enable people to tap into the complete, positive potentiality given to them by the Creator* (Akbar, 1994; Asante, 1990; Diop, 1991; Karenga, 1989; Van Sertima, 1989). By cultivating the beliefs that humans have great potential to tap into the spirit and essence of the

Creator and that science should not be separated from this pursuit, the African ancients are thought to have possessed the moral ingredients for creating a society wherein human interactions and ideals are undergirded by mutual respect, a concern for collective well-being, spirituality, and a striving toward excellence.

3. *Each idea or theory uniquely adds to a different understanding of the totality of the human experience.* Afrocentric social work research asserts that no one theory is, or can be, robust enough to explain all or most dimensions of social and human phenomena. Rather, theories are conceived as uniquely different ways in which social and human phenomena can be described and explained. They are unique in that they reflect interpretations held by one individual or a cadre of like-minded individuals. Each theory serves to contribute a unique piece of understanding that can be used to construct a complete picture of social life that limits or prevents knowledge hegemony. To this extent, I disagree with Horton's (1993) contention that the consensual mode of theorizing is distinctive in that "members of a community . . . share a *single overarching framework* [italics mine] of . . . assumptions" (p. 328) in which intellectual innovation is executed. It can be maintained that to the degree that social theorizing is a cultural phenomenon, confirming and reflecting the various strains within a particular cultural setting, then all theorizing within a specific cultural setting can be said to mirror that setting's single overarching framework or worldview (i.e., the philosophical entity that distinguishes one cultural setting from another). Inconsistent with Horton's description, the Western, or Eurocentric, perspective of theorizing also can be said to operate within a single overarching worldview (Ani, 1994; Asante, 1987; Baldwin and Hopkins, 1990; Kambon, 1992), despite the competitiveness that camouflages its unity.

What may be critically different between social theorizing in the Afrocentric and Eurocentric overarching frameworks is the Afrocentric framework does not require the fierce competition of ideas that occurs within the Eurocentric framework. The consensual character within Afrocentric knowledge development requires knowledge disseminators to mutually respect the uniqueness and integrity of divergent ideas, while simultaneously identifying commonalities, without imposing superior/inferior designations. To designate hierarchical assessments of various ideas, there must be universal standards to which the various originators of ideas agree. And, whereas universal standards that evaluate an idea's or a theory's moral capacity are essential from an Afrocentric framework (Akbar, 1984, 1994; Karenga, 1989), universal standards that seek to evaluate other aspects of an idea are dissuaded. One could contend, however, that any aspect of a theory or idea has moral implications. The point here is that the Afrocentric view on knowledge development encourages cross-cultural consensus in affirming values and practices that prevent and arrest the exploitation of people.

However, because knowledge evaluations in social work and the general American society have been based largely on standards set by European/European-American culture, often defaming the cultural integrity and traditions of people of African descent (Baldwin, 1985; Schiele, 1996), Afrocentric knowledge development is compelled to come out of its natural state of consensus to challenge ideas that support and maintain Eurocentric knowledge hegemony. In this way, cultural oppression, and the political and economic inequality with which it is associated, upsets the free-flowing process of knowledge development based on consensus.

Knowledge Inquiry As Value Laden and Interchangeable

The Afrocentric paradigm posits that since research or knowledge inquiry is a "people made" activity, it, as with additional human creations and activities, is influenced by, and imbued with, human values (Akbar, 1994; Asante, 1990; Semmes, 1981). These values not only influence the process of a particular knowledge inquiry and development paradigm but also shape the very structure and philosophical tenets that undergird the process. Unlike the positivist/post-positivist paradigm, the Afrocentric paradigm does not posit the superiority or hierarchy of methods. The Afrocentric paradigm rejects Kerlinger's (1979) assertion that "procedures of science are objective—not the scientist" (p. 264), because this exaggerates methodology's power to remove subjectivity from knowledge inquiry and development. Methods are developed by people, and the Afrocentric paradigm contends that all knowledge inquiry methods are subjective, reflecting the ideas about knowledge inquiry and development held by their creators.

The Afrocentric paradigm also repudiates Popper's (1972) notion that objectivity is a system of organized/mutual critique—that science is objective because of the willingness of the scientist to have his or her work critiqued by colleagues. Although Popper (1969) contends that it is rare for the social scientist to be value free, he still implies, similar to Kerlinger, that objectivity lies in some sort of method (in his case, the critical method), thus again separating the method from the people who create and subscribe to it. The notion that the critical thinking method in some way suspends the scientist's values while the scientist forms a critique is unfounded, Afrocentrically. Although the critical thinking method appears to be value neutral because of its focus on identifying the pros and cons of an idea, all critiques are permeated with the philosophical and ideological preferences of the evaluator. Furthermore, critical analysis is itself a value, in that it demonstrates the preference for a more subdued form of debate: by identifying the pros and cons of an idea uneffusively, one is misled into believing that one's assessment of the idea is objective or at least fair.

At the core of the Afrocentric vision that knowledge inquiry and development are value laden is the belief that objectivity is an illusion (Akbar, 1984; Ani, 1994). It is believed to be illusionary because Afrocentricity disagrees with the notion of objectification, the belief that the knower should, and can, emotionally detach himself or herself from that which he or she is attempting to know—even if the targeted entities are humans and their social environments. This, of course, nurtures the well-discussed "subject/object" duality. From an Afrocentric viewpoint, this duality is inappropriate because "in the pure Africanized worldview of the unity of [people] and the phenomenal world, there is no empty perceptual space between the self and phenomena" (Dixon, 1976, p. 70). Further, this duality fosters and reinforces a process of knowing that is sterile and incomplete.

The process is sterile and incomplete in that the knower, by attempting to remove himself or herself emotionally from that which is observed, fails to connect to the vitality—the *life force*—of those who are being observed. This life force is a spiritual substance, which can be nurtured or retarded by culture, that gives people a sense of being, integrity, and identity as human beings. Although universal, each person's life force is different, and this difference is attributed to various factors, mainly to the way the individual interprets and experiences the world around him or her. Tapping into this life force requires more than just cognitive understanding; it requires the willingness to vicariously assume the life force of another in a way that emotionally connects the observer to the observed. This emotional connection, unlike emotional detachment, allows the observer greater insight into the thoughts, feelings, and behaviors of the observed because the observer, while connecting to the observed's life force, simultaneously remains in touch with his or her own life force, which renders the knowledge inquiry and development process more complete and authentic.

To the degree that the observer acknowledges his or her life force in the knowledge inquiry process and recognizes the interconnectedness of the life forces between the observer and observed, he or she is comfortable with and encourages the interchangeability of the roles of observer and observed. In this more complete process of knowledge inquiry, there is little demarcation, if any, between observer and observed. To place it in the words of the antifoundationalists, the observer-observed relationship is a subject-subject relationship in which both parties learn from each other in a mutual process of information exchange and role interchangeability.

This interchangeability of roles of observer/observed is important in social work because it is consistent with the values of reciprocity and equality in social work practice. These values reflect the belief that the helping process, and by extension the knowledge inquiry process, should not be based on elitism and condescension. This is vital in knowledge inquiry and development because the extent to which the observer separates himself or herself from that which he or she observes, and defines the roles of each without any feedback from those he observes, is the extent to which social and social work research can be viewed as implicitly oppressive (Blauner and Wellman, 1973; Holmes, 1992).

The Interconnectedness of Realism and Relativity

One of the salient characteristics of Eurocentric knowledge inquiry and development is the debate over realism and relativity. Realism posits that there are absolute truths that should be sought and that these truths are independent of, or have nothing to do with, the feelings and values of the knower. The belief in realism has inevitably led to the bifurcation in traditional empiricist/positivist thinking of facts from opinions (Smith, 1993). Within this bifurcation, facts are considered to be phenomena perceived via the five senses, and for which there is considerable agreement, that exist separate from the personal world of the knower's thoughts, feelings, and interests. To the degree that facts are agreed-upon phenomena that can be sensed, quantified, and occur independent of the knower, they are deemed true. Opinions are defined as values or beliefs that people have regarding phenomena. They are thought to constitute the personal and provincial world of the knower; therefore, they are considered subjective, restricted, and inferior to facts in traditional empiricist/positivist thinking. Facts are considered supreme because (1) they represent the "truths" of the public milieu or wider social environment, and (2) they are directly observable and quantifiable. Also, because individuals rarely quantify their experiences, these experiences are believed to be too vague, lacking a sense of precision and specificity. Thus, as Smith (1993) asserts, the philosophy of empiricism depends heavily on the belief in facts or realism, which ultimately supports the value of objectivity.

Relativity or relativism is at the other end of the continuum and can be defined as the belief that reality—or what is considered the truth—varies significantly from one individual to the next. There is no absolute truth (realism) because reality is determined by the unique interpretations of individuals. Within this conceptual framework, there is no need to separate facts from opinions because all facts are considered opinions. A knowledge hierarchy is absent, and no distinction is made between bad and good knowledge. To strike a balance between the impossibility of certitude (realism) and the undesirability of relativism, some have begun to use the terms critical or sophisticated realism, but they still subscribe to an objective and independent reality (Smith, 1993). The critical difference between realism and relativity, however, is that realism accentuates knowledge that transcends, and is assumed to be separate from, the personal milieu of an individual's interpretations and experiences, whereas relativity accentuates knowledge that emanates from those unique experiences and interpretations.

Recently, the concepts of critical realism, sophisticated realism, or fallabilistic realism have emerged in postpositivist/postempiricist literature (Fraser, 1993; Smith, 1993). Each acknowledges that the social world can never be fully knowable, but they still subscribe to an objective, independent reality. Each also accepts that social reality is patternistic, but, within these patterns, there are crinkles that cause uncertainty. Fallabilistic realism further maintains that because of the imperfectability of social work research methods and the nonexhaustiveness of most research studies, mistakes can be made in determining and knowing social reality. In short, the critical, sophisticated, and fallabilistic realism of postpositivists/postempiricists attempts to strike a balance between the impossibility of certitude and the undesirability of relativism (Smith, 1993).

Afrocentric social work research maintains that knowledge which transcends the milieu of individuals and knowledge which emanates from the personal experiences of individuals are equally important, and that they do not have to be conceived as oppositional. As Geertz (1979) contends, social researchers should rely on both "experience-near" knowledge (knowledge that reflects the individual's experience and interpretation) and "experience-distant" knowledge (knowledge that extends beyond the individual's experience and interpretation) to achieve a more complete understanding of human and social behavior. Afrocentric social work research agrees with this but also adds that the two should not be thought of as independent of each other; they should be considered interconnected and transparent sides of the same coin.

As interconnected and transparent sides of the same coin, the Afrocentric paradigm assumes that social reality is never independent of individuals because individuals (i.e., the actions, thoughts, and feelings of a collection of individuals) create social reality. The experiences and conditions of one individual are a piece or component of a broader set of individual experiences and conditions that constitute the totality of social reality. Suppose, for example, that the research question at hand is "How prevalent is homelessness in the United States?" To fully answer this question, one would have to take into account the specific and individual living conditions and interpretations of the experiences of all involved. Because of the diversity of these conditions and interpretations, homelessness could be viewed as a jigsaw puzzle, and, as with all jigsaw puzzles, to achieve a comprehensive grasp, one must connect the individual pieces, that is, the individual conditions and interpretations. In addition, before the pieces of a jigsaw puzzle are connected, there appears to be no relationship or connection between and among the pieces. But when connected, one discerns how each piece is related to the others and that each is vital to comprehending the total puzzle, or, in this case, the reality about homelessness. Thus, the dichotomy between experience-near and experience-distant reality is a false one if we conceive reality as a coalescence of diverse and idiographic component experiences and interpretations.

With this in mind, Afrocentric social work research maintains that certitude is only possible when the experiences and interpretations of all within a sociocultural context are known, and, even then, one cannot be completely confident because of the indeterminacy and fluidity of human actions, feelings, and thoughts. Afrocentric social work research contends that although collective human actions, feelings, and thoughts can be discerned as patterns sometimes, these patterns vary significantly by not only the perceiver of the pattern but also the sociocultural setting in which the actions, feelings, and thoughts occur. Moreover, much research today primarily focuses on dominant patterns and conceives less dominant patterns as outliers (Gilgun, 1994). Within this framework, understanding of "divergent singulars" is lost. The loss of this information, from an Afrocentric viewpoint, encourages incomplete understanding of the diversity of experiences and interpretations of the manifold consumers, potential consumers, and deliverers of social work services, and how these experiences and interpretations are similar but yet different.

Since Afrocentric social work research acknowledges the adversities of cultural oppression, it critically questions claims of universal, absolute, and relativistic truth. A primary criticism of realism and relativity within the context of cultural oppression is that, often, claims of absolute or relative truth emerge from the knowledge inquiry strategies, experiences, and interpretations of the cultural group in power, thereby limiting the exposure of knowledge claims from additional cultural groups. From an Afrocentric viewpoint, in the context of a multicultural society, there are multiple definitions and interpretations of reality and each validates the experiences and cultural ethos of the group from which it arises. In a multicultural society such as the United States, instead of speaking of universal social realities or truths, it may be more appropriate to speak of multiple group realities or, better yet, *pluriversal social realities* (see Keto, 1989). To the extent that reality reflects the collective experiences and interpretations of a group, Afrocentric social work research supports the notion that reality is an expression of group consensus. The problem in a society that practices cultural hegemony is that the agreement of which people speak is often an imposition of the consensus of the cultural group in power. Afrocentrically, this means that the consensus about social reality in America is what Asante (1987) calls the *collective subjectivity* of European Americans. I would add the term *multiple subjectivities* of European Americans.

Legitimacy of a Multidimensional, Polysense Orientation to Data Collection

In Afrocentric social work research, a multidimensional or polysense orientation to data collection is validated and employed. This polysense orientation reflects Afrocentricity's epistemological orientation that embraces the material and spiritual realms equally (Kambon, 1992; Myers, 1988). In other words, the unseen is just as important in Afrocentric knowledge inquiry and development as is the seen (Akbar, 1994; Kambon, 1992). As Akbar (1991) states, "What is tangible is only a reflection of a higher intangible reality" (p. x) in the Afrocentric paradigm.

The unseen or intangible reality is said to be tapped by what Gyekye (1995) calls a *paranormal cognitive epistemology*. This epistemology is predicated on the assumptions "that perception does not wholly or exclusively occur through the physical senses, and that human beings are not entirely subject to the limitations of time and space" (Gyekye, 1995, p. 346). The notion that perception does not exclusively occur via the physical senses underscores the belief in the power of individuals to transcend the boundaries of the physical. Thus, phenomena can be felt, sensed, or forecasted by means of extrasensory perception, such as psychokinesis, precognition, intuition, spirit mediation, and vibes (Gyekye, 1995; Kambon, 1992). Although these methods would be considered absurd within traditional Eurocentric social science, the researcher in Afrocentric social work research is encouraged to use these methods because it is believed that to attain a more holistic viewpoint of human behavior, one must go beyond the limitations of the physical instruments of knowing. Further, the use of a polysense mode of gaining knowledge is believed to give Afrocentricity greater *knowledge absorption* capacities (Asante, 1990), that is, a knowledge paradigm's ability to know all that is potentially knowable, or at least potentially interpretable. An Afrocentric social work researcher relies on these polysense methods to gain a greater understanding of and the ability to eliminate the various social problems faced by consumers and deliverers of social work services. The researcher can attempt to develop skills in these methods or consult others who may already possess the skills.

The assumption that human beings are not restricted to the boundaries of time and space affirms Afrocentricity's belief in the existence of a world of ancestral spirits (Ezeabasili, 1977; Gyekye, 1995; Mbiti, 1970; Nobles, 1980; Zahan, 1979). The person never dies but lives on in this spiritual world. The ancestral spiritual world is believed to influence the behavior of those of us in the material world (Gyekye, 1995; Zahan, 1979). This is because in traditional African philosophy, the powers of the spiritual world are considered to be greater than those of the material world (Gyekye, 1995; Mbiti, 1970; Zahan, 1979). The material world, though important to comprehend in isolation, is thought to be better understood in its relationship with the spiritual world. When attempting to interpret events in the material realm, the Afrocentric social work researcher is encouraged to extend explanations of material events into the spiritual realm. For example, an Afrocentric social work researcher attempting to explain marital dissolution would not only examine interpersonal and broader sociocultural factors but also might consider factors such as a couple's willingness to tap into the positive energy of their ancestors or the possibility that the couple's tension is a material continuation of conflict among their ancestors.

It is critical to note that the focus on using the spiritual realm to explain material reality in the Afrocentric paradigm is contrary to the use of spiritual and theological explications to disparage the poor and explain poverty. These explications only justify the existence of material oppression that, from an Afrocentric viewpoint, is inconsistent with the tenets of spirituality (Ani, 1994; Myers, 1988). Rather, emphasis on the connection of the spiritual and the material in Afrocentric social work research is used as an aid to construct and maintain societies that manifest justice, equality, and compassion in their social relationships. Underscoring the importance of the unseen in the Afrocentric paradigm is viewed as an essential mode through which people can, and should, acknowledge the invisible universal substance that connects all human beings to one another and to a Creator (Akbar, 1984; Schiele, 1996).

Emphasis on Diunital or Holistic Logic

Consistent with the application and acknowledgment of a multidimensional, polysense orientation to data collection and interpretation, Afrocentric social work research legitimizes the use of diunital or holistic logic to make sense of the social world and human problems. Diunital logic views apparent and conflictual opposites as interdependent and complementary. It is holistic in that phenomena are seen both in their parts and, mainly, in their entirety (Baldwin, 1981; Nichols, 1987). Because of this focus, a circle is used to symbolize diunital logic (Burgest, 1982). The circle, unlike the line that has been employed to characterize the Western analytic tradition, encompasses greater space and envelops that space as a whole unit. A circle also symbolizes reciprocity—what goes around comes around. Thus, causes are not so rigidly separated from effects, and ideas and events are viewed as reciprocal and interchangeable.

Within diunital logic, left hemisphere brain functions, which regulate the ability to analyze or fragment, are not deemed oppositional or separate from right hemisphere brain functions that control affect and intuition (Bell, 1994; Schiele, 1991). As Bell (1994) notes, the hemispheric integration perspective underlies the existence and use of diunital logic. This hemispheric integration paradigm fosters a more balanced and complete understanding of social phenomena because the social scientist is encouraged to rely on analytic and holistic cognitive functions concurrently. Moreover, one brain function is not seen as superior to the other because both are conceived as equal partners in explanation and interpretation. A hemispheric fragmentation paradigm tends to be oblivious to the unity of the functions, and, too often in Eurocentric societies, the analytic function is considered superior to the holistic/affective/intuitive function. The reliance on this separatist/conflict-oriented view of brain functions has created uniperceptual and monocognitive orientations to data collection in most Eurocentric social sciences that depend heavily on the ocular sense and linear, analytic logic to explain human behavior.

The emphasis on diunital logic is similar in some ways to Hegelian dialectics. Indeed, some have asserted that since Hegelian dialectics is based heavily on Aristotelian ideas, and since Aristotle and many other Greek philosophers were trained in ancient Egypt (Kemet), the origins of dialectics can be attributed to ancient Egyptian (Kemetic) philosophy that was stolen and/or adapted by the Greeks (Diop, 1991; James, 1954). Dialectics in ancient Egyptian (Kemetic) philosophy was known as the "laws of opposites" (Diop, 1991). Later on, Karl Marx and Friedrich Engels (see Tucker, 1978) applied the dialectic tradition in German philosophy to historical materialism, often critiquing Hegel and others at that time for not adapting their dialectics to "material" reality. Unfortunately, this debate over the use of dialectics helped create an extreme and unnecessary dichotomy in Western social science between the importance of ideas (i.e., rationalism/idealism) and that of the material world (i.e., empiricism). The Afrocentric viewpoint merges the extreme idealism of the Eurocentric tradition with the extreme materialist/empiricist standpoint of the Eurocentric tradition. The Afrocentric paradigm asserts that reality is both idea and action simultaneously, and that both the idea and the action are based on the interpretation of not only the individual but also the collective interpretation of the social group to which the individual belongs. Moreover, Marx's and Engels's version of dialectics has created the belief over the last one hundred and fifty years or so that dialectics inherently implies conflict. This emphasis on conflict, which is used as a paradigm to explain and create economic, cultural, and social change, is often referred to as "dialectic tension." The exclusive application of dialectical thinking in a conflictual way is essentially Eurocentric (Asante, 1990). Whereas viewing opposites as mutually dependent and potentially bringing about a new force is Afrocentric, viewing opposites exclusively as conflictual or as creating tension is not.

Some might interpret from this discussion that the Afrocentric approach to knowledge inquiry and development is nonrational, that rationality does not fit into the equation of Afrocentric social work research. Afrocentric social work research is rational to the extent that it considers consequences of behavior and options in decision making; it does not, however, advocate a view of rationality that is devoid of, downplays, or is separate from emotion or feeling. Rationality occurs in the Afrocentric paradigm without the reliance on, or acceptance of, the value of objectification. As Akbar (1984) observes, the consequences of the lack or suppression of emotions in the social sciences are grave. This can lead to a form of indifference or passive insensitivity on the part of the scientist that allows or condones horrific social events such as the enslavement of Africans by Europeans, the Jewish holocaust (Akbar, 1984), or other systems of oppression and human degradation. This passive insensitivity is supported not only by suppressing emotions but also by relying on the process of identifying the "pros" or benefits of an event or idea, even when that idea or event has caused considerable human suffering. Identifying the pros of an idea or event, even in the face of that idea's or event's relationship with human destruction, is valued in most Eurocentric social science because it demonstrates the scientist's objectivity, his or her ability or willingness to disconnect his or her emotions from observations of the social environment.

The Afrocentric paradigm does not encourage the separation of reason from emotions but recognizes them as two transparent and interdependent sides of the same coin (Schiele, 1996). Instead of emotions hindering social work researchers' activity, Afrocentric social work research maintains that emotions can help in the inquiry enterprise because they are the most direct experiences of self (Akbar, 1984) and can conduce scientists to a more authentic understanding of their social environment that is intimately reflected in them. In essence, while observing others in their social milieu, researchers ultimately observe themselves (Babbie, 1986; Akbar, 1984).

Application of Both Quantitative and Qualitative Modes of Observation

Afrocentric social work research recognizes the importance of both quantitative and qualitative modes of observation in explaining and interpreting human behavior and in advancing societies. However, of the two, Afrocentric social work research claims that qualitative methods are better structured to elicit the deeper and more authentic experiences of human beings (Asante, 1990). This is because qualitative methods utilize procedures that allow individuals to be observed in their natural settings, they involve strategies to tap people's personal narratives, which can be elicited over time, and they hinge less on the quantification of observations (Mark, 1996). Although qualitative methods may do a better job at eliciting in-depth aspects of an individual's or group's interpretation of the world than quantitative methods, qualitative methods also are restricted in their ability to know and interpret human behavior. This is partly because most current qualitative methods, similar to quantitative methods, share the same underlying assumptions regarding knowledge/scientific inquiry that originate from Eurocentric culture; they are as follows:

1. Human bias and emotion should be controlled, reduced, or eliminated in human inquiry.
2. There should be separate expectations for the observer and the observed, even if their reciprocity is acknowledged. In other words, the observer and observed are usually viewed as separate entities, oftentimes with mutually exclusive roles.
3. When collecting, processing, and coding information, phenomena should be reduced to their simplest forms (i.e., reductionism).
4. Directly observable (i.e., material) phenomena are deemed the most legitimate forms of reality. In other words, deemphasis is placed on unseen or spiritual aspects of reality.
5. Rational, linear, and dichotomous thinking are the primary modes through which human behavior is understood and interpreted.

Though these assumptions are less obvious in some qualitative methods, qualitative and quantitative methods are complementary (Harrison,

1994; Werner, 1994) representing two sides of the same coin: whereas qualitative methods tap deep but narrow aspects of social life, quantitative methods tap shallow but broad aspects (Werner, 1994). Furthermore, as Mark (1996) contends, the concepts qualitative and quantitative refer more to types of measurements as opposed to distinctly different research paradigms. The Afrocentric paradigm agrees that qualitative and quantitative methods of inquiry should be viewed as complementary, but adds that they should be predicated on different cultural assumptions of inquiry that emphasize (1) the importance and necessity of human emotion in human inquiry, (2) the union or interchangeability of the roles of observer/observed, (3) a deemphasis on the need to reduce phenomena to their simplest forms (i.e., reductionism), (4) legitimation and inclusion of the spiritual or unseen, and (5) the use and integration of diunital/reciprocal logic (i.e., logic that underscores unity in polarity).

Because the Afrocentric paradigm affirms the legitimacy of both qualitative and quantitative methods, it also posits deduction and induction as equal partners in the pursuit of logic. As noted previously, the Afrocentric paradigm conceives logic as circular rather than linear (Bell, 1994; Burgest, 1981). In this sense, induction and deduction would not be viewed as polarities but as interchangeable and nonsequential ways through which researchers and people generally can make sense of the world. This circular or reciprocal logic is believed, within Afrocentric social work research, to more appropriately capture the essence of the interconnectedness of human behavior, human problems, and the social environment.

The Afrocentric paradigm of knowledge inquiry and development contends that quantification is an important feature of social work research but recognizes the shortcomings of a count-and-measure system to explain and interpret human behavior. Counting human problems and phenomena can be restrictive and misleading, not only when certain consumer groups and circumstances are omitted or distorted, but also when numbers become the exclusive driving force for change, making the process of change sterile and perfunctory. Though not always intentional, an exclusive reliance on numbers can dehumanize and oversimplify the deplorable conditions in which many consumers of human services find themselves daily.

Measuring human problems and phenomena, that is, determining their intensity and duration, also can be problematic, especially when measuring latent or obscure variables. First, the levels of variable measurement—nominal, ordinal, interval, ratio—employed in much research today tend not to fit the multidimensionality and fluidity of human thought and action. The practice, for example, of placing a construct such as self-esteem on an ordinal or interval scale, albeit efficient, seems not to take into consideration the possibility that human constructs and problems may not conform to the requirements of these measurement scales. Second, since the basis for counting and measuring human problems and phenomena in social work research is conceptualization and operationalization, the problem of defining constructs is critical. From an Afrocentric perspective, the prevailing view of conceptualization and operationalization is problematic for two reasons: (1) their basis in reductionism tends to oversimplify the sundry and mutable meanings of constructs, and (2) because we live in a multicultural society that practices cultural oppression, the definitions of constructs in social work research can omit additional cultural meanings and reinforce a cultural/political hegemony in social work. To prevent this, the Afrocentric paradigm recommends that when there is disagreement about the meaning of a construct, and when meaning is subject to different cultural interpretations, persons from diverse cultural groups, whether they be researchers, practitioners, or potential research participants, should be consulted for their interpretations of the construct's meaning. Although this strategy is less time efficient, it would generate greater validity of concepts.

In this regard, validity is extremely important in Afrocentric social work research. Though reliability is essential, it is validity that deals with the question of whether a measure or method actually elicits the kind of information one seeks. To augment the relevance and meaning of reliability in human behavior, Afrocentric social work research expands the concept of reliability to include both consistent and inconsistent human responses. Because human behavior is both predictive and indeterminate, reliability in Afrocentric social work research does not value behavioral consistency over behavioral inconsistency, or vice versa.

Last, the Afrocentric social work paradigm advocates for the diversification of the cadre of quantitative, as well as qualitative, social researchers. The selection of research topics, questions, theoretical frameworks, and operational definitions reflects the interests, experiences, and values of the researchers (Harding, 1991; Heineman-Pieper, 1989; Tyson, 1995). In the United States, scant numbers of researchers are people of color. In academia, gender and race have been found to contribute significantly to those most likely to conduct research (Long and Fox, 1995), with European Americans and men more likely to conduct research than people of color and women. This perhaps implies that most social and social work research promotes the interests, values, and experiences of European-American men.

This Eurocentric research interest also may affect funding patterns for research. For example, in an article describing some impediments to research opportunities for black scholars and black organizations, Hill (1980) offers several factors for the institutional barriers that blacks experience when seeking funding for research projects. These factors can be placed in two categories: attitudinal factors and structural factors. Some of the attitudinal factors that Hill describes are (1) the belief held by whites that blacks are nonrational and nonscientific human beings, (2) the belief among whites that blacks find it arduous to be detached and objective, and (3) the belief that blacks are incapable of carrying out scientific research. A few of the structural factors that Hill identifies are as follows: First, blacks are less likely than whites to serve on research panels, review boards, and commissions. As Hill observes, this is significant because these positions bring with them the opportunity to have considerable say about the allocation of research resources and the definition of "quality" research. Hill maintains that this factor impedes the funding of black proposals because of the "buddy system": often institutions who have representatives on funding panels frequently receive the bulk of the resources and funds allocated by a panel. A second structural factor identified by Hill is that quotas restrict the number of blacks on review panels. A third structural factor is that blacks are denied access to knowledge regarding the system and process of obtaining research funding. Here, Hill notes that white researchers are more likely than black researchers to receive "sole source" or noncompetitive contracts (i.e., contracts that are awarded to a researcher without having to compete with other researchers for the funding). Although Hill's assumptions are not substantiated by empirical findings, researchers exploring sex discrimination in academia have documented similar findings concerning women (see, for example, Astin, 1984; Astin and Davis, 1985; Long and Fox, 1995).

With their research interests generally being different from their white counterparts, social and social work researchers of color are likely to find it more difficult to obtain research funding from Eurocentrically oriented funding sources. If social and social work researchers of color are to feel freer in the framing of their research topics and questions, it may be essential for people of color, especially persons of color in the business community, to establish their own research foundations that will fund research of interest to them and that advances their research agendas. In addition, there is a need to establish periodicals and publishing companies that address the specific concerns of people of color. These recommendations are especially relevant in social work academia because it has been found that social work academics of color overwhelmingly feel that both funding sources and editorial boards of professional journals are insensitive to their research and scholarly interests (Schiele and Francis, 1996).

Chapter 11

Conclusion:
Threats to the Survival and Continuation
of the Afrocentric Paradigm

There are at least seven threats to the survival and expansion of the Afrocentric paradigm of human services: (1) trends toward the privatization of human services, (2) the dominance of postpositivist epistemology in academia, (3) continued uneasiness with spirituality, (4) the ascendency of postmodernism, (5) continued cultural misorientation among people of African descent, (6) the African oral tradition, and (7) the Afrocentric paradigm's association with black people.

THE TREND TOWARD PRIVATIZATION

As discussed in Chapter 9, the privatization and federal devolution of human services can pose opportunities for African-American human service workers to establish human service organizations that apply ideas and values found in the Afrocentric paradigm. Privatization also offers these human service professionals the opportunity to become more autonomous from human service organizations that are controlled and funded exclusively by those outside of the African-American community. Despite these opportunities, many of the themes upon which the privatization of human services is based affirm and accentuate capitalistic modes of organizational activities that tend to place more value on the profit motive than on human self-worth and positive human transformation. As examined in Chapter 7, capitalistic ideas are believed to be an outgrowth of the Eurocentric worldview, from an Afrocentric perspective. The focus on affecting human transformation through labor-efficient methods to expand profits is contrary to the Afrocentric vision that conceives positive human change as an end in itself.

Many of those who support the privatization of human services note that, not only is it a reality increasingly faced by human service professionals but also it has the potential to significantly improve the quality of human services delivery (see Karger and Stoesz, 1998; Stoesz, 1994). This idea is based on the assumption that privatization creates more incentives for human service organizations to provide quality services. For the providers of human services, privatization and the devolution of the hegemonic grip of state-sponsored human services will create greater opportunities for the development of a more diversified human service market in which participants can compete against one another for consumers. The competition for more consumers, which generates greater profits and resources for human service organizations, can serve as a catalyst for human service professionals to devise services that will be more effective and convenient for consumers to access. Also for consumers, privatization can expand their choices and offer more diverse service technologies, as they decide which human service organization to select. Some proponents of privatization argue that the increase in choices will lead to more "educated consumers." Educated human service consumers can shop around and identify the best service for the best price, which is thought to empower consumers by offering them greater control over the selection of human services.

Although the Afrocentric paradigm of human services does not oppose effective services and consumer choice, it is concerned with the greater commodification of human need for the sake of profit or other material incentives inherent in capitalism. It echoes the concern raised by Karger (1994) who asks, "Is it morally correct to allow for profit companies to make a profit off the hardship of others?" (p. 112). From an Afrocentric perspective, the answer is no. This is because a critical belief of Afrocentric moral philosophy is that the relationship between human beings and material items is not stronger than relationships between and among human beings themselves (Gyekye, 1987; Mbiti, 1970). Thus, the Afrocentric paradigm would conclude that privatization of human services increasingly places consumers of human services at risk of being objectified and assisted primarily for the wealth, resources, and status that can accrue to human service organizations and those who run them.

There is a second and closely related problem with the for-profit privatization movement, from an Afrocentric perspective. This problem is the notion that private, for-profit human services are inherently superior and more effective than public human services. The Afrocentric paradigm would assume that the glorification of privatization and market principles, over state-sponsored interventions and organizations, reflects a deep suspiciousness of governmental authority found in European-American political thought (see Jansson, 1997; Kohl, 1989; Quadagno, 1994). This cynicism can be said to stem not only from the concerns eighteenth-century American revolutionaries had over the hegemonic regime of Great Britain but also from a deeper cultural value that embraces individualism and stretches the boundaries of individual liberties. From this logic, that which is good or better is interpreted as that which is controlled by the individual or a smaller, localized number of people. It is believed to be better because it allows the individual, or fewer people, to exercise greater control over his or her destiny.

The Afrocentric paradigm is certainly not adverse to people controlling their life destinies. However, if one juxtaposes the profit motive alongside the need to exert greater control, the privatization of human services may be a method by which human service professionals can increase professional autonomy while generating greater personal wealth. Instead of continuing to critique and attempting to change a social system that produces the desire and necessity to possess more personal wealth, human service professionals are retreating from a reform agenda and increasingly being lured into the benefits of a market economy based heavily on cultural themes of the Eurocentric worldview.

Finally, privatization increases the risk of leaving large numbers of poor and dispossessed persons who need human services without access to these services. This is a particular concern of the Afrocentric paradigm since African Americans are disproportionately found in this population. The privatization of human services might eventually require that persons have some kind of insurance plan or be able to pay out of pocket to obtain human services. If the medical model represents a harbinger for the human services, then perhaps increasingly in the future larger numbers of persons in need of human services will not have the insurance necessary to access such services. This could result in increased psychosocial pain, diminished human potential, and limited access to resources essential not only to prosper but also to survive. Therefore, if greater numbers of African Americans are at risk of biological destruction, what impact will this have on the survival of the Afrocentric worldview in the future? Although the service gaps provided by privatization might provide copious opportunities for African-American human service professionals, who, consistent with the self-help thrust of the Afrocentric paradigm, should avail themselves of this prospect, a few critical questions emerge concerning this trend for African Americans and the perpetuation of the Afrocentric worldview:

1. Since most black-owned businesses of any kind are sole proprietor-
   ships (see Herbert, 1998), and since African Americans, relative to
   many other groups, have less wealth and start-up capital (U.S. Bureau of the Census, 1998), what capacity do black, privately owned
   and operated human service organizations, alone, have to deal with
   the enormous social, psychological, and health problems that afflict
   many members of the African-American community?
2. If Eurocentric domination remains a reality in the near and distant
   future, to what extent will it affect the distribution of resources (e.g.,
   technology, equipment, property) to human service organizations
   that are privately owned and managed by African Americans?
3. As more African-American human service professionals contem-
   plate and establish privately owned, for-profit human service organizations, to what extent will the benefits of enhanced profits and
   personal wealth compromise not only their commitment to continue
   to service African-American consumers but also their commitment
   to the values of collectivity and spirituality thought to be the cornerstones of the Afrocentric worldview, not only in the abstract sense,
   but also as practiced personally by many of their parents, grandparents, and great grandparents who socialized them?
4. To what extent will the move toward greater privatization of human
   services within the African-American community increasingly provide some with greater evidence and justification to argue for a more
   diminished role of federal, state, and local governments in protecting
   the civil rights of African Americans and in financially compensat-
   ing them for the injustices they suffered in the past and continue to
   suffer in the present?

What these questions indicate is that increasingly more in the future,
African Americans will have to consider whether and/or how to maintain a
balance between advocating for state-sponsored and privately sponsored
solutions to their social problems. For far too long, these debates have
fractured and disunified African-American struggles toward liberation and
advancement.

THE DOMINANCE OF POSTPOSITIVIST
EPISTEMOLOGY IN ACADEMIA

Although inroads have been made in academia, generally, and in social
work academia, specifically, to challenge the epistemological model of
postpositivism, it still remains the dominant mode of understanding social

events and solving human problems. As examined in Chapter 10, post-positivism is an attempt to balance some of the old aspects of positivism with recent acknowledgment by quantitative types of the fallibility of the notion of absolute certitude and the shortcomings of quantitative measures and analysis. Despite this recognition, those wedded to the postpositivist model continue to believe—though subtly at times—that it, compared to other ways of knowing, is a more superior and systematic epistemological method. Indeed, it is the systematic, methodological quality that some suggest render it a more superior (i.e., objective) way of inquiry (see Judd, Smith, and Kidder, 1991; Kerlinger, 1979). This dominant attitude, although increasingly challenged in academia, makes it arduous to advance Afrocentric epistemology in academia. As identified in Chapter 10, this epistemology places significant emphasis on a more subjective, affective, and holistic style of knowing that equally validates realism and relativity and both quantitative and qualitative modes of research. Many postpositivists, though realizing the importance of subjective dimensions and qualitative strategies in the knowledge inquiry and validation process, continue to have a preference for more quantitative, and supposedly more objective, procedures of knowledge inquiry and development (Smith, 1993; Tyson, 1995).

Because postpositivists exert considerable control in academia and in human service work, they wield substantive power over ideas about what knowledge is valid. In academia, this can be manifested in the questioning and devaluation of a colleague whose scholarship is generally more "conceptual" than "quantitative," more "subjective" than "objective." For those who rely more on Afrocentric ways of knowing, this type of critique may prevent the professor from being promoted and tenured, both of which are needed to elevate the status of the professor and his or her ability to exert more influence over academic decisions and curriculum policy. The hegemony of postpositivism in academia also can encourage human service students, in various fields, to uncritically accept the notion that postpositivist methods are the only strategies for inquiring about solutions to human suffering.

Along these lines, the postpositivist model has ascended in recent years as the prominent model through which the effectiveness of human service interventions are evaluated (see Bloom, Fischer, and Orme, 1995). Although many in the postpositivist cadre maintain that postpositivist methods are beneficial to consumers because they more effectively and systematically help to identify interventions that do not work than other knowledge inquiry models, this claim has not been consistently substantiated to dismiss additional epistemological styles. Because of its dominance, even what is "consistently substantiated" would probably be subjected to a postpositivist litmus test. From an Afrocentric viewpoint, the pervasiveness of the postpositivist paradigm in both academia and in human service work can be conceived as a subtle, yet effective, approach to suppress the most important quality of additional human service or social science paradigms: ideas about how social events and human problems can be best known and understood.

CONTINUED UNEASINESS WITH SPIRITUALITY

Although much more attention is being devoted to spirituality in both the human service and social science literature, Eurocentric social science's discomfort and general denial of the significance of the unseen in comprehending human behavior is one of the major obstacles to the advancement and viability of the Afrocentric human service paradigm. The uneasiness with spirituality concepts is in part due to the reliance on the postpositivist paradigm just discussed. Because it insists on extremely reductionistic, materialistic, or behavioralistic definitions of social events and human problems, postpositivism's ability and willingness to validate and grapple with seemingly abstruse, vague, and unmeasurable constructs is circumscribed. Since the Afrocentric paradigm is well designed to accommodate unseen and ostensibly vague constructs, it is subject to criticisms of being unscientific. This enhances the chances of it being construed as polemical and impractical by those convinced that science and materialism are synonymous. As long as there remains a wide divide between science, religion, and philosophy in Eurocentric human service work and social science, the validity and viability of the Afrocentric paradigm always will be questioned.

THE ASCENDANCY OF POSTMODERNISM

Though many versions of the postmodernist paradigm currently exist in academia, a prominent concept found in much of the postmodernist literature is that of a disunified subject with multiple and ephemeral identities that can be equally important in determining the individual's self-concept and self-definition. This aspect of postmodernism can cause some to question the claims, found consistently throughout Afrocentric literature, that, notwithstanding the diversity within and among them, people of African descent are adversely affected by Eurocentric cultural and political domination. Postmodernism would suggest that this "grand narrative" about people of African descent undercuts and repudiates the multiple and ephemeral ways people of African descent view themselves and construct their own identities. Not all people of African descent, postmodernists would argue, construct their identities around racial oppression, or race at all. Many postmodernists contend that, often, more localized or immediate social identities take precedence over racial identity. Some examples of these identities could be the identity of single-motherhood, of a football coach, of a member of a movie audience, of a subway or airplane passenger, or of an employee. Moreover, many postmodernists maintain that there are larger, more inclusive social identities that significantly undermine the grand narrative of racial identity, such as gender, social class, geographic region, or nation-state identities.

The problem with this analysis, as it pertains to the Afrocentric paradigm's goal of collective advancement for people of African descent, is that a core and critical ingredient of liberation struggles is the identification of common experiences and conditions of members of an oppressed group (Freire, 1970; Wilson, 1993). It is these experiences and conditions, produced by oppression, that help to forge social identities that are not precisely uniform across the African diaspora or, more specifically, the African-American community, but that significantly intersect enough to collectively hinder the full manifestation of positive potentiality by people of African descent. As Harris (1993) contends, the postmodernist critique strips the oppressed of the agency necessary to coalesce its members' efforts toward resisting oppression.

Another problem with much of the postmodernist critique is found in the remedies advanced to disrupt human hegemony. Many of these remedies center around enhancing the validity of the narratives of those whose stories have been suppressed. This is best seen in Foucault's (1977) *Power/Knowledge* and in the writings of the American postmodernist Steve Seidman. In discussing how problems of domination can be resolved, Seidman (1994) suggests that postmodernism's "broader social significance would lie in encouraging unencumbered open public moral and social debate and in deepening the notion of public discourse" (p. 137). Although the Afrocentric paradigm is not against expanding public discourses to include and validate a broader range of social narratives and critiques, it contends that there also must be substantive endeavors aimed at toppling the institutional themes and structures which continue hegemonic social relationships and which reproduce drastic, unequal material conditions. Although the insurrection of the narratives that describe how people of African descent have been victimized, abused, and stigmatized by racial oppression is important, these narratives alone will not alter the current institutional themes and structures so that all may have an equal chance of realizing their vast human possibility.

CONTINUED CULTURAL MISORIENTATION

Throughout the book, Kambon's (1992) construct of cultural misorientation was used to describe a psychocultural condition in which people of African ancestry fail to acknowledge and seek information that legitimates their African cultural traditions, values, and visions. Instead, as Fanon (1961) and Cabral (1973) suggest, these persons culturally identify with the oppressor and view their past and unique cultural attributes as inferior or nonexistent. Although Kambon posits a normal, bell curve distribution to hypothesize about how people of African ancestry are distributed along the cultural misorientation construct, with most falling in the middle or moderate ranges, the current mutation of Eurocentric domination away from domination by terror toward domination by seduction (see Schiele, in press) may place greater numbers of people of African descent in jeopardy of denying their African cultural origins and identity. Domination by seduction differs from domination by terror in two important ways: (1) In domination by seduction, though the dominant group does not completely liquidate its overt and explicit means of control, its methods of domination mutate to cloak and conceal underlying intentions of exploitation and oppression (Bauman, 1992; Marcuse, 1964). (2) Instead of relying exclusively on violence, terror, intimidation, and overt legal discrimination, domination by seduction draws on tactics of cultural absorption (i.e., absorption of alternatives), inordinate consumerism, political and economic co-optation, and symbolic racism (Bauman, 1992; Marcuse, 1964; Rothenberg, 1990).

Fundamentally, domination by seduction may create unhealthy illusions among people of African descent that suggest that the current system works on behalf of their collective interests. This may cause people of African descent to feel less compelled to seek information about, and perpetuate traditions that originate from, their African cultural heritage. If this is so, then how is the Afrocentric paradigm to survive and reproduce itself in future generations? In this regard, how can African-American human service workers acquire the aspiration to construct human service interventions based on cultural values and practices emerging from a traditional African/African-American worldview? In addition, if the blurring of cultural differences and the suppression of cultural alternatives are to continue, how can people of African ancestry develop and sustain a critical consciousness that some say is necessary for the collective advancement and mobilization of an oppressed group?

The latter observation is especially relevant to the consumers of human services, many of whom are disproportionately black and poor. If, as Marcuse (1964) contends, the effects of science and technology continue to have a perceptually equalizing effect across social classes by promoting conceptual one-dimensionality, but yet continue material inequality, increasing numbers of the black poor may be at risk of not conceding the severity of their socioeconomic and psychosocial conditions. This disavowal may not only influence noncompliance with, and lack of participation in, human service interventions that may be beneficial but also obviate grassroots organizing among the black poor and with other progressive people to chip away at oppressive elements of the social system.

THE AFRICAN ORAL TRADITION

Another threat to the survival and advancement of the Afrocentric paradigm of human services is the exclusive and primary reliance, among African-American human service professionals, on an oral transmission of knowledge. Although many traditional African societies relied on scripts to transmit knowledge and ideas, a major cultural theme in these societies was the predominance of oral modes of communication and of recording historical events (Asante, 1990; Finnegan, 1970; Horton, 1993; Okpewho, 1992). Both Finnegan (1970) and Okpewho (1992) refer to this tradition as *oral literature,* and within it, selected individuals were trained in various aspects of information storage, retrieval, and dissemination that relied exclusively on memory and oral communications. These persons were trained, for example, to memorize and store copious data about a group's past events, experiences, and struggles that could extend back many years (Finnegan, 1970; Okpewho, 1992). Referred to as *babalawo* by the Yoruba of West Africa, these traditional oral artists were masters of storytelling and poetry and could be considered, in present-day Eurocentric vernacular, journalists, scholars, or intellectuals.

Because of the emphasis in many traditional African societies on social intercourse imbued with intense and extemporaneous expressions of affect, the oral tradition was well suited because it requires, as compared to written communications, person-to-person interaction in which audience participation is encouraged. The mutual and often impromptu oral exchange and validation of ideas in the African/African-American tradition is referred to as the *call and response* phenomenon, perhaps best preserved in the exchange of ideas found in many African-American churches and other religious organizations (Walker, 1995).

If the validity of the assumptions of the Afrocentric paradigm is accepted, it could be hypothesized that many African Americans today, although able to read and write, may have a cultural preference for expressing ideas orally and that this preference may preclude African Americans, particularly African-American human service professionals, from relying extensively on written modes of communication. Burgest (1981) used this logic to suggest that this cultural preference may be a primary impediment to the publication productivity of African-American academics. Since writing requires long periods of solitude devoid of a live audience that can provide immediate feedback, Burgest asserts that the written mode of communication may not fit well within an African/African-American cultural ethos.

To test Burgest's (1981) assumption, Schiele (1991) developed an orality scale to examine its relationship to the publication productivity of a national sample of 264 African-American social work academics. The orality scale was comprised of six items that elicited the degree to which respondents preferred to communicate ideas orally rather than in writing. The higher the score, the greater the preference for expressing ideas orally. Schiele's (1991) analysis indicated that although orality did not exert a statistically significant effect on publication productivity when other variables were simultaneously controlled or considered, it did exert a statistically significant effect on productivity at the bivariate level, that is, when only the relationship between it and productivity were examined. Also, though the correlation between orality and publication productivity was relatively weak ($r = -.209$), the direction of the relationship indicated that higher preferences for orality were associated with lower levels of publication productivity. This finding corroborates Burgest's (1981) ideas about the effects of the African oral tradition on the publication productivity of African-American academics.

Burgest's theory and Schiele's finding have significant implications for the ability of the Afrocentric paradigm to survive and advance. Although many studies of scholarly productivity report that a large amount of the publications by social work academics are produced by a small number of faculty (see, for example, Baker and Wilson, 1992; Green, Hutchison, and Sar, 1992; Johnson and Hull, 1995; Schiele and Francis, 1996), the publication distribution of African-American social work academics is more uneven, indicating that a larger number of African-American social work academics are not publishing at all. For example, a comparison made by Schiele (1991) of the publication distributions of his sample of African-American social work faculty with a wider sample of social work faculty who were overwhelmingly white (see Green, Hutchison, and Sar, 1990) showed that 20 percent of the wider social work academic sample had never published a journal article, whereas almost a third (32.3 percent) of African-American social work academics had not.

Limited participation of African-American social work faculty in publication productivity means that there is less of an opportunity for them to interject and advance their perspectives in the scholarly literature. Though the African oral tradition should be maintained by African-American social work faculty and other human service professionals of African descent, these professionals should recognize that codifying and recording a group's perspectives in writing can help increase that group's political power in society. In this technological age, in which written, computer transmissions from e-mails to online publications are becoming more ordinary than not, exclusive or primary dependence on the African oral tradition will not be sufficient to politically advance the Afrocentric paradigm now and in the near future.

THE AFROCENTRIC PARADIGM'S ASSOCIATION WITH BLACK PEOPLE

Perhaps the most important threat to the survival and progression of the Afrocentric paradigm of human services is its association with people of African ancestry. As with most other concepts, practices, and organizations that emerge from, and are sanctioned primarily by, people of African descent, there is a tendency to devalue them and interpret them as inferior cultural and/or organizational products. This is because of the devaluation of black people, generally, and their African origins, specifically, that began in the transatlantic slave trade and, as some suggest, even before then (see Dove, 1995; Williams, 1987). As long as people, specifically people of African descent, continue to psychologically embrace debilitating stereotypes about blackness and Africa, the Afrocentric paradigm's ability to be deemed a credible model to explain and solve the social problems of our times, as well to as expand positive human potentiality, will be confined.

FINAL THOUGHTS

Human service professionals, and society and the world in general, cannot afford to dismiss paradigms that may contribute to the positive potentiality of the human family. In recent history, the horrors of the transatlantic slave trade, the extermination of native or First Nation peoples in the Americas, the insanity of Hitler's Third Reich, and the 1990s ethnic-cleansing atrocities that occurred in Kosovo, Bosnia, and Liberia all indicate a dire need to consider and implement alternative ways of conceiving humanity and constructing future societies. Grounded in the ideology of domination and xenophobia, these historical human calamities demonstrate the worst in human beings and their respective cultural products.

Although many human service professionals grapple with human problems on a smaller scale, these problems nonetheless involve many of the themes of domination and xenophobia found in the larger theater of social relationships. The Afrocentric paradigm of human services is one important mode through which human service professionals, and the human family in general, can illuminate and undermine the vestiges of a paradigm that repeatedly has failed at eliciting the best in human beings. To this extent, the ultimate Afrocentric vision is to nurture social relationships that elicit the full, positive potentiality of human beings so that the divine quality in humans, recognized and cultivated by the world's first civilizations, can be restored.

References

Chapter 1

Akbar, N. (1976). Rhythmic patterns in African personality. In L. King, V. Dixon, and W. Nobles (Eds.), *African philosophy: Assumptions and paradigms for research on black people* (pp. 175-189). Los Angeles, CA: Fanon Center Publications.

Akbar, N. (1979). African roots of black personality. In W.D. Smith, H. Kathleen, M.H. Burlew, and W.M. Whitney (Eds.), *Reflections on black psychology* (pp. 79-87). Washington, DC: University Press of America.

Akbar, N. (1984). Afrocentric social sciences for human liberation. *Journal of Black Studies*, 14(4), 395-414.

Akbar, N. (1994). *Light from ancient Africa*. Tallahassee, FL: Mind Productions and Associates.

Akbar, N. (1996). *Breaking the chains of psychological slavery*. Tallahassee, FL: Mind Productions and Associates.

Ani, M. (1994). *Yurugu: An African-centered critique of European cultural thought and behavior*. Trenton, NJ: Africa World Press.

Asante, M.K. (1980). International/intercultural relations. In M.K. Asante and A. Vandi (Eds.), *Contemporary black thought* (pp. 43-58). Beverly Hills, CA: Sage.

Asante, M.K. (1987). *The Afrocentric idea*. Philadelphia, PA: Temple University Press.

Asante, M.K. (1988). *Afrocentricity*. Trenton, NJ: Africa World Press.

Asante, M.K. (1990). *Kemet, Afrocentricity, and knowledge*. Trenton, NJ: Africa World Press.

Asante, M.K. (1992). The painful demise of Eurocentrism. *World and I*, April, 305-317.

Baldwin, J. (1981). Notes on an Afrocentric theory of black personality. *The Western Journal of Black Studies*, 5(3), 172-179.

Baldwin, J. (1985). Psychological aspects of European cosmology in American society. *The Western Journal of Black Studies*, 9(4), 216-223.

Baldwin, J. and Hopkins, R. (1990). African-American and European-American cultural differences as assessed by the worldviews paradigm: An empirical analysis. *The Western Journal of Black Studies*, 14(1), 38-52.

Bekerie, A. (1994). The four corners of a circle: Afrocentricity as a model of synthesis. *Journal of Black Studies*, 25(2), 131-149.

Billingsley, A. (1970). Black families and white social science. *Journal of Social Issues*, 26(3), 127-142.

Blauner, R. (1972). *Racial oppression in America*. New York: Harper & Row.

Boykin, W. (1983). The academic performance of Afro-American children. In J. Spence (Ed.), *Achievement and achievement motives* (pp. 324-371). San Francisco, CA: W. Freeman.

Brisbane, F.L. and Womble, M. (1991). *Working with African Americans: The professional's handbook*. Chicago, IL: HRDI International Press.

Cabral, A. (1973). *Return to the source: Selected speeches by Amilcar Cabral*. New York: Monthly Review Press.

Canda, E.R. (1988). Spirituality, religious diversity, and social work practice. *Social Casework*, 69(4), 238-247.

Canda, E.R. (Ed.) (1998). *Spirituality in social work: New directions*. Binghamton, NY: The Haworth Press, Inc.

Carruthers, J. (1972). *Science and oppression*. Chicago, IL: Northeastern Illinois University, Center for Inner City Studies.

Chau, K.L. (1991). Social work with ethnic minorities: Practice issues and potentials. *Journal of Multicultural Social Work*, 1(1), 23-39.

Chavez, L. (Ed.) (1994). *Alternatives to Afrocentrism*. New York: Manhattan Institute.

Cook, N. and Kono, S. (1977). Black psychology: The third great tradition. *The Journal of Black Psychology*, 3(2), 18-20.

Daly, A., Jennings, J., Beckett, J., and Leashore, B. (1995). Effective coping strategies of African Americans. *Social Work*, 40(2), 240-248.

Descartes, R. (1641/1986). *Meditations on first philosophy*. New York: Cambridge University Press.

Devore, W. and Schlesinger, E. (1981). *Ethnic-sensitive social work practice*. St. Louis, MO: C.V. Mosby.

Dixon, V. (1976). World views and research methodology. In L. King, V. Dixon, and W. Nobles (Eds.), *African philosophy: Assumptions and paradigms for research on black persons*, (pp. 51-93). Los Angeles, CA: Fanon Center Publications.

English, R. (1984, November). *The challenge for mental health: Minorities and their world views*. Paper presented at the second annual Robert L. Sutherland lecture, University of Texas at Austin, Austin, TX.

English, R. (1991). Diversity of world views among African Americans. In J.E. Everett, S.S. Chipungu, and B.R. Leashore (Eds.), *Child welfare: An Afrocentric perspective* (pp. 19-35). New Brunswick, NJ: Rutgers University Press.

Everett, J.E., Chipungu, S.S., and Leashore, B.R. (Eds.) (1991). *Child welfare: An Afrocentric perspective*. New Brunswick, NJ: Rutgers University Press.

Fraser, M.W. (1993, January). *Scholarship in social work: Imperfect methods, approximate truths, and emerging challenges*. Paper presented at the 6th National Symposium on Doctoral Research and Social Work Practice, Ohio State University, College of Social Work, Columbus, Ohio.

Green, J.W. (1982). *Cultural awareness in the human services*. Englewood Cliffs, NJ: Prentice-Hall.

Hale-Benson, J. (1982). *Black children: Their roots, culture, and learning styles.* Provo, UT: Brigham Young University Press.

Hegel, G.W.F. (1837/1956). *The philosophy of history.* New York: Dover Publications, Inc.

Herskovits, M.J. (1941). *The myth of the Negro past.* New York: Harper & Row.

Hilliard, A.G. (1989). Kemetic concepts in education. In I.V. Sertima (Ed.), *Nile Valley civilizations* (pp. 153-162). Atlanta, GA: Morehouse College.

Hilliard, A.G. (1995). *The maroon within us: Selected essays on African American community socialization.* Baltimore, MD: Black Classic Press.

Hutnik, N. (1991). *Ethnic minority identity: A social psychological perspective.* Oxford: Clarendon Press.

Jeff, M.F.X. (1994). Afrocentrism and African-American male youths. In R.B. Muncy (Ed.), *Nurturing young black males* (pp. 99-118). Washington, DC: The Urban Institute Press.

Kambon, K. (1992). *The African personality in America: An African-centered framework.* Tallahassee, FL: Nubian Nation Publication.

Karenga, M. (1993). *Introduction to black studies* (Second edition). Los Angeles, CA: University of Sankore.

Karenga, M. (1996). The nguzo saba (the seven principles): Their meaning and message. In M.K. Asante and A.S. Abarry (Eds.), *African intellectual heritage* (pp. 543-554). Philadelphia, PA: Temple University Press.

Kershaw, T. (1992). Afrocentrism and the Afrocentric method. *The Western Journal of Black Studies,* 16(3), 160-168.

Khatib, S., Akbar, N., McGee, D., and Nobles, W. (1979). Voodoo or IQ: An introduction to African psychology. In W.D. Smith, K.H. Burlew, M.H. Mosley, and W.M. Whitney (Eds.), *Reflections on black psychology* (pp. 61-67). Washington, DC: University Press of America.

Lum, D. (1992). *Social work practice and people of color: A process-stage approach* (Second edition). Pacific Grove, CA: Brooks/Cole.

Martin, E.P. and Martin, J.M. (1995). *Social work and the black experience.* Washington, DC: National Association of Social Workers.

Myers, L.J. (1988). *Understanding an Afrocentric world view: Introduction to an optimal psychology.* Dubuque, IA: Kendall/Hunt Publishing Company.

Nobles, W.W. (1974). African root and American fruit: The black family. *Journal of Social and Behavioral Sciences,* 20, 66-75.

Nobles, W.W. (1978). *African consciousness and liberation struggles: Implications for the development and construction of scientific paradigms.* Unpublished manuscript presented at Fanon Research and Development Conference, Port of Spain, Trinidad.

Nobles, W.W. (1980). African philosophy: Foundations for black psychology. In R. Jones (Ed.) (Second edition), *Black psychology* (pp. 23-35). New York: Harper & Row.

Phillips, F.B. (1990). NTU psychotherapy: An Afrocentric approach. *The Journal of Black Psychology,* 17(1), 55-74.

Rose, S.M. (1990). Advocacy/empowerment: An approach to clinical practice for social work. *Journal of Sociology and Social Welfare*, 17(2), 41-50.

Rothenberg, P. (1990). The construction, deconstruction, and reconstruction of difference. *Hypatia*, 5(1), 42-57.

Saleebey, D. (Ed). (1992). *The strengths perspective in social work practice.* New York: Longman.

Saleebey, D. (1996). The strengths perspective in social work practice: Extensions and cautions. *Social Work*, 41(3), 296-305.

Schiele, J.H. (1993). Cultural oppression, African Americans, and social work practice. *Black Caucus: Journal of the National Association of Black Social Workers*, Fall(2), 20-34.

Schiele, J.H. (1994). Afrocentricity as an alternative world view for equality. *Journal of Progressive Human Services*, 5(1), 5-25.

Schiele, J.H. (1996). Afrocentricity: An emerging paradigm in social work practice. *Social Work*, 41(3), 284-294.

Schiele, J.H. (1997). The contour and meaning of Afrocentric social work. *Journal of Black Studies*, 27(6), 800-819.

Schlesinger, A. (1991). *The disuniting of America: Reflections on a multicultural society.* New York: Norton.

Semmes, C.E. (1981). Foundations of an Afrocentric social science: Implications for curriculum-building, theory, and research in black studies. *Journal of Black Studies*, 12(1), 3-17.

Sermabeikian, P. (1994). Our clients, ourselves: The spiritual perspective and social work practice. *Social Work*, 39(2), 178-183.

Smith, J.K. (1993). *After the demise of empiricism.* Norwood, NJ: Ablex Publishing Company.

Sue, D.W. (1977). Counseling the culturally different: A conceptual analysis. *The Personnel and Guidance Journal*, 55(7), 422-425.

Swigonski, M.E. (1996). Challenging privilege through Afrocentric social work practice. *Social Work*, 41(2), 153-161.

Verharen, C.C. (1995). Afrocentrism and acentrism: A marriage of science and philosophy. *Journal of Black Studies*, 26(1), 62-76.

Welsh-Asante, K. (1985). Commonalities in African dance: An aesthetic foundation. In M.K. Asante and K. Welsh-Asante (Eds.), *African culture: The rhythms of unity* (pp. 71-82). Westport, CT: Greenwood.

Woodson, C.G. (1933). *The miseducation of the negro.* Washington, DC: Associated Publishers.

Young, I.M. (1990). *Justice and the politics of difference.* Princeton, NJ: Princeton University Press.

Chapter 2

Akbar, N. (1979). African roots of black personality. In W.D. Smith, H. Kathleen, M.H. Burlew, and W.M. Whitney (Eds.), *Reflections on black psychology* (pp. 79-87). Washington, DC: University Press of America.

Akbar, N. (1984). Afrocentric social sciences for human liberation. *Journal of Black Studies*, 14(4), 395-414.

Akbar, N. (1994). *Light from ancient Africa*. Tallahassee, FL: Mind Productions and Associates.

Akbar, N. (1996). *Breaking the chains of psychological slavery*. Tallahassee, FL: Mind Productions and Associates.

Akinyela, M.M. (1995). Rethinking Afrocentricity: The foundation of a theory of critical Afrocentricity. In A. Darder (Ed.), *Culture and difference: Critical perspectives on the bicultural experience in the United States* (pp. 21-39). New York: Bethon and Garvey Press.

Ameen, R.U.N. (1990). *Metu neter* (Volume 1). Bronx, NY: Khamit Corporation.

Ani, M. (1994). *Yurugu: An African-centered critique of European cultural thought and behavior*. Trenton, NJ: Africa World Press.

Appiah, K.A. (1992). *In my father's house: Africa in the philosophy of culture*. New York: Oxford University Press.

Asante, M.K. (1980). International/intercultural relations. In M.K. Asante and A. Vandi (Eds.), *Contemporary black thought* (pp. 43-58). Beverly Hills, CA: Sage.

Asante, M.K. (1987). *The Afrocentric idea*. Philadelphia, PA.: Temple University Press.

Asante, M.K. (1988). *Afrocentricity*. Trenton, NJ: Africa World Press.

Asante, M.K. (1990). *Kemet, Afrocentricity, and knowledge*. Trenton, NJ: Africa World Press.

Baldwin, J. (1981). Notes on an Afrocentric theory of black personality. *The Western Journal of Black Studies*, 5(3), 172-179.

Baldwin, J. (1985). Psychological aspects of European cosmology in American society. *The Western Journal of Black Studies*, 9(4), 216-223.

Baldwin, J. and Bell, Y. (1985). The African self-consciousness scale: An Afrocentric personality questionnaire. *The Western Journal of Black Studies*, 9(2), 62-68.

Baldwin, J.A., Brown, R. and Rackley, R. (1990). Some socio-behavioral correlates of African self-consciousness in African-American college students. *The Journal of Black Psychology*, 17(1), 1-17.

Baldwin, J.A., Duncan, J.A., and Bell, Y.R. (1987). Assessment of African self-consciousness among black students from two college environments. *The Journal of Black Psychology*, 13(2), 27-41.

Baldwin, J. and Hopkins, R. (1990). African-American and European-American cultural differences as assessed by the worldviews paradigm: An empirical analysis. *The Western Journal of Black Studies*, 14(1), 38-52.

Bell, Y.R. (1994). A culturally sensitive analysis of black learning style. *Journal of Black Psychology*, 20(1), 47-61.

Bell, Y.R., Bouie, C.L. and Baldwin, J.A. (1990). Afrocentric cultural consciousness and African-American male-female relationships. *Journal of Black Studies*, 21(2), 162-189.

Ben-Jochannon, Y. (1971). *Africa: Mother of western civilization.* New York: Alkebulan Publishing Company.

Biebuyck, D. (1964). Land holding and social organization. In M. Herskovits and M. Harwitz (Eds.), *Economic transition in Africa* (pp. 99-112). Evanston, IL: Northwestern University Press.

Bolling, J.L. (1990). *The heart of soul: An Afrocentric approach to psycho-spiritual wholeness.* New York: Mandala Rising Press.

Boykin, W. (1983). The academic performance of Afro-American children. In J. Spence (Ed.), *Achievement and achievement motives* (pp. 324-371). San Francisco, CA: W. Freeman.

Boykin, W. and Toms, F. (1985). Black child socialization: A conceptual framework. In H.P. McAdoo (Ed.), *Black children.* Beverly Hills, CA: Sage.

Brisbane, F.L. and Womble, M. (1991). *Working with African Americans: The professional's handbook.* Chicago, IL: HRDI International Press.

Cabral, A. (1973). *Return to the source.* New York: Monthly Review Press.

Cann, R. (1987). Mitachondrial DNA and human evolution. *Nature,* 325(1), 31-36.

Carruthers, J.H. (1972). *Science and oppression.* Chicago, IL: The Center for Inner City Studies.

Chapin, R.K. (1995). Social policy development: The strengths perspective. *Social Work,* 40(4), 506-514.

Chavez, L. (Ed.) (1994). *Alternatives to Afrocentrism.* New York: The Manhattan Institute.

Chazan, N. (1993). Between liberalism and statism: African political cultures and democracy. In L. Diamond (Ed.), *Political culture and democracy in developing countries* (pp. 67-105). Boulder, CO: Lynne Rienner.

Cheatham, H.E., Tomilinson, S.M., and Ward, T.J. (1990). The African self-consciousness construct and African-American students. *Journal of College Student Development,* 31(6), 492-499.

Clarke, J.H. (1991). *Africans at the crossroads: Notes for an African world revolution.* Trenton, NJ: Africa World Press.

Crouch, S. (1996). The Afrocentric hustle. *The Journal of Blacks in Higher Education,* Winter (10), 77-82.

Davidson, B. (1969). *The African genius: An introduction to African cultural and social history.* Boston, MA: Little, Brown and Company.

Dei, G.J. (1994). Afrocentricity: A cornerstone of pedagogy. *Anthropology and Education Quarterly,* 25(1), 3-28.

Diop, C.A. (1974). *The African origin of civilization: Myth or reality.* Westport, CT: Lawrence Hill and Company.

Diop, C.A. (1978). *The cultural unity of black Africa.* Chicago, IL: Third World Press.

Diop, C.A. (1987). *Precolonial black Africa: A comparative study of the political and social systems of Europe and black Africa.* Brooklyn, NY: Lawrence Hill Books.

Diop, C.A. (1991). *Civilization or barbarism.* Brooklyn, NY: Lawrence Hill Books.

Dixon, V. (1976). World views and research methodology. In L. King, V. Dixon, and W. Nobles (Eds.), *African philosophy: Assumptions and paradigms for research on black persons* (pp. 51-93). Los Angeles, CA: Fanon Center Publications.

Dubois, W.E.B. (1965). *The world and Africa.* New York: International Publishers.

Fallers, L.A. (1964). Social stratification and economic progress. In M. Herskovits and M. Harwitz (Eds.), *Economic transition in Africa* (pp. 113-130). Evanston, IL: Northwestern University Press.

Farrar, T. (1997). The queenmother, matriarchy, and the question of female political authority in precolonial West African monarchy. *Journal of Black Studies*, 27(5), 579-597.

Finch, C.S. (1982). The works of Gerald Massey: Studies in Kamite origins. *Journal of African Civilizations*, 4(2), 55-67.

Franklin, J.H. (1980). *From slavery to freedom: A history of negro Americans* (Fifth edition). New York: Alfred A. Knopf.

Gyekye, K. (1987). *An essay on African philosophical thought: The Akan conceptual scheme.* New York: Cambridge University Press.

Gyekye, K. (1992). Person and community in African thought. In K. Wiredu and K. Gyekye (Eds.), *Person and community: Ghanaian philosophical studies, I* (pp. 101-122). Washington, DC: The Council for Research in Values and Philosophy.

Hale-Benson, J. (1982). *Black children: Their roots, culture, and learning styles.* Provo, UT: Brigham Young University Press.

Harvey, A.R. and Rauch, J.B. (1997). A comprehensive Afrocentric rites of passage program for black male adolescents. *Health and Social Work*, 22(1), 30-37.

Herskovits, M.J. (1941). *The myth of the negro past.* New York: Harper & Row.

Hilliard, A.G. (1989). Kemetic concepts in education. In I. Van Sertima (Ed.), *Nile Valley civilizations* (pp. 153-162). Atlanta, GA: Morehouse College.

Horton, R. (1993). *Patterns of thought in Africa and the west: Essays on magic, religion and science.* New York: Cambridge University Press.

Hyden, G. (1983). *No shortcuts to progress: African development management in perspective.* Berkeley, CA: University of California Press.

Jackson, J.G. (1990). *Introduction to African civilizations.* New York: Carol Publishing Group.

James, G.M. (1954). *Stolen legacy.* New York: Philosophical Library.

Kambon, K. (1992). *The African personality in America: An African-centered framework.* Tallahassee, FL: Nubian Nation Publication.

Karenga, M. (1993a). *Introduction to black studies* (Second edition). Los Angeles, CA: University of Sankore Press.

Karenga, M. (1993b). Towards a sociology of Maatian ethics: Literature and context. In I. Van Sertima (Ed.), *Egypt revisited* (pp. 352-395). New Brunswick, NJ: Transaction Publishers.

Karenga, M. and Carruthers, J. (Eds.) (1986). *Kemet and the African worldview: Research, rescue, and restoration.* Los Angeles, CA: University of Sankore Press.

Keita, L. (1978). African philosophical systems—A rational reconstruction. *The Philosophical Forum*, 9(2/3), 169-189.

Lemelle, S.J. (1994). The politics of cultural existence: Pan-Africanism, historical materialism, and Afrocentricity. In S.J. Lemelle and R. Kelley (Eds.), *Imagining home: Class, culture, and nationalism in the African diaspora* (pp. 331-350). New York: Verso.

Madu, O.V. (1978). Kinship and social organization. In C. Mojekwu, V. Uchendu, and L. Van Hoey (Eds.), *African society, culture, and politics: An introduction to African studies* (pp. 76-90). Lanham, MD: University Press of America.

Martin, J.M. and Martin, E.P. (1985). *The helping tradition in the black family and community.* Silver Spring, MD: National Association of Social Workers.

Mazrui, A. (1986). *The Africans: A reader.* New York: Greenwood Publishing Company.

Mbiti, J. (1970). *African religions and philosophy.* Garden City, NY: Anchor Books.

Mbiti, J. (1991). *Introduction to African religion* (Second edition). Portsmouth, NH: Heinemann Educational Books, Inc.

Montagu, A. (1958). *Man: His first million years.* New York: Mentor Books.

Myers, L.J. (1985). Transpersonal psychology: The role of the afrocentric paradigm. *The Journal of Black Psychology*, 12(1), 31-42.

Myers, L.J. (1988). *Understanding an Afrocentric world view: Introduction to an optimal psychology.* Dubuque, IA: Kendall/Hunt Publishing Company.

Nkrumah, K. (1970). *Consciencism: Philosophy and ideology for decolonization.* New York: Monthly Review Press.

Nobles, W.W. (1980). African philosophy: Foundations for black psychology. In R. Jones (Ed.). *Black psychology* (Third edition) (pp. 23-35). New York: Harper & Row.

Nyerere, J. (1968). *Ujamaa—Essays on socialism.* London: Oxford University Press.

Oyebade, B. (1990). African studies and the Afrocentric paradigm: A critique. *Journal of Black Studies*, 21(2), 233-238.

Paris, P.J. (1995). *The spirituality of African peoples.* Minneapolis, MN: Fortress Press.

Phillips, F.B. (1990). NTU psychotherapy: An Afrocentric approach. *The Journal of Black Psychology*, 17(1), 55-74.

Radcliffe-Brown, A.R. and Forde, D. (1967). *African systems of kinship and marriage.* London: Oxford University Press.

Rodney, W. (1980). *How Europe underdeveloped Africa.* Washington, DC: Howard University Press.

Saleebey, D. (1996). The strengths perspective in social work practice: Extensions and cautions. *Social Work*, 41(3), 296-305.

Schiele, J.H. (1990). Organizational theory from an Afrocentric perspective. *Journal of Black Studies*, 21(2), 145-161.

Schiele, J.H. (1994). Afrocentricity as an alternative world view for equality. *Journal of Progressive Human Services*, 5(1), 5-25.

Schiele, J.H. (1996). Afrocentricity: An emerging paradigm in social work practice. *Social Work*, 41(3), 284-294.

Schiele, J.H. (1997). The contour and meaning of Afrocentric social work. *Journal of Black Studies*, 27(6), 800-819.

Schiele, J.H. (1999). The team approach to black liberation. In J.L Conyers and A.P. Barnett (Eds.), *African American sociology: A social study of the pan-African diaspora,* (pp. 144-163). Chicago, IL: Nelson-Hall Publishers.

Senghor, L.S. (1964). *On African socialism.* New York: Frederic A. Praeger.

Serequeberhan, T. (1991). *African philosophy: The essential readings.* New York: Paragon House.

Stokes, J.E., Murray, C.B., Peacock, M.J., and Kaiser, R.T. (1994). Assessing the reliability, factor structure, and validity of the African self-consciousness scale in a general population of African Americans. *The Journal of Black Psychology*, 20(1), 62-74.

Sudarkasa, N. (1988). Interpreting the African heritage in Afro-American family organization. In H.P. McAdoo (Ed.), *Black families* (Second edition) (pp. 27-43). Beverly Hills, CA: Sage.

Van Sertima, I. (Ed.) (1989). *Nile Valley civilizations.* Atlanta, GA: Morehouse College.

Weems, L. (1974). Black community research needs: Methods, model, and modalities. In L.E. Gary (Ed.), *Social research and the black community: Selected issues and priorities* (pp. 25-38). Washington, DC: Institute for Urban Affairs.

Williams, C. (1987). *The destruction of black civilization.* Chicago, IL: Third World Press.

Williams, C. (1993). *The rebirth of African civilization.* Chicago, IL: Third World Press.

Zahan, D. (1979). *The religion, spirituality, and thought of traditional Africa.* Chicago, IL: University of Chicago Press.

Chapter 3

Akbar, N. (1994). *Light from ancient Africa.* Tallahassee, FL: Mind Productions and Associates.

Appiah-Kubi, K. (1993). Traditional African healing system versus western medicine in southern Ghana: An encounter. In J.K. Olupona and S.S. Nyang (Eds.), *Religious plurality in Africa: Essays in honor of John S. Mbiti* (pp. 95-107). Belin: Mouton de Gruyter Press.

Atwell, I. and Azibo, D. (1991). Diagnosing personality disorder in Africans (blacks) using the Azibo nosology: Two case studies. *Journal of Black Psychology*, 17(2), 1-22.

Azibo, D. (1991). Towards a metatheory of African personality. *Journal of Black Psychology*, 17(2), 37-45.

Biebuyck, D. (1964). Land holding and social organization. In M. Herskovits and M. Harwitz (Eds.), *Economic transition in Africa* (pp. 99-112). Evanston, IL: Northwestern University Press.

Billingsley, A. (1968). *Black families in white America*. Englewood Cliffs, NJ: Prentice-Hall.

Billingsley, A. (1994). *Climbing Jacob's ladder: The enduring legacy of African families*. New York: Simon and Schuster.

Billingsley, A. and Caldwell, C.H. (1995). The social relevance of the contemporary black church. *National Journal of Sociology*, 8(1/2), 1-23.

Brisbane, F.L. and Womble, M. (1991). *Working with African Americans: The professional's handbook*. Chicago, IL: HRDI International Press.

Carlton-LaNey, I. (1994). The career of Birdye Henrietta Haynes, a pioneer settlement house worker. *Social Service Review*, 68(2), 254-273.

Carruthers, J.H. (1981). Reflections on the history of the Afrocentric worldview. *Black Books Bulletin*, 7(1), 4-7.

Chazan, N. (1993). Between liberalism and statism: African political cultures and democracy. In L. Diamond (Ed.), *Political culture and democracy in developing countries* (pp. 67-105). Boulder, CO: Lynne Rienner.

Cone, J.H. (1969). *Black theology and black power*. New York: Seabury Press.

Conyers, J.E. (1988). Biographical portraits of four black sociologists: Dubois, Johnson, Frazier, and Cox. *The Western Journal of Black Studies*, 12(3), 150-156.

Davidson, B. (1969). *The African genius: An introduction to African cultural and social history*. Boston, MA: Little, Brown and Company.

Davis, L.G. (1980). The politics of black self-help in the United States: A historical overview. In L.S. Yearwood (Ed.), *Black organizations* (pp. 37-50). Lanham, MD: University Press of America.

Day, P.J. (1997). *A new history of social welfare* (Second edition). Boston, MA: Allyn and Bacon.

Dei, G.J. (1994). Afrocentricity: A cornerstone of pedagogy. *Anthropology and Education Quarterly*, 25(1), 3-28.

Diop, C.A. (1978). *The cultural unity of black Africa*. Chicago, IL: Third World Press.

Diop, C.A. (1987). *Precolonial black Africa: A comparative study of the political and social systems of Europe and black Africa*. Brooklyn, NY: Lawrence Hill Books.

Edwards, G.F. (1968). *E. Franklin Frazier on race relations*. Chicago, IL: University of Chicago Press.

Ezeabasili, N. (1977). *African science: Myth or reality?* New York: Vantage Press.

Fallers, L.A. (1964). Social stratification and economic progress. In M. Herskovits and M. Harwitz (Eds.), *Economic transition in Africa* (pp. 113-130). Evanston, IL: Northwestern University Press.

Farrar, T. (1997). The queenmother, matriarchy, and the question of female political authority in precolonial West African monarchy. *Journal of Black Studies*, 27(5), 579-597.

Franklin, J.H. (1980). *From slavery to freedom: A history of Negro Americans* (Fifth edition). New York: Alfred A. Knopf.

Frazier, E.F. (1924a). Social work in race relations. *The Crisis*, 27(6), 252-254.

Frazier, E.F. (1924b). Discussion. *Opportunity*, 2(20), 239.

Frazier, E.F. (1926). Three scourges of the Negro family. *Opportunity*, 4(43), 210-213, 234.

Frazier, E.F. (1927). Is the Negro family a unique sociological unit? *Opportunity*, 5(6), 165-166.

Frazier, E.F. (1939). *The Negro family in the United States*. Chicago, IL: University of Chicago Press.

Frazier, E.F. (1957). *Black bourgeoisie: The rise of a new middle class in the United States*. New York: Collier Books.

Frazier, E.F. (1964). *The Negro church in America*. New York: Schocken Books.

Griaule, M. (1978). *Conversations with Ogotemmeli*. New York: Oxford University Press.

Gutman, H.G. (1976). *The black family in slavery and freedom, 1750-1925*. New York: Pantheon Books.

Gyekye, K. (1987). *An essay on African philosophical thought: The Akan conceptual scheme*. New York: Cambridge University Press.

Gyekye, K. (1992). Person and community in African thought. In K. Wiredu and K. Gyekye (Eds.), *Person and community: Ghanaian philosophical studies, I* (pp. 101-122). Washington, DC: The Council for Research in Values and Philosophy.

Harvey, A.R. (Ed.) (1985). *The black family: An Afrocentric perspective*. New York: United Church of Christ, Commission for Racial Justice.

Herskovits, M.J. (1941). *The myth of the Negro past*. New York: Harper & Row.

Hilliard, A.G. (1989). Kemetic concepts in education. In I. Van Sertima (Ed.), *Nile Valley civilizations* (pp. 153-162). Atlanta, GA: Morehouse College.

Horton, R. (1993). *Patterns of thought in Africa and the west: Essays on magic, religion and science*. New York: Cambridge University Press.

Jackson, W.S., Rhone, J.V., and Sanders, C.L. (1973). *Social service delivery system in the black community during the ante-bellum period (1619-1860)*. Atlanta, GA: Alton M. Children Services.

Johnson, C.S. (1936). *A preface to racial understanding*. New York: Friendship Press.

Jones, B.A. (1974). The tradition of sociology teaching in black colleges: The unheralded professionals. In J.E. Blackwell and M. Janowitz (Eds.), *Black sociologists: Historical and contemporary perspectives* (pp. 121-163). Chicago, IL: University of Chicago Press.

Kalu, O.U. (1991). The African perception of his world. In E.M. Uka (Ed.), *Readings in African traditional religion* (pp. 11-37). New York: Peter Lang.

Kambon, K. (1992). *The African personality in America: An African-centered framework*. Tallahassee, FL: Nubian Nation Publication.

Karenga, M. (1993). *Introduction to black studies* (Second edition). Los Angeles, CA: University of Sankore Press.

Karenga, M. (1996). The nguzo saba (the seven principles): Their meaning and message. In M.K. Asante and A.S. Abarry (Eds.), *African intellectual heritage* (pp. 543-554). Philadelphia, PA: Temple University Press.

Khatib, S., Akbar, N., McGee, D. and Nobles, W. (1979). Voodoo or IQ: An introduction to African psychology. In W.D. Smith, K.H. Burlew, M.H. Mosley, and W.M. Whitney (Eds.), *Reflections on black psychology*. Washington, DC: University Press of America.

King, N.Q. (1986). *African cosmos: An introduction to religion in Africa*. Belmont, CA: Wadsworth Publishing Company.

Lincoln, C.E. and Mamiya, L.H. (1990). *The black church in the African American experience*. Durham, NC: Duke University Press.

Lubove, R. (1983). *The professional altruist: The emergence of social work as a career*. New York: Atheneum.

Madu, O.V. (1978). Kinship and social organization. In C. Mojekwu, V. Uchendu, and L. Van Hoey (Eds.), *African society, culture, and politics: An introduction to African studies* (pp. 76-90). Lanham, MD: University Press of America.

Martin, E.P. and Martin, J.M. (1978). *The black extended family*. Chicago, IL: University of Chicago Press.

Martin, E.P. and Martin, J.M. (1995). *Social work and the black experience*. Washington, DC: National Association of Social Workers.

Martin, J.M. and Martin, E.P. (1985). *The helping tradition in the black family and community*. Silver Spring, MD: National Association of Social Workers.

Mbiti, J. (1970). *African religions and philosophy*. Garden City, NY: Anchor Books.

Menkiti, I.A. (1984). Person and community in African traditional thought. In R.A. Wright (Ed.), *African philosophy: An introduction* (pp. 171-181). Lanham, MD: University Press of America.

Moore, J.T. (1981). *A search for equality: The national urban league, 1910-1961*. University Park, PA: Pennsylvania State University Press.

Nobles, W.W. (1974). Africanity: Its role in black families. *The Black Scholar*, 5(9), 10-17.

Nobles, W.W. (1980). African philosophy: Foundations for black psychology. In R. Jones (Ed.) *Black psychology* (Second edition) (pp. 23-35). New York: Harper & Row.

Okonjo, K. (1976). The dual-sex political system in operation: Igbo women and community politics in midwestern Nigeria. In N.J. Hafkin and E.G. Bay (Eds.), *Women in Africa: Studies in social and economic change* (pp. 45-58). Stanford, CA: Stanford University Press.

Paris, P.J. (1995). *The spirituality of African peoples*. Minneapolis, MN: Fortress Press.

Pollard, W.L. (1978). *A study of black self-help*. San Francisco, CA: R&E Associates.

Radcliffe-Brown, A.R. and Forde, D. (1967). *African systems of kinship and marriage*. London: Oxford University Press.

Ray, B.C. (1976). *African religions*. Englewood Cliffs, NJ: Prentice-Hall.

Robbins, R. (1974). Charles S. Johnson. In J.E. Blackwell and M. Janowitz (Eds.), *Black sociologists: Historical and contemporary perspectives* (pp. 56-84). Chicago, IL: University of Chicago Press.

Ross, E. (1978). *The black heritage in social welfare, 1860-1930.* Metuchen, NJ: Scarecrow Press.

Schiele, J.H. (1997). An Afrocentric perspective on social welfare philosophy and policy. *Journal of Sociology and Social Welfare*, 24(2), 21-39.

Stampp, K.M. (1956). *The peculiar institution: Slavery in the ante-bellum south.* New York: Vintage Books.

Stoeltje, B.J. (1994). Asante queenmothers: A study in identity and continuity. In M. Reh and G. Ludwar-Ene (Eds.), *Gender and identity in Africa* (pp. 15-32). Munster: Hamburg.

Stuckey, S. (1987). *Slave culture: Nationalist theory and the foundations of black culture.* New York: Oxford University Press.

Sudarkasa, N. (1988). Interpreting the African heritage in Afro-American family organization. In H.P. McAdoo (Ed.) *Black families* (Second edition) (pp. 27-43). Beverly Hills, CA: Sage.

Sudarkasa, N. (1989). The status of women in indigenous African societies. In L. Richardson and V. Taylor (Eds.), *Feminist frontiers II: Rethinking sex, gender, and society* (pp. 152-158). New York: McGraw-Hill.

Sudarkasa, N. (1997). African American families and family values. In H.P. McAdoo (Ed.), *Black families* (Third edition) (pp. 9-40). Thousand Oaks, CA: Sage.

Washington, F.B. (1925). What professional training means to the social worker. *Annals of the American Academy of Political and Social Science*, 121(September), 165-169.

Washington, F.B. (1935). The need and education of Negro social workers. *Journal of Negro Education*, 4(1), 76-93.

Welsing, F.C. (1991). *The Isis papers: The keys to the colors.* Chicago, IL: Third World Press.

Wenocur, S. and Reisch, M. (1989). *From charity to enterprise: The development of American social work in a market economy.* Urbana, IL: University of Illinois Press.

Williams, C. (1987). *The destruction of black civilization.* Chicago, IL: Third World Press.

Williams, C. (1993). *The rebirth of African civilization.* Chicago, IL: Third World Press.

Zahan, D. (1979). *The religion, spirituality, and thought of traditional Africa.* Chicago, IL: University of Chicago Press.

Chapter 4

Akbar, N. (1984). Afrocentric social sciences for human liberation. *Journal of Black Studies*, 14(4), 395-414.

Akbar, N. (1994). *Light from ancient Africa.* Tallahassee, FL: Mind Productions and Associates.

Ameen, R.U.N. (1990). *Metu neter* (Volume 1). Bronx, NY: Khamit Corporation.

Ani, M. (1994). *Yurugu: An African-centered critique of European cultural thought and behavior.* Trenton, NJ: Africa World Press.

Asante, M.K. (1980). International/intercultural relations. In M.K. Asante and A. Vandi (Eds.), *Contemporary black thought* (pp. 43-58). Beverly Hills, CA: Sage.

Asante, M.K. (1987). *The Afrocentric idea.* Philadelphia, PA: Temple University Press.

Asante, M.K. (1988). *Afrocentricity.* Trenton, NJ: Africa World Press.

Asante, M.K. (1990). *Kemet, Afrocentricity, and knowledge.* Trenton, NJ: Africa World Press.

Asante, M.K. (1992). The painful demise of Eurocentrism. *World and I*, April, 305-317.

Bailey, R. (1992). The slave(ry) trade and the development of capitalism in the United States: The textile industry in New England. In J.E. Inikori and S.L. Engerman (Eds.), *The Atlantic slave trade: Effects on economies, societies, and peoples of Africa, the Americas, and Europe* (pp. 205-246). Durham, NC: Duke University Press.

Baldwin, J. (1985). Psychological aspects of European cosmology in American society. *The Western Journal of Black Studies*, 9(4), 216-223.

Baldwin, J. and Hopkins, R. (1990). African-American and European-American cultural differences as assessed by the worldviews paradigm: An empirical analysis. *The Western Journal of Black Studies*, 14(1), 38-52.

Barbosa, L.C. (1990). Dependencia, environmental imperialism and human survival: A critical essay on the global environmental crisis. *Humanity and Society*, 14(4), 329-344.

Bazargan, M. (1996). Self-reported sleep disturbance among African-American elderly: The effects of depression, health status, exercise, and social support. *International Journal of Aging and Human Development*, 42(2), 143-160.

Bekerie, A. (1994). The four corners of a circle: Afrocentricity as a model of synthesis. *Journal of Black Studies*, 25(2), 131-149.

Bell, Y.R., Bouie, C.L., and Baldwin, J.A. (1990). Afrocentric cultural consciousness and African-American male-female relationships. *Journal of Black Studies*, 21(2), 162-189.

Ben-Jochannon, Y. (1971). *Africa: Mother of western civilization.* New York: Alkebulan Publishing Company.

Bensley, R.J. (1991). Defining spiritual health: A review of the literature. *Journal of Health Education*, 22(5), 287-290.

Berman, M. (1981). *The reenchantment of the world.* Ithaca, NY: Cornell University Press.

Blaut, J.M. (1993). *The colonizer's model of the world.* New York: Guilford Press.

Bolling, J.L. (1990). *The heart of soul: An afrocentric approach to psycho-spiritual wholeness.* New York: Mandala Rising Press.

Boykin, W. (1983). The academic performance of Afro-American children. In J. Spence (Ed.), *Achievement and achievement motives* (pp. 324-371). San Francisco, CA: W. Freeman.

Burgest, D.R. (1981). Theory on white supremacy and black oppression. *Black Books Bulletin*, 7(2), 26-30.

Cann, R. (1987). Mitochondrial DNA and human evolution. *Nature*, 325(1), 31-36.

Capra, F. (1982). The turning point: A new vision of reality. *The Futurist*, December, 19-24.

Chaffin, M., Kelleher, K., and Hollenberg, J. (1996). Onset of physical abuse and neglect: Psychiatric, substance abuse, and social risk factors from prospective community data. *Child Abuse and Neglect,* 20(3), 191-203.

Chandler, C.K., Holden, J.M., and Kolander, C.A. (1992). Counseling for spiritual wellness: Theory and practice. *Journal of Counseling and Development*, 71(2), 168-175.

Clarke, J.H. (1991). *Africans at the crossroads: Notes for an African world revolution.* Trenton, NJ: Africa World Press.

Cohen, G. (1996). Toward a spirituality based on justice and ecology. *Social Policy*, 26(3), 6-18.

Diop, C.A. (1974). *The African origin of civilization: Myth or reality?* Westport, CT: Lawrence Hill and Company.

Diop, C.A. (1991). *Civilization or barbarism.* Brooklyn, NY: Lawrence Hill Books.

Dixon, V. (1976). World views and research methodology. In L. King, V. Dixon, and W. Nobles (Eds.), *African philosophy: Assumptions and paradigms for research on black persons* (pp. 51-93). Los Angeles, CA: Fanon Center Publications.

Elkins, D.N. (1995). Psychotherapy and spirituality: Toward a theory of the soul. *Journal of Humanistic Psychology*, 35(2), 78-88.

Finch, C.S. (1982). The works of Gerald Massey: Studies in Kamite origins. *Journal of African Civilizations*, 4(2), 55-67.

Fromm, E. (1941). *Escape from freedom.* New York: Rinehart and Company.

Gary, L.E. (1985). Depressive symptoms and black men. *Social Work Research and Abstracts*, 21(4), 21-29.

Harkness, G. (1957). *Christian ethics.* New York: Abingdon Press.

Harris, D.B. (1997). The duality complex: An unresolved paradox in African American politics. *Journal of Black Studies*, 27(6), 783-799.

Harvey, P.D., Stokes, J.L., Lord, J., and Pogge, D.L. (1996). Neurocognitive and personality assessment of adolescent substance abusers: A multidimensional approach. *Assessment*, 3(3), 241-253.

Havelock, E.A. (1963). *Preface to Plato.* Cambridge, MA: Harvard University Press.

Hekman, S.J. (1986). *Hermeneutics and the sociology of knowledge.* Notre Dame, IN: University of Notre Dame Press.

Hobson, J.A. (1949). *The evolution of modern capitalism.* New York: Macmillan.

James, G.M. (1954). *Stolen legacy*. New York: Philosophical Library.

Jansson, B.S. (1993). *The reluctant welfare state: A history of American social welfare policies* (Second edition). Pacific Grove, CA: Brooks/Cole.

Karenga, M. (1993). *Introduction to black studies* (Second edition). Los Angeles, CA: University of Sankore Press.

Khatib, S., Akbar, N., McGee, D. and Nobles, W. (1979). Voodoo or IQ: An introduction to African psychology. In W.D. Smith, K.H. Burlew, M.H. Mosley, and W.M. Whitney (Eds.), *Reflections on black psychology* (pp. 61-87). Washington, DC: University Press of America.

Kohl, L.F. (1989). *The politics of individualism: Parties and the American character in the Jacksonian era*. New York: Oxford University Press.

Ladd, A.E. (1988). Toward a brave new technocracy: Rationality or ecocide? *Sociological Viewpoints*, 4(2), 31-43.

Leonard, P. (1995). Postmodernism, socialism, and social welfare. *Journal of Progressive Human Services,* 6(2), 3-19.

Levenson, D. (1997, February). Anxiety: It's not just "all in your head." *National Association of Social Workers News*, 42(2), 3.

Lovejoy, A.O. (1966). *The great chain of being: A study of a history of an idea*. Cambridge, MA: Harvard University Press.

MacPherson, C.B. (1962). *The political theory of possessive individualism: Hobbes to Locke*. London: Oxford University Press.

Malmquist, C.P. (1995). Depression and homicidal violence. *International Journal of Law and Psychiatry*, 18(2), 145-162.

Marcuse, H. (1964). *One dimensional man*. Boston, MA: Beacon Press.

May, R. (1975). Values, myths, and symbols. *American Journal of Psychiatry*, 132(7), 703-706.

May, R. (1977). *The meaning of anxiety*. New York: W.W. Norton and Company.

May, R. (1983). *The discovery of being*. New York: Van Nostrand Reinhold.

McGuire, M.B. (1993). Health and spirituality as contemporary concerns. *Annals of the American Academy of Political and Social Science*, 527(May), 144-154.

Montagu, A. (1958). *Man: His first million years*. New York: Mentor Books.

Mosse, G.L. (1978). *Toward the final solution: A history of European racism*. New York: Howard Fertig.

Myers, L.J. (1988). *Understanding an Afrocentric world view: Introduction to an optimal psychology*. Dubuque, IA: Kendall/Hunt Publishing Company.

National Opinion Research Center (1994). *General social survey*. Chicago, IL: National Opinion Research Center.

Plato (1992). *Republic* (G.M.A. Grube, Trans.). Indianapolis, IN: Hackett Publishing Company.

Rose, N. (1989). The political economy of welfare. *Journal of Sociology and Social Welfare*, 16(2), 87-108.

Rothenberg, P. (1990). The construction, deconstruction, and reconstruction of difference. *Hypatia*, 5(1), 42-57.

Schiele, J.H. (1993). Cultural oppression, African Americans, and social work practice. *Black Caucus: Journal of the National Association of black Social Workers*, Fall(2), 20-34.

Schiele, J.H. (1994). Afrocentricity as an alternative world view for equality. *Journal of Progressive Human Services*, 5(1), 5-25.

Schiele, J.H. (1996). Afrocentricity: An emerging paradigm in social work practice. *Social Work*, 41(3), 284-294.

Schiele, J.H. (1997). The contour and meaning of Afrocentric social work. *Journal of Black Studies*, 27(6), 800-819.

Sermabeikian, P. (1994). Our clients, ourselves: The spiritual perspective and social work practice. *Social Work*, 39(2), 178-183.

Smith, J.K. (1993). *After the demise of empiricism*. Norwood, NJ: Ablex Publishing Company.

Swigonski, M.E. (1996). Challenging privilege through Afrocentric social work practice. *Social Work*, 41(2), 153-161.

Turner, J.H., Singleton, R., and Musick, D. (1984). *Oppression: A socio-history of black-white relations in America*. Chicago, IL: Nelson-Hall.

Van Sertima, I. (Ed.) (1989). *Nile Valley civilizations*. Atlanta, GA: Morehouse College.

Verharen, C.C. (1995). Afrocentrism and acentrism: A marriage of science and philosophy. *Journal of Black Studies*, 26(1), 62-76.

Wakefield, J.C. (1993). Is altruism part of human nature? Toward a theoretical foundation for the helping professions. *Social Service Review*, 67(3), 406-458.

Wayne, J. (1986). The function of social welfare in a capitalist economy. In J. Dickinson and B. Russell (Eds.), *Family, economy, and state: The social reproduction process under capitalism* (pp. 56-84). London: Croom Helm, Ltd.

West, C. (1982). *Prophesy deliverance*. Louisville, KY: Westminster Press.

Westgate, C.E. (1996). Spiritual wellness and depression. *Journal of Counseling and Development*, 75(1), 26-35.

Williams, E. (1944). *Capitalism and slavery*. Chapel Hill, NC: University of North Carolina.

Wolk, S.I. and Weissman, M.M. (1996). Suicidal behavior in depressed children grown up: Preliminary results of a longitudinal study. *Psychiatric Annals*, 26(6), 331-335.

Young, I.M. (1990). *Justice and the politics of difference*. Princeton, NJ: Princeton University Press.

Chapter 5

Akbar, N. (1981). Mental disorder among African Americans. *Black Books Bulletin*, 7(2), 18-25.

Akbar, N. (1984). Afrocentric social sciences for human liberation. *Journal of Black Studies*, 14(4), 395-414.

Akbar, N. (1991). *Visions for black men*. Nashville, TN: Winston-Derek Publishers, Inc.

Akbar, N. (1996). *Breaking the chains of psychological slavery.* Tallahassee, FL: Mind Productions and Associates.

Amato, P.R. and Rezac, S.J. (1994). Contact with nonresident parents, interparental conflict, and children's behavior. *Journal of Family Issues*, 15(2), 191-207.

Amy, D.J. (1993). *Real choices/new voices: The case for proportional representation elections in the United States.* New York: Columbia University Press.

Ani, M. (1994). *Yurugu: An African-centered critique of European cultural thought and behavior.* Trenton, NJ: Africa World Press.

Asante, M.K. (1988). *Afrocentricity.* Trenton, NJ: Africa World Press.

Asante, M.K. (1991). The Afrocentric idea in education. *Journal of Negro Education*, 60(2), 170-180.

Azibo, D. (1991). Towards a metatheory of African personality. *Journal of Black Psychology*, 17(2), 37-45.

Baldwin, J. (1985). Psychological aspects of European cosmology in American society. *The Western Journal of Black Studies*, 9(4), 216-223.

Baldwin, J. (1991, October). *An Afrocentric perspective on health and social behavior of African American males.* Paper presented at the National Conference on Health and Social Behavior of African American Males, Institute for Urban Affairs and Research, Washington, DC.

Baldwin, J.A. and Bell, Y. (1985). The African self-consciousness scale: An Afrocentric personality questionnaire. *The Western Journal of Black Studies*, 9(2), 62-68.

Baldwin, J. and Hopkins, R. (1990). African-American and European-American cultural differences as assessed by the worldviews paradigm: An empirical analysis. *The Western Journal of Black Studies*, 14(1), 38-52.

Belgrave, F.Z., Cherry, V.R., Cunningham, D., Walwyn, S., Letlaka-Rennert, K., and Phillips, F. (1994). The influence of Africentric values, self-esteem, and black identity on drug attitudes among African American fifth graders: A preliminary study. *The Journal of Black Psychology*, 20(2), 143-156.

Bell, Y.R. (1994). A culturally sensitive analysis of black learning style. *Journal of Black Psychology*, 20(1), 47-61.

Bell, Y.R., Bouie, C.L., and Baldwin, J.A. (1990). Afrocentric cultural consciousness and African-American male-female relationships. *Journal of Black Studies*, 21(2), 162-189.

Bensley, R.J. (1991). Defining spiritual health: A review of the literature. *Journal of Health Education*, 22(5), 287-290.

Billingsley, A. (1968). *Black families in white America.* Englewood Cliffs, NJ: Prentice-Hall.

Billingsley, A. (1970). Black families and white social science. *Journal of Social Issues*, 26(3), 127-142.

Billingsley, A. (1994). *Climbing Jacob's ladder: The enduring legacy of African families.* New York: Simon and Schuster.

Bowman, P.J. (1995). Family structure and marginalization of black men: Policy implications/commentary. In M.B. Tucker and C. Mitchell-Kernan (Eds.), *The decline of marriage among African Americans: Causes, consequences, and policy implications* (pp. 309-323). New York: Russell Sage.

Bradley, M. (1991). *The iceman inheritance: Prehistoric sources of western man's racism, sexism, and aggression.* New York: Kayode Publications LTD.

Brookins, C.C. (1996). Promoting ethnic identity development in African American youth: The role of rites of passage. *Journal of Black Psychology*, 22(3), 388-417.

Brown, D.R., Gary, L.E., Greene, A.D., and Milburn, N.G. (1992). Patterns of social affiliation as predictors of depressive symptoms among urban blacks. *Journal of Health and Social Behavior*, 33(September), 242-253.

Burgest, D.R. (1981). Theory on white supremacy and black oppression. *Black Books Bulletin*, 7(2), 26-30.

Canda, E.R. (Ed.) (1998). *Spirituality in social work: New directions.* Binghamton, NY: The Haworth Press, Inc.

Carten, A.J. and Dumpson, J. (1998). *Removing risks from children: Shifting the paradigm for the 21ˢᵗ century.* Silver Spring, MD: Beckham House Press.

Centerwall, B.S. (1984). Race, socioeconomic status, and domestic homicide, Atlanta, 1971-2. *American Journal of Public Health*, 74(8), 813-815.

Charren, P. (1995). A public policy perspective on televised violence and youth: From a conversation with Peggy Charren. *Harvard Educational Review*, 65(2), 282-291.

Cohen, G. (1996). Toward a spirituality based on justice and ecology. *Social Policy*, 26(3), 6-18.

Daly, A., Jennings, J., Beckett, J., and Leashore, B. (1995). Effective coping strategies of African Americans. *Social Work*, 40(2), 240-248.

Day, P.J. (1997). *A new history of social welfare* (Second edition). Boston, MA: Allyn and Bacon.

Diop, C.A. (1978). *The cultural unity of black Africa: The domains of patriarchy and of matriarchy in classical antiquity.* Chicago, IL: Third World Press.

Dixon, V. (1976). World views and research methodology. In L. King, V. Dixon, and W. Nobles (Eds.), *African philosophy: Assumptions and paradigms for research on black persons*, (pp. 51-93). Los Angeles, CA: Fanon Center Publications.

Dove, N. (1996). Understanding education for cultural affirmation. In E.K. Addae (Ed.), *To heal a people: African scholars defining a new reality* (pp. 269-298). Columbia, MD: Kujichagulia Press.

DuCharme, J., Koverola, C., and Battle, P. (1997). Intimacy development: The influence of abuse and gender. *Journal of Interpersonal Violence*, 12(4), 590-599.

Dudley, J. (1991). Increasing our understanding of fathers who have infrequent contact with their children. *Journal of Family Relations*, 4(3), 281-291.

Fanon, F. (1961). *Black skin, white masks.* New York: Grove Press.

Fergusson, D.M. and Lynskey, M.T. (1997). Physical punishment/maltreatment during childhood and adjustment in young adulthood. *Child Abuse and Neglect*, 21(7), 617-630.

Gary, L.E. (Ed.) (1981). *Black men.* Thousand Oaks, CA: Sage.

Gary, L.E. (1985). Depressive symptoms and black men. *Social Work Research and Abstracts*, 21(4), 21-29.

Gary, L.E. and Booker, C.B. (1992, October). Empowering African Americans to achieve academic success. *NASSP Bulletin*, 50-55.

Gary, L.E. and Leashore, B.R. (1982). High-risk status of black men. *Social Work*, 27(1), 54-58.

Gelles, R.J. (1989). Child abuse and violence in single parent families: Parent absence and economic deprivation. *American Journal of Orthopsychiatry*, 59(4), 492-502.

Gelles, R.J. and Conte, J.R. (1990). Domestic violence and sexual abuse of children: A review of research in the eighties. *Journal of Marriage and the Family*, 52(4), 1045-1058.

Ghee, K.L. (1990). Enhancing educational achievement through cultural awareness in young black males. *The Western Journal of Black Studies*, 14(2), 77-89.

Hale-Benson, J. (1982). *Black children: Their roots, culture, and learning styles*. Provo, UT: Brigham Young University Press.

Hall, L.K. (1981). Support systems and coping patterns. In L.E. Gary (Ed.), *Black men* (pp. 159-167). Thousand Oaks, CA: Sage.

Harvey, A.R. and Rauch, J.B. (1997). A comprehensive Afrocentric rites of passage program for black male adolescents. *Health and Social Work*, 22(1), 30-37.

Hill, H.M., Soriano, F.I., Chen, S.A., and LaFromboise, T.D. (1994). Sociocultural factors in the etiology and prevention of violence among ethnic minority youth. In L.D. Eron and J.H. Gentry (Eds.), *Reason to hope: A psychosocial perspective on violence and youth* (pp. 59-97). Washington, DC: American Psychological Association.

Hilton, N.Z., Harris, G.T., and Rice, M.E. (1998). On the validity of self-reported rates of interpersonal violence. *Journal of Interpersonal Violence*, 13(1), 58-72.

Jackson, A.P. (1999). The effects of nonresident father involvement on single black mothers and their young children. *Social Work*, 44(2), 156-166.

Jagers, R.J. and Owens-Mock, L. (1993). Culture and social outcomes among inner-city African American children: An afrographic exploration. *The Journal of Black Psychology*, 19(4), 391-405.

Jansson, B.S. (1994). *Social policy: From theory to policy practice* (Second edition). Pacific Grove, CA: Brooks/Cole.

Jansson, B.S. (1997). *The reluctant welfare state: A history of American social welfare policies* (Third edition)). Pacific Grove, CA: Brooks/Cole.

Jeff, M.F.X. (1994). Afrocentrism and African-American male youths. In R.B. Muncy (Ed.), *Nurturing young black males* (pp. 99-118). Washington, DC: The Urban Institute Press.

Jewell, K.S. (1988). *Survival of the black family: The institutional impact of American social policy*. New York: Praeger.

Jung, M. (1996). Family-centered practice with single-parent families. *Families in Society*, 77(9), 583-590.

Kambon, K. (1992). *The African personality in America: An African-centered framework*. Tallahassee, FL: Nubian Nation Publication.

Karenga, M. (1993). *Introduction to black studies* (Second edition). Los Angeles, CA: University of Sankore Press.

Karenga, M. (1996). The nguzo saba (the seven principles): Their meaning and message. In M.K. Asante and A.S. Abarry (Eds.), *African intellectual heritage* (pp. 543-554). Philadelphia, PA: Temple University Press.

Kershaw, T. (1992). Afrocentrism and the Afrocentric method. *The Western Journal of Black Studies*, 16(3), 160-168.

King, A.E. (1997). Understanding violence among young African American males: An Afrocentric perspective. *Journal of Black Studies*, 28(1), 79-96.

King, V. (1994). Variation in the consequences of nonresident father involvement for children's well-being. *Journal of Marriage and the Family*, 56(4), 963-972.

Kotz, D.M. (1995). Lessons for a future socialism from the Soviet collapse. *Review of Radical Political Economics*, 27(3), 1-11.

Kunjufu, J. (1984). *Countering the conspiracy to destroy black boys* (Volume 1) Chicago, IL: African American Images.

Lemelle, A.J. (1991). "Betcha cain't reason with 'em": Bad black boys in America. In B.P. Bowser (Ed.), *Black male adolescents: Parenting and education in community context* (pp. 91-128). Lanham, MD: University Press of America.

Litty, C.G., Kowalski, R., and Minor, S. (1996). Moderating effects of physical abuse and perceived social support on the potential to abuse. *Child Abuse and Neglect*, 20(4), 305-314.

Longres, J.F. (1995). *Human behavior in the social environment* (Second edition). Itasca, IL: F.E. Peacock.

Lowry, R., Sleet, D., Duncan, C., Powell, K., and Kolbe, L. (1995). Adolescents at risk for violence. *Educational Psychology Review*, 7(1), 7-39.

Madhubuti, H.R. (1990). *Black men obsolete, single, dangerous? Afrikan American families in transition: Essays in discovery, solution, and hope*. Chicago, IL: Third World Press.

Majors, R. and Billson, J.M. (1992). *Cool pose: The dilemmas of black manhood in America*. New York: Lexington Books.

Myers, L.J. (1988). *Understanding an Afrocentric world view: Introduction to an optimal psychology*. Dubuque, IA: Kendall/Hunt Publishing Company.

Myers, S.L. and Drescher, P.J. (1994, March). *The economics of violent crime*. Paper presented at the annual black Family Conference, Hampton University, Hampton, VA.

Newman, B.M. and Newman, P.R. (1991). *Development through life: A psychosocial approach*. Pacific Grove, CA: Brooks/Cole.

Nobles, W.W. (1974). Africanity: Its role in black families. *The Black Scholar*, 5(9), 10-17.

Nobles, W.W. (1980). African philosophy: Foundations for black psychology. In R. Jones (Ed.), *Black psychology* (Third edition) (pp. 23-35). New York: Harper & Row.

Ogbu, J.U. (1978). *Minority education and caste: The American system in cross-cultural perspective*. New York: Academic Press.

Ogbu, J.U. (1988). Black education: A cultural-ecological perspective. In H.P. McAdoo (Ed.), *Black families* (Second edition) (pp. 169-184). Thousand Oaks, CA: Sage.

Oliver, W. (1989). Black males and social problems: Prevention through Afrocentric socialization. *Journal of Black Studies*, 20(1), 15-39.

Price, J.H. and Everett, S.A. (1997). A national assessment of secondary school principals' perceptions of violence in schools. *Health Education and Behavior*, 24(2), 218-229.

Rodriquez, N., Ryan, S.W., Vande Kemp, H., and Foy, D.W. (1997). Post-traumatic stress disorder in adult female survivors of child sexual abuse: A comparison study. *Journal of Consulting and Clinical Psychology*, 65(1), 53-59.

Sampson, R.J. (1993). The community context of violent crime. In W.J. Wilson (Ed.), *Sociology and the public agency* (pp. 259-286). Thousand Oaks, CA: Sage.

Schiele, J.H. (1994). Afrocentricity as an alternative world view for equality. *Journal of Progressive Human Services*, 5(1), 5-25.

Schiele, J.H. (1996). Afrocentricity: An emerging paradigm in social work practice. *Social Work*, 41(3), 284-294.

Schiele, J.H. (1998). Cultural alignment, African-American male youths, and violent crime. *Journal of Human Behavior in the Social Environment*, 1(2/3), 165-181.

Schooler, C. and Flora, J.A. (1996). Pervasive media violence. *Annual Review of Public Health*, 17, 275-299.

Sermabeikian, P. (1994). Our clients, ourselves: The spiritual perspective and social work practice. *Social Work*, 39(2), 178-183.

Shujaa, M. (Ed.) (1994). *Too much schooling, too little education*. Lawrenceville, NJ: Africa World Press.

Steele, D.R. (1996). Between immorality and unfeasibility: The market socialist predicament. *Critical Review*, 10(3), 307-331.

Strasburger, V. (1995). *Adolescents and the media: Medical and psychological impact*. Thousand Oaks, CA: Sage.

Sudarkasa, N. (1997). African American families and family values. In H.P. McAdoo (Ed.), *Black families* (Third edition) (pp. 9-40). Thousand Oaks, CA: Sage.

Thomas, G., Farrell, M.P., and Barnes, G.M. (1996). The effects of single-mother families and nonresident fathers on delinquency and substance abuse in black and white adolescents. *Journal of Marriage and the Family*, 58(4), 884-894.

Trattner, W.I. (1994). *From poor law to welfare state* (Fifth edition). New York: The Free Press.

U.S. Bureau of the Census (1998). *Statistical abstract of the United States, 1998*. Washington, DC: U.S. Government Printing Office.

U.S. Department of Justice, Federal Bureau of Investigation (1998). *Uniform crime reports for the United States, 1997*. Washington, DC: U.S. Government Printing Office.

Vosler, N.R. and Proctor, E.K. (1991). Family structure and stressors in a child guidance clinic population. *Families in Society*, 72(3), 164-173.

Ward, J.V. (1995). Cultivating a morality of care in African American adolescents: A culture-based model of violence prevention. *Harvard Educational Review*, 65(2), 175-188.

Warfield-Coppock, N. (1992). The rites of passage movement: A resurgence of African-centered practices for socializing African American youth. *Journal of Negro Education*, 61(4), 471-482.

Wass, H., Raup, J., and Sisler, H. (1989). Adolescents and death on television: A follow-up study. *Death Studies*, 13(2), 161-173.

Webber, J. (1997). Comprehending youth violence: A practicable perspective. *Remedial and Special Education*, 18(2), 94-104.

Welsing, F.C. (1991). *The Isis papers: The keys to the colors*. Chicago, IL: Third World Press.

Wilson, A.N. (1990). *Black-on-black violence: The psychodynamics of black self-annihilation in the service of white domination*. New York: Afrikan World Infosystems.

Wilson, A.N. (1992). *Understanding black adolescent male violence: Its remediation and prevention*. New York: Afrikan World Infosystems.

Wilson, W.J. (1996). *When work disappears: The world of the new urban poor*. New York: Knopf.

Young, I.M. (1990). *Justice and the politics of difference*. Princeton, NJ: Princeton University Press.

Zastrow, C. and Kirst-Ashman, K. (1997). *Understanding human behavior and the social environment* (Fourth edition). Chicago, IL: Nelson-Hall.

Zimmerman, J.D. (1996). A prosocial media strategy: "Youth against violence: Choose to de-fuse." *American Journal of Orthopsychiatry*, 66(3), 354-362.

Zimmerman, M.A. and Maton, K.I. (1992). Lifestyle and substance use among male African-American urban adolescents: A cluster analytic approach. *American Journal of Community Psychology*, 20(1), 121-138.

Zimmerman, M.A., Salem, D.A., and Maton, K.I. (1995). Family structure and psychosocial correlates among urban African-American adolescent males. *Child Development*, 66(December), 1598-1613.

Chapter 6

Abdullah, A.K. (1998). *A comparative analysis of adolescent African American drug users and drug dealers on the benefits and liabilities of drugs and locus of control*. Doctoral dissertation, Howard University, Washington, DC.

Akbar, N. (1984). *Chains and images of psychological slavery*. Jersey City, NJ: New Mind Productions and Associates.

Akbar, N. (1991). *Visions for black men*. Nashville, TN: Winston-Derek Publishers, Inc.

Akbar, N. (1994). *Light from ancient Africa.* Tallahassee, FL: Mind Productions and Associates.

Akbar, N. (1996). *Breaking the chains of psychological slavery.* Tallahassee, FL: Mind Productions and Associates.

Ameen, R.U.N. (1990). *Metu neter,* Volume 1. Bronx, NY: Khamit Corporation.

Ani, M. (1994). *Yurugu: An African-centered critique of European cultural thought and behavior.* Trenton, NJ: Africa World Press.

Asante, M.K. (1987). *The Afrocentric idea.* Philadelphia, PA: Temple University Press.

Asante, M.K. (1988). *Afrocentricity.* Trenton, NJ: Africa World Press.

Asante, M.K. (1990). *Kemet, Afrocentricity, and knowledge.* Trenton, NJ: Africa World Press.

Assagioli, R. (1965). *Psychosynthesis: A manual of principles and techniques.* New York: Viking Penguin.

Bachman, J.G., Wallace, J.M, O'Malley, P.M., Johnston, L.D., Kurth, C.L., and Neighbors, H.W. (1991). Racial/ethnic differences in smoking, drinking, and illicit drug use among American high school seniors, 1976-1989. *American Journal of Public Health,* 81(3), 372-377.

Barnes, C.W. and Kingsnorth, R. (1996). Race, drug, and criminal sentencing: Hidden effects of the criminal law. *Journal of Criminal Justice,* 24(1), 39-55.

Belgrave, F.Z., Cherry, V.R., Cunningham, D., Walwyn, S., Letlaka-Rennert, K., and Phillips, F. (1994). The influence of Afrocentric values, self-esteem, and black identity on drug attitudes among African American fifth graders: A preliminary study. *The Journal of Black Psychology,* 20(2), 143-156.

Bell, D. (1992). *Faces at the bottom of the well.* New York: Basic Books.

Block, C.J. and Carter, R.T. (1996). White racial identity attitude theories: A rose by any other name is still a rose. *Counseling Psychologist,* 24(2), 326-334.

Block, C.J. and Carter, R.T. (1998). White racial identity: Theory, research, and implications for organizational contexts. In A. Daly (Ed.), *Workplace diversity, issues, and perspectives* (pp. 265-280). Washington, DC: National Association of Social Workers.

Bourgois, P. (1995). *In search of respect: Selling crack in el barrio.* New York: Cambridge University Press.

Brisbane, F.L. and Womble, M. (Ed.) (1985). *Treatment of black alcoholics.* Binghamton, New York: The Haworth Press, Inc.

Brisbane, F.L. and Womble, M. (1991). *Working with African Americans: The professional's handbook.* Chicago, IL: HRDI International Press.

Brookins, C.C. (1996). Promoting ethnic identity development in African American youth: The role of rites of passage. *Journal of Black Psychology,* 22(3), 388-417.

Caetano, R. and Clark, C.L. (1998a). Trends in alcohol-related problems among whites, Blacks, and Hispanics: 1984-1995. *Alcoholism: Clinical and Experimental Research,* 22(2), 534-538.

Caetano, R. and Clark, C.L. (1998b). Trends in alcohol consumption patterns among whites, Blacks, and Hispanics: 1984-1995. *Journal of Studies on Alcohol*, 59(6), 659-668.

Carroll, S. (1993). Spirituality and purpose in life in alcoholism recovery. *Journal of Studies on Alcohol*, 54(3), 297-301.

Chandler, C.K., Holden, J.M., and Kolander, C.A. (1992). Counseling for spiritual wellness: Theory and practice. *Journal of Counseling and Development*, 71(2), 168-175.

Chen, K. and Kandel, D.B. (1995). The natural history of drug use from adolescence to the mid-thirties in a general population sample. *American Journal of Public Health*, 85(1), 41-47.

Chickerneo, N.B. (1993). *Portraits of spirituality in recovery: The use of art in recovery from co-dependency and/or chemical dependency*. Springfield, IL: Charles C Thomas.

Christmon, K. (1995). Historical overview of alcoholism in the African American community. *Journal of Black Studies*, 25(3), 318-330.

Day, P.J. (1997). *A new history of social welfare* (Second edition). Boston, MA: Allyn and Bacon.

Dixon, P. and Azibo, D. (1998). African self-consciousness, misorientation behavior, and a self-destructive disorder: African American male crack-cocaine users. *Journal of Black Psychology*, 24(2), 226-247.

Dubois, W.E.B. (1935). *Black reconstruction in America—1860-1880*. New York: Russell and Russell.

Eckersley, R.M. (1993). The West's deepening cultural crisis. *The Futurist*, 27(6), 8-12.

Elkins, D.N. (1995). Psychotherapy and spirituality: Toward a theory of the soul. *Journal of Humanistic Psychology*, 35(2), 78-88.

Foulks, E.F., and Pena, J.M. (1995). Ethnicity and psychotherapy: A component in the treatment of cocaine addiction in African Americans. *The Psychiatric Clinics of North America*, 18(3), 607-620.

Franklin, D.L. (1997). *Ensuring inequality: The structural transformation of the African American family*. New York: Oxford University Press.

Free, M.D. (1997). The impact of federal sentencing reforms on African Americans. *Journal of Black Studies*, 28(2), 268-286.

Fromm, E. (1941). *Escape from freedom*. New York: Rinehart and Company.

Fudge, R.C. (1996). The use of behavioral therapy in the development of ethnic consciousness: A treatment model. *Cognitive and Behavioral Practice*, 3(2), 317-335.

Gary, L.E. and Berry, G.L. (1985). Predicting attitudes toward substance use in a black community: Implications for prevention. *Community Mental Health Journal*, 21(1), 42-51.

Goodman, J., Lovejoy, P.E., and Sherratt, A. (Eds.) (1995). *Consuming habits: Drugs in history and anthropology*. New York: Routledge and Kegan Paul.

Gordon, D.M. (1996). Underpaid workers, bloated corporations: Two pieces in the puzzle of U.S. economic decline. *Dissent*, 43(2), 23-34.

Grant, D., Martinez, D.G., and White, B.W. (1998). Substance abuse among African American children: A developmental framework for identifying intervention strategies. *Journal of Human Behavior in the Social Environment*, 1(2/3), 137-163.

Hall, M.F. (1997). The "war on drugs": A continuation of the war on the African American family. *Smith College Studies in Social Work*, 67(3), 609-621.

Haronian, F. (1972). *Repression of the sublime*. New York: Psychosynthesis Research Foundation.

Harvey, A.R., and Rauch, J.B. (1997). A comprehensive Afrocentric rites of passage program for black male adolescents. *Health and Social Work*, 22(1), 30-37.

Helms, J.E. (Ed.) (1990a). *Black and white racial identity: Theory, research, and practice*. New York: Greenwood Press.

Helms, J.E. (1990b). Toward a model of white racial identity development. In J.E. Helms (Ed.), *Black and white racial identity: Theory, research, and practice* (pp. 49-66). New York: Greenwood Press.

Henderson, E.A. (1997). The lumpenproletariat as vanguard? The black panther party, social transformation, and Pearson's analysis of Huey Newton. *Journal of Black Studies*, 28(2), 171-199.

Horton, R. (1993). *Patterns of thought in Africa and the west: Essays on magic, religion and science*. New York: Cambridge University Press.

Jackson, M.S. (1995). Afrocentric treatment of African American women and their children in a residential chemical dependency program. *Journal of Black Studies*, 26(1), 17-30.

Jackson, M.S., Stephens, R.C., and Smith, R.L. (1997). Afrocentric treatment in residential substance abuse care. *Journal of Substance Abuse Treatment*, 14(1), 87-92.

Jacobs, C.C. and Bowles, D.D. (Eds.) (1988). *Ethnicity and race: Critical concepts in social work*. Washington, DC: National Association of Social Workers.

Jansson, B.S. (1997). *The reluctant welfare state: A history of American social welfare policies* (Third edition). Pacific Grove, CA: Brooks/Cole.

Jeff, M.F.X. (1994). Afrocentrism and African-American male youths. In R.B. Muncy (Ed.), *Nurturing young black males* (pp. 99-118). Washington, DC: The Urban Institute Press.

Jhally, S. and Lewis, J. (1992). *Enlightened racism: The Cosby Show, audiences, and the myth of the American dream*. Boulder, CO: Westview Press.

Johnson, D. (1994). Stress, depression, substance abuse, and racism. *American Indian and Alaska Native Mental Health Research*, 6(1), 29-33.

Johnston, L., O'Malley, P., and Bachman, J. (1998). *National survey results on drug use from the monitoring the future study, 1975-1998*. Washington, DC: National Institute on Drug Abuse.

Kallan, J.E. (1998). Drug abuse-related mortality in the United States: Patterns and correlates. *American Journal of Drug and Alcohol Abuse*, 24(1), 103-117.

Kambon, K. (1992). *The African personality in America: An African-centered framework*. Tallahassee, FL: Nubian Nation Publication.

Karenga, M. (1986). Social ethics and the black family: An alternative analysis. *The Black Scholar*, 17(5), 41-54.

Karenga, M. (1993). *Introduction to black studies* (Second edition). Los Angeles, CA: University of Sankore Press.

Kasee, C.R. (1995). Identity, recovery, and religious imperialism: Native American women and the new age. *Women and Therapy*, 16(2/3), 83-93.

Labouvie, E., Bates, M.E., and Pandina, R.J. (1997). Age of first use: Its reliability and predictive utility. *Journal of Studies on Alcohol*, 58(6), 638-643.

Lemelle, A.J. (1995). *Black male deviance*. Westport, CT: Praeger.

Lewis, O. (1969). The culture of poverty. In D.P. Moynihan (Ed.), *On understanding poverty: Perspectives from the social sciences* (pp. 187-200). New York: Basic Books.

Li, G.H., Keyl, P.M., Rothman, R., Chanmugam, A., and Kelen, G.D. (1998). Epidemiology of alcohol-related emergency department visits. *Academic Emergency Medicine*, 5(8), 788-795.

Linsky, A.S., Colby, J.P., and Straus, M.A. (1987). Social stress, normative constraints and alcohol problems in American states. *Social Science and Medicine*, 24(10), 875-883.

Longshore, D., Grills, C., Annon, K., and Grady, R. (1998). Promoting recovery from drug abuse: An Afrocentric intervention. *Journal of Black Studies*, 28(3), 319-333.

Lusane, C. (1991). *Pipe dream blues: Racism and the war on drugs*. Boston, MA: South End Press.

Martin, J.M. and Martin, E.P. (1985). *The helping tradition in the black family and community*. Washington, DC: National Association of Social Workers.

Mathew, R.J., Georgi, J., Wilson, W.H., and Mathew, G.V. (1996). A retrospective study of the concept of spirituality as understood by recovering individuals. *Journal of Substance Abuse Treatment*, 13(1), 67-73.

Maton, K.I. and Zimmerman, M.A. (1992). Psychosocial predictors of substance use among urban black male adolescents: Cross-sectional and prospective analyses. *Drugs and Society*, 6, 79-113.

Mauer, M. (1997). *Intended and unintended consequences: State racial disparities in imprisonment*. Washington, DC: The Sentencing Project.

Mauer, M. (1999, March 3). Prisons and drugs (e-mail communication). Washington, DC: The Sentencing Project.

Mauer, M. and Huling, T. (1995). *Young black Americans and the criminal justice system: Five years later*. Washington, DC: The Sentencing Project.

May, R. (1977). *The meaning of anxiety*. New York: W.W. Norton and Company.

Mbiti, J. (1970). *African religions and philosophy*. Garden City, NY: Anchor Books.

Moore, S.E. (1995). Adolescent black males' drug trafficking and addiction: Three theoretical perspectives. *Journal of Black Studies*, 26(2), 99-116.

Morell, C. (1996). Radicalizing recovery: Addiction, spirituality, and politics. *Social Work*, 41(3), 306-312.

Muhammad, E. (1965). *Message to the black man.* Chicago, IL: The Nation of Islam.

Myers, L.J. (1988). *Understanding an Afrocentric world view: Introduction to an optimal psychology.* Dubuque, IA: Kendall/Hunt Publishing Company.

Ngozi-Brown, S. (1997). The Us organization, Maulana Karenga, and conflict with the black panther party: A critique of sectarian influences on historical discourse. *Journal of Black Studies,* 28(2), 157-170.

Nobles, W.W. (1984). Alienation, human transformation and adolescent drug use: Toward a reconceptualization of the problem. *Journal of Drug Issues,* 14(2), 243-252.

Nobles, W.W. (1986). Ancient Egyptian thought and the renaissance of African (black) psychology. In M. Karenga and J.H. Carruthers (Eds.), *Kemet and the African worldview: Research, rescue, and restoration* (pp. 100-118). Los Angeles, CA: University of Sankore Press.

Novak, J. (1989). *How to meditate.* Nevada City, CA: Crystal Clarity.

Oliver, W. (1989). Black males and social problems: Prevention through Afrocentric socialization. *Journal of Black Studies,* 20(1), 15-39.

O'Reilly, K. (1989). *"Racial matters": The FBI's secret file on black America, 1960-1972.* New York: The Free Press.

Pfeil, F. (1997). Sympathy for the devils: Notes on some white guys in the ridiculous class war. In M. Hill (Ed.), *Whiteness: A critical reader* (pp. 21-34). New York: New York University Press.

Philleo, J., Brisbane, F.L., and Epstein, L. (1997). *Cultural competence in substance abuse prevention.* Washington, DC: National Association of Social Workers.

Phillips, F.B. (1990). NTU psychotherapy: An Afrocentric approach. *The Journal of Black Psychology,* 17(1), 55-74.

Prendergast, M.L., Austin, G.A., Maton, K.I., and Baker, R. (1989). Substance abuse among black youth. *Prevention Research Update,* 4(1), 1-27.

Quadagno, J. (1994). *The color of welfare: How racism undermined the war on poverty.* New York: Oxford University Press.

Reese, L.E., Vera, E.M., and Paikoff, R.L. (1998). Ethnic identity assessment among inner-city African American children: Evaluating the applicability of the multigroup ethnic identity measure. *Journal of Black Psychology,* 24(3), 289-304.

Rifkin, J. (1995). *The end of work: The decline of the global labor force and the dawn of the post-market era.* New York: G.P. Putnam's Sons.

Riley, K.J. (1997). *Crack, powder cocaine, and heroin: Drug purchase and use patterns in six U.S. cities.* Washington, DC: National Institute of Justice and Office of National Drug Control Policy.

Rowe, D. and Grills, C. (1993). African-centered drug treatment: An alternative conceptual paradigm for drug counseling with African-American clients. *Journal of Psychoactive Drugs,* 25(1), 21-33.

Rowe, W., Bennett, S.K., and Atkinson, D.R. (1994). White racial identity models: A critique and alternative proposal. *Counseling Psychologist*, 22(1), 129-146.

Schiele, J.H. (1996). Afrocentricity: An emerging paradigm in social work practice. *Social Work*, 41(3), 284-294.

Schiele, J.H. (1997). The contour and meaning of Afrocentric social work. *Journal of Black Studies*, 27(6), 800-819.

Schiele, J.H. (1998). The personal responsibility act of 1996: The bitter and the sweet for African American families. *Families in Society*, 79(4), 424-432.

Semmes, C.E. (1993). Religion and the challenge of Afrocentric thought. *The Western Journal of Black Studies*, 17(3), 158-163.

The Sentencing Project (1997). *On the latest proposals to adjust the disparity in crack and powder cocaine sentencing: Political process highlights arbitrary character of legislated mandatory minimum sentences.* Washington, DC: The Sentencing Project.

Shine, C. and Mauer, M. (1993). *Does the punishment fit the crime? Drug users and drunk drivers: Questions of race and class.* Washington, DC: The Sentencing Project.

Tart, C.T. (1990). Adapting eastern spiritual teachings to western culture. *Journal of Transpersonal Psychology*, 22(2), 149-166.

U.S. Bureau of the Census (1998). *Statistical abstract of the United States, 1998.* Washington, DC: U.S. Government Printing Office.

U.S. Department of Justice, Federal Bureau of Investigation (1995a). *Uniform crime reports for the United States, 1994.* Washington, DC: U.S. Government Printing Office.

U.S. Department of Justice, Federal Bureau of Investigation (1995b). *Supplementary homicide reports, 1994.* Washington, DC: U.S. Government Printing Office.

U.S. Department of Justice, Federal Bureau of Investigation (1996). *Uniform crime reports for the United States, 1995.* Washington, DC: U.S. Government Printing Office.

U.S. Sentencing Commission (1995). *Special report to congress: Cocaine and federal sentencing policy.* Washington, DC: U.S. Government Printing Office.

Walker, W.T. (1995). *Somebody's calling my name.* New York: Judson Press.

Walters, R. (1995). The impact of *bell curve* ideology on African American public policy. *American Behavioral Scientist*, 39(1), 98-108.

Ward, J.V. (1995). Cultivating a morality of care in African American adolescents: A culture-based model of violence prevention. *Harvard Educational Review*, 65(2), 175-188.

Watkins, E. (1997). Essay on spirituality. *Journal of Substance Abuse Treatment*, 14(6), 581-583.

Webb, G. (1996, August 18). America's "crack" plague has roots in Nicaragua war: Colombia-San Francisco bay area drug pipeline helped finance CIA-backed contras. *Mercury Center and San Jose Mercury News.*

Welsing, F.C. (1991). *The Isis papers: The keys to the colors.* Chicago, IL: Third World Press.

Westermeyer, J. (1995). Cultural aspects of substance abuse and alcoholism: Assessment and management. *The Psychiatric Clinics of North America*, 18(3), 589-605.

Willhelm, S. (1970). *Who needs the Negro?* Cambridge, MA: Schenkman Press.

Williams, R.L. (Ed.) (1973). *Ebonics: The true language of black folks.* St Louis, MO: Robert L. Willams and Associates.

Williams, R.L. (1997). The ebonics controversy. *Journal of Black Psychology*, 23(3), 208-214.

Wilson, A.N. (1990). *Black-on-black violence: The psychodynamics of black self-annihilation in service of white domination.* New York: Afrikan World Infosystems.

Wilson, W.J. (1987). *The truly disadvantaged: The inner city, the underclass, and public policy.* Chicago, IL: University of Chicago Press.

Wilson, W.J. (1996). *When work disappears: The world of the new urban poor.* New York: Knopf.

Zimmerman, M.A. and Maton, K.I. (1992). Lifestyle and substance use among male African-American urban adolescents: A cluster analytic approach. *American Journal of Community Psychology*, 20(1), 121-138.

Chapter 7

Abramovitz, M. (1996). *Regulating the lives of women: Social welfare policy from colonial times to the present* (Revised edition.). Boston, MA: South End Press.

Akbar, N. (1984). Afrocentric social sciences for human liberation. *Journal of Black Studies*, 14(4), 395-414.

Akbar, N. (1994). *Light from ancient Africa.* Tallahassee, FL: Mind Productions and Associates.

Akbar, N. (1996). *Breaking the chains of psychological slavery.* Tallahassee, FL: Mind Productions and Associates. and Associates.

Allen, R.L. (1998). Past due: The African American quest for reparations. *Black Scholar*, 28(2), 2-17.

Amott, T.L. and Matthaei, J.A. (1991). *Race, gender, and work: A multicultural economic history of women in the United States.* Boston, MA: South End Press.

Ani, M. (1994). *Yurugu: An African-centered critique of European cultural thought and behavior.* Trenton, NJ: Africa World Press.

Anonymous (1994, April 25). Florida legislature to pay $2.1 million to victims of 1923 racist massacre in Rosewood. *Jet Magazine*, 12.

Anonymous (1995, January 16). State of Florida to award each Rosewood massacre survivor $100,000 more. *Jet Magazine*, 18.

Anonymous (1997, March 24). "Rosewood" tells story of how white mob destroyed a black town in 1923. *Jet Magazine*, 56-59.

Asante, M.K. (1988). *Afrocentricity.* Trenton, NJ: Africa World Press.

Asante, M.K. (1990). *Kemet, Afrocentricity, and knowledge.* Trenton, NJ: Africa World Press.

Asante, M.K. (1991). The Afrocentric idea in education. *Journal of Negro Education,* 60(2), 170-180.

Asante, M.K. (1992). The painful demise of Eurocentrism. *The World and I,* April, 305-317.

Asante, M.K. (1997). *The Afrocentric idea* (Revised edition). Philadelphia, PA: Temple University Press.

Bailey, R. (1992). The slave(ry) trade and the development of capitalism in the United States: The textile industry in New England. In J.E. Inikori and S.L. Engerman (Eds.), *The Atlantic slave trade: Effects on economies, societies, and peoples of Africa, the Americas, and Europe* (pp. 205-246). Durham, NC: Duke University Press.

Baldwin, J. (1980). The psychology of oppression. In M.K. Asante and A. Vandi (Eds.), *Contemporary black thought: Alternative analyses in social and behavioral science* (pp. 95-110). Beverly Hills, CA: Sage.

Baldwin, J. (1985). Psychological aspects of European cosmology in American society. *The Western Journal of Black Studies,* 9(4), 216-223.

Baldwin, J. and Hopkins, R. (1990). African-American and European-American cultural differences as assessed by the worldviews paradigm: An empirical analysis. *The Western Journal of Black Studies,* 14(1), 38-52.

Baraka, A. (1998). The case for reparations. *Black Collegian,* 29(1), 26-27.

Bauman, Z. (1992). *Intimations of postmodernity.* New York: Routledge.

Bell, D. (1992). *Faces at the bottom of the well.* New York: Basic Books.

Bell, Y.R. (1994). A culturally sensitive analysis of black learning style. *Journal of Black Psychology,* 20(1), 47-61.

Bell, Y.R., Bouie, C.L., and Baldwin, J.A. (1990). Afrocentric cultural consciousness and African-American male-female relationships. *Journal of Black Studies,* 21(2), 162-189.

Bennett, L. (1966). *Before the Mayflower: A history of the Negro in America, 1619-1964.* Chicago, IL: Johnson Publishing Company.

Biebuyck, D. (1964). Land holding and social organization. In M. Herskovits and M. Harwitz (Eds.), *Economic transition in Africa* (pp. 99-112). Evanston, IL: Northwestern University Press.

Blau, J. (1999). *Illusions of prosperity: America's working families in an age of economic insecurity.* New York: Oxford University Press.

Blaut, J.M. (1993). *The colonizer's model of the world.* New York: Guilford Press.

Bowen, W.G. and Bok, D. (1998). *The shape of the river: Long-term consequences of considering race in college and university admissions.* Princeton, NJ: Princeton University Press.

Boykin, W. (1983). The academic performance of Afro-American children. In J. Spence (Ed.), *Achievement and achievement motives* (pp. 324-371). San Francisco, CA: W. Freeman.

Bradley, M. (1991). *The iceman inheritance: Prehistoric sources of western man's racism, sexism, and aggression.* New York: Kayode Publications LTD.

Brisbane, F.L. and Womble, M. (1991). *Working with African Americans: The professional's handbook*. Chicago, IL.: HRDI International Press.

Burgest, D.R. (1981). Theory on white supremacy and black oppression. *Black Books Bulletin*, 7(2), 26-30.

Cabral, A. (1973). *Return to the source*. New York: Monthly Review Press.

Cahn, S.M. (1995). Introduction. In S.M. Cahn (Ed.), *The affirmative action debate* (pp. xi-xii). New York: Routledge.

Chenoweth, K. (1997). A measurement of what? *black Issues in Higher Education*, 14(14), 18-22, 25.

Clarke, J.H. (1991). *Africans at the crossroads: Notes for an African world revolution*. Trenton, NJ: Africa World Press.

Connerly, W. (1996, April 29). Up from affirmative action. *The New York Times*, sec. A, 27.

Cowan, X. (1995). Inverse discrimination. In. S.M. Cahn (Ed.), *The affirmative action debate*. New York: Routledge.

Davis, L.G. (1980). The politics of black self-help in the United States: A historical overview. In L.S. Yearwood (Ed.), *Black organizations* (pp. 37-50). Lanham, MD: University Press of America.

Diop, C.A. (1978). *The cultural unity of black Africa: The domains of patriarchy and of matriarchy in classical antiquity*. Chicago, IL: Third World Press.

Diop, C.A. (1987). *Precolonial black Africa: A comparative study of the political and social systems of Europe and black Africa*. Brooklyn, NY: Lawrence Hill Books.

Dove, N. (1995). An African-centered critique of Marx's logic. *Western Journal of Black Studies*, 19(4), 260-271.

Dubois, W.E.B. (1935). *Black reconstruction in America—1860-1880*. New York: Russell and Russell.

Ehrenreich, J.H. (1985). *The altruistic imagination: A history of social work and social policy in the United States*. Ithaca, NY: Cornell University Press.

Faryna, S., Stetson, B., and Conti, J.G. (Eds.) (1997). *Black and right: The bold new voice of black conservatives in America*. Westport, CT: Praeger.

Feagin, J.R. (1975). *Subordinating the poor*. Englewood Cliffs, NJ: Prentice-Hall, Inc.

Florida House of Representatives (1994). *Special master's final report on Rosewood case*. Tallahassee, FL: State of Florida Printing Office.

Franklin, J.H. (1980). *From slavery to freedom: A history of Negro Americans* (Fifth edition). New York: Alfred A. Knopf.

Franks, G. (1996). *Searching for the promised land: An African American's optimistic odyssey*. New York: Regan Books.

Frazier, E.F. (1927). Is the Negro family a unique sociological unit? *Opportunity*, 5(6), 165-166.

Frazier, E.F. (1939). *The Negro family in the United States*. Chicago, IL: University of Chicago Press.

Gilligan, C. (1989). Woman's place in man's life cycle. In L. Richardson and V. Taylor (Eds.), *Feminist frontiers II: Rethinking sex, gender, and society* (pp. 31-42). New York: McGraw-Hill, Inc.

Gingrich, N. and Connerly, W. (1997, June 15). Face the failure of racial preferences. *The New York Times*, sec. 4, 15.

Glazer, N. (1975). *Affirmative action, ethnic inequality, and public policy.* New York: Columbia University Press.

Gonzalez, V. (1996). Do you believe in intelligence? Sociocultural dimensions of intelligence assessment in majority and minority students. *Educational Horizons*, 75(1), 45-52.

Gould, S.J. (1981). *The mismeasure of man.* New York: W.W. Norton and Company.

Gutman, H.G. (1976). *The black family in slavery and freedom, 1750-1925.* New York: Pantheon Books.

Hacker, A. (1992). *Two nations: Black and white, separate, hostile, unequal.* New York: Charles Scribner's Sons.

Hale-Benson, J. (1982). *Black children: Their roots, culture, and learning styles.* Provo, UT: Brigham Young University Press.

Herrnstein, R.J. and Murray, C. (1994). *The bell curve: Intelligence and class structure in American life.* New York: The Free Press.

Hilliard, A.G. (1987). The ideology of intelligence and IQ magic in education. *The Negro Educational Review,* 38(2/3), 136-145.

Hobson, J.A. (1949). *The evolution of modern capitalism.* New York: Macmilan.

Horkheimer, M. (1972). *Critical theory: Selected essays.* New York: Herder and Herder.

Jansson, B.S. (1997). *The reluctant welfare state: A history of American social welfare policies* (Third edition). Pacific Grove, CA: Brooks/Cole.

Jerome, R. and Sider, D. (1995, January 16). A measure of justice. *People Weekly*, 46-49.

Kadushin, G. and Kulys, R. (1995). Job satisfaction among social work discharge planners. *Health and Social Work*, 20(3), 174-186.

Kambon, K. (1992). *The African personality in America: An African-centered framework.* Tallahassee, FL: Nubian Nation Publication.

Kambon, K. and Hopkins, R., (1993). An African-centered analysis of Penn et al.'s critique of the own-race preference assumption underlying Afrocentric models of personality. *Journal of Black Psychology*, 19(3), 342-349.

Karenga, M. (1986). Social ethics and the black family: An alternative analysis. *The Black Scholar*, 17(5), 41-54.

Karenga, M. (1993). *Introduction to black studies* (Second edition). Los Angeles, CA: University of Sankore Press.

Karenga, M. (1996). The nguzo saba (the seven principles): Their meaning and message. In M.K. Asante and A.S. Abarry (Eds.), *African intellectual heritage* (pp. 543-554). Philadelphia, PA: Temple University Press.

Karger, H.J. and Stoesz, D. (1998). *American social welfare policy: A pluralist approach* (Third edition). New York: Longman.

Keller, D. (1994). The effects of college grade adjustment on the predictive validity and utility of SAT scores. *Research in Higher Education*, 35(2), 195-208.

Kershaw, T. (1992). Afrocentrism and the Afrocentric method. *The Western Journal of Black Studies*, 16(3), 160-168.

Knoop, R. (1995). Influence on participative decision making on job satisfaction and organizational commitment of school principles. *Psychological Reports*, 76(2), 379-382.

Kohl, L.F. (1989). *The politics of individualism: Parties and the American character in the Jacksonian era*. New York: Oxford University Press.

Kunjufu, J. (1985). *Countering the conspiracy to destroy black boys* (Volume 1) Chicago, IL: African American Images.

Kunjufu, J. (1991). *Black economics: Solutions for economic and community empowerment*. Chicago, IL: African American Images.

Leonard, P. (1995). Postmodernism, socialism, and social welfare. *Journal of Progressive Human Services,* 6(2), 3-19.

Linn, R.L. (1990). Admissions testing: Recommended uses, validity, differential prediction, and coaching. *Applied Measurement in Education*, 3(4), 297-318.

Lumumba, C., Obadele, I.M., and Taifa, N. (1993). *Reparations yes! The legal and political reasons why new Afrikans—black people in the United States—should be paid now for the enslavement of our ancestors and for war against us after slavery* (Third edition). Baton Rouge, LA: House of Songhay Commission for Positive Education.

MacKenzie, D. (1981). *Statistics in Great Britain: 1885-1930*. Edinburgh, Scotland: Edinburgh University Press.

Mahubuti, H. (1998, October 6). *Speech given at the Clark Atlanta University 10th annual convocation ceremonies*. Atlanta, GA.

Marcuse, H. (1964). *One dimensional man*. Boston, MA: Beacon Press.

Martin, E.P. and Martin, J.M. (1995). *Social work and the black experience*. Washington, DC: National Association of Social Workers.

Martin, T. (Ed.) (1986). *Message to the people: The course of African philosophy by Marcus Garvey*. Dover, MA: The Majority Press.

McAdoo, H.P. (1997), *Black families* (Third edition). Thousand Oaks, CA: Sage.

McAdoo, H.P. and McAdoo, J.L. (Eds.) (1985). *Black children: Social, educational, and parental environments*. Thousand Oaks, CA: Sage.

McCall, N. (1997). *What's going on: Personal essays*. New York: Random House.

McGregor, D. (1960). *The human side of enterprise*. New York: McGraw-Hill.

Meyer, E.L. (1991, December 9). Demographics shift, much stays the same. *Washington Post*, sec. A, 18.

Mills, C.W. (1959). *The sociological imagination*. New York: Oxford University Press.

Muhammad, E. (1965). *Message to the black man*. Chicago, IL: The Nation of Islam.

Murray, C. (1984). *Losing ground: American social policy, 1950-1980*. New York: Basic Books.

Newman, B.M. and Newman, P.R. (1991). *Development through life: A psycho-social approach*. Pacific Grove, CA: Brooks/Cole.

Nichols, E. (1987, September). *Counseling perspectives for a multi-ethnic and pluralistic work force*. Paper presented at the National Association of Social Workers Annual Conference, New Orleans, LA.

Nkrumah, K. (1970). *Consciencism: Philosophy and ideology for decolonization*. New York: Monthly Review Press.

Nobles, W.W. (1974). Africanity: Its role in black families. *The Black Scholar*, 5(9), 10-17.

Nobles, W.W. (1978). Toward an empirical and theoretical framework for defining black families. *Journal of Marriage and the Family*, 40(4), 679-688.

Novak, M. (1982). *The spirit of democratic capitalism*. New York: Touchstone.

Nyerere, J. (1968). *Ujamaa—Essays on socialism*. London: Oxford University Press.

Ogbu, J.U. (1978). *Minority education and caste: The American system in cross-cultural perspective*. New York: Academic Press.

Ogbu, J.U. (1988). Black education: A cultural-ecological perspective. In H.P. McAdoo (Second edition), *Black families* (pp. 169-184). Thousand Oaks, CA: Sage.

Pinderhughes, E. (1989). *Understanding race, ethnicity and power*. New York: The Free Press.

Piven, F.F. and Cloward, R.A. (1971). *Regulating the poor: The functions of public welfare*. New York: Random House.

Piven, F.F. and Cloward, R. (1982). *The new class war*. New York: Pantheon.

Rashad, A. (1991). *Aspects of Euro-centric thought: Racism, sexism, and imperialism*. Hampton, VA: United Brothers and Sisters Communications Systems.

Robinson, L. (1997, February). Righting a wrong. *Emerge Magazine*, 8(4), 42-49.

Rothenberg, P. (1990). The construction, deconstruction, and reconstruction of difference. *Hypatia*, 5(1), 42-57.

Rubin, A. and Babbie, E. (1993). *Research methods for social work* (Second edition). Pacific Grove, CA: Brooks/Cole.

Schiele, J.H. (1990). Organizational theory from an Afrocentric perspective. *Journal of Black Studies*, 21(2), 145-161.

Schiele, J.H. (1994). Afrocentricity as an alternative world view for equality. *Journal of Progressive Human Services*, 5(1), 5-25.

Schiele, J.H. (1997a). An Afrocentric perspective on social welfare philosophy and policy. *Journal of Sociology and Social Welfare*, 24(2), 21-39.

Schiele, J.H. (1997b). The contour and meaning of Afrocentric social work. *Journal of Black Studies*, 27(6), 800-819.

Schiele, J.H. (1998). Cultural alignment, African American male youths, and violent crime. *Journal of Human Behavior in the Social Environment*, 1(2/3), 165-181.

Schiele, J.H. (in press). Mutations of Eurocentric domination and their implications for African American families. In J. Young and L. Fenwick (Eds.), *Our children, youth, and families: What we must do*. Thousand Oaks, CA.: Sage.

Shujaa, M. (Ed.) (1994). *Too much schooling, too little education.* Lawrenceville, NJ: Africa World Press.

Solomon, B. (1976). *Black empowerment: Social work with oppressed communities.* New York: Columbia University Press.

Sowell, T. (1989, December). Affirmative action: A worldwide disaster. *Commentary,* 88(6).

Stampp, K.M. (1956). *The peculiar institution: Slavery in the ante-bellum south.* New York: Vintage Books.

Staples, R. (1994). *The black family* (Fifth edition). Belmont, CA: Wadsworth.

Starr, P. (1994). *The logic of health care reform: Why and how the president's plan will work.* New York: Penguin Books.

Steele, S. (1990). *The content of our character: A vision of race and reason in America.* New York: St. Martin's Press.

Stuckey, S. (1987). *Slave culture: Nationalist theory and the foundations of black culture.* New York: Oxford University Press.

Thernstrom, S. and Thernstrom, A. (1999). Racial preferences: What we now know. *Commentary,* 107(2), 44-50.

Thomas, A. and Sillen, S. (1972). *Racism and psychiatry.* New York: Brunner/Mazel Publishers.

Trattner, W.I. (1994). *From poor law to welfare state* (Fifth edition). New York: The Free Press.

Turner, J.H., Singleton, R., and Musick, D. (1984). *Oppression: A socio-history of black-white relations in America.* Chicago, IL: Nelson-Hall.

U.S. House of Representatives (1989). *Commission to study reparation proposals for African Americans Act—HR 3745.* Washington, DC: U.S. Government Printing Office.

U.S. House of Representatives, House Committee on Ways and Means (1993). *The green book.* Washington, DC: U.S. Government Printing Office.

Watson, E. (1998). Guess what came to American politics?—Contemporary black conservatism. *Journal of Black Studies,* 29(1), 73-92.

Weber, M. (1958). *The Protestant ethic and the spirit of capitalism.* New York: Charles Scribner.

Williams, C. (1993). *The rebirth of African civilization.* Chicago, IL: Third World Press.

Williams, E. (1944). *Capitalism and slavery.* Chapel Hill, NC: University of North Carolina Press.

Wilson, A.N. (1980). *The developmental psychology of the black child* (Fifth edition). New York: Africana Research Publications.

Wilson, A.N. (1993). *The falsification of Afrikan consciousness: Eurocentric history, psychiatry and the politics of white supremacy.* New York: Afrikan World Infosystems.

Wilson, W.J. (1987). *The truly disadvantaged: The inner city, the underclass, and public policy.* Chicago, IL: University of Chicago Press.

Wilson, W.J. (1996). *When work disappears: The world of the new urban poor.* New York: Knopf.

Woodruff, P. (1995). What's wrong with discrimination? In. S.M. Cahn (Ed.), *The affirmative action debate* (pp. 39-42). New York: Routledge.

Wright, B.E. (1984). *The psychopathic racial personality.* Chicago, IL: Third World Press.

Wyche, L.G. and Novick, M. (1985). Standards for educational and psychological testing: The issue of testing bias from the perspective of school psychology and psychometrics. *Journal of Black Psychology,* 11(2), 43-48.

Young, I.M. (1990). *Justice and the politics of difference.* Princeton, NJ: Princeton University Press.

Chapter 8

Abramovitz, M. (1996). *Regulating the lives of women: Social welfare policy from colonial times to the present* (Revised edition). Boston, MA: South End Press.

Alger, D. (1998). *Megamedia: How giant corporations dominate mass media, distort competition, and endanger democracy.* Lanham, MD: Rowman and Littlefield.

Amy, D.J. (1993). *Real choices/new voices: The case for proportional representation elections in the United States.* New York: Columbia University Press.

Ani, M. (1994). *Yurugu: An African-centered critique of European cultural thought and behavior.* Trenton, NJ: Africa World Press.

Asante, M.K. (1988). *Afrocentricity.* Trenton, NJ: Africa World Press.

Asante, M.K. (1997). *The Afrocentric idea* (Revised edition). Philadelphia, PA: Temple University Press.

Axinn, J. and Levin, H. (1982). *Social welfare: A history of the American response to need* (Second edition). New York: Harper & Row.

Bauman, Z. (1992). *Intimations of postmodernity.* New York: Routledge.

Bennett, L. (1966). *Before the Mayflower: A history of the Negro in America, 1619-1964.* Chicago, IL: Johnson Publishing Company.

Blau, J. (1989). Theories of the welfare state. *Social Service Review,* 63(1), 26-38.

Blau, J. (1994). Can workfare programs bring large numbers of people out of poverty? No. In H.J. Karger and J. Midgley (Eds.), *Controversial issues in social policy* (pp. 244-248). Boston, MA: Allyn and Bacon.

Blau, J. (1999). *Illusions of prosperity: America's working families in an age of economic insecurity.* New York: Oxford University Press.

Bloomfield, M.W. (1976). A brief history of the English language. In W. Morris (Ed.), *The American heritage dictionary of the English language* (pp. xiv-xviii). Boston, MA: Houghton Mifflin Company.

Casse, D. (1997). Why welfare reform is working. *Commentary,* 104(3), 36-42.

Canda, E.R and Chambers, D. (1994). Should spiritual principles guide social policy? Yes. In H.J. Karger and J. Midgley (Eds.), *Controversial issues in social policy* (pp. 63-69). Boston, MA: Allyn and Bacon.

Chapin, R.K. (1995). Social policy development: The strengths perspective. *Social Work,* 40(4), 506-514.

Children's Defense Fund and National Coalition for the Homeless (1998). *Welfare to what? Early findings on family hardship and well-being.* Washington, DC: Children's Defense Fund.

Copeland, V.C. and Wexler, S. (1995). Policy implementation in social welfare: A framework for analysis. *Journal of Sociology and Social Welfare*, 22(3), 51-68.

Day, P.J. (1997). *A new history of social welfare* (Second edition). Boston, MA: Allyn and Bacon.

Dinitto, D.M. (1995). *Social welfare: Politics and public policy* (Fourth edition). Boston, MA: Allyn and Bacon.

Diop, C.A. (1978). *The cultural unity of black Africa: The domains of patriarchy and of matriarchy in classical antiquity.* Chicago, IL: Third World Press.

Dobelstein, A.W. (1996). *Social welfare: Policy and analysis.* Chicago, IL: Nelson-Hall Publishers.

Ehrenreich, J.H. (1985). *The altruistic imagination: A history of social work and social policy in the United States.* Ithaca, NY: Cornell University Press.

Gilbert, N. and Specht, H. (1986). *Dimensions of social welfare policy* (Second edition). Englewood Cliffs, NJ: Prentice-Hall.

Gill, D.G. (1992). *Unraveling social policy* (Fifth edition). Rochester, VT: Schenkman Books.

Guinier, L. (1994). *The tyranny of the majority: Fundamental fairness in representative democracy.* New York: The Free Press.

Gyekye, K. (1992). Person and community in African thought. In K. Wiredu and K. Gyekye (Eds.), *Person and community: Ghanaian philosophical studies, I* (pp. 101-122). Washington, DC: The Council for Research in Values and Philosophy.

Haskins, R. (1999). Welfare reform is working for the poor and taxpayers both. *The American Enterprise*, 10(1), 62-65.

Henderson, E.A. (1995). *Afrocentrism and world politics: Towards a new paradigm.* Westport, CT: Praeger.

Horkheimer, M. (1972). *Critical theory: Selected essays* (English translation). New York: Herder and Herder.

Jagers, R.J. and Owens-Mock, L. (1993). Culture and social outcomes among inner-city African American children: An afrographic exploration. *The Journal of Black Psychology*, 19(4), 391-405.

Jansson, B.S. (1997). *The reluctant welfare state: A history of American social welfare policies* (Third edition). Pacific Grove, CA: Brooks/Cole.

Jhally, S. and Lewis, J. (1992). *Enlightened racism: The Cosby Show, audiences, and the myth of the American dream.* Boulder, CO: Westview Press.

Karenga, M. (1996). The nguzo saba (the seven principles): Their meaning and message. In M.K. Asante and A.S. Abarry (Eds.), *African intellectual heritage* (pp. 543-554). Philadelphia, PA: Temple University Press.

Karger, H.J. (1994). Is privatization a positive trend in social services? No. In H.J. Karger and J. Midgley (Eds.), *Controversial issues in social policy* (pp. 110-116). Boston, MA: Allyn and Bacon.

Karger, H.J. and Stoesz, D. (1993). Retreat and retrenchment: Progressives and the welfare state. *Social Work*, 38(2), 212-220.

Karger, H.J. and Stoesz, D. (1998). *American social welfare policy: A pluralist approach* (Third edition). New York: Longman.

Kellner, D. (1990). *Television and the crisis of democracy.* Boulder, CO: Westview Press.

Kennedy, D. (1982). Legal education as training for hierarchy. In D. Kairys (Ed.), *The politics of law: A progressive critique* (pp. 40-61). New York: Pantheon Books.

Leonard, P. (1995). Postmodernism, socialism, and social welfare. *Journal of Progressive Human Services,* 6(2), 3-19.

Leven-Epstein, J. (1996, November). *Teen parent provisions in the new law.* Washington, DC: Center for Law and Social Policy.

Licht, R.A. (Ed.) (1992). *The framers and fundamental rights.* Washington, DC: The American Enterprise Institute.

Louthan, W.C. (1979). *The politics of justice: A study in law, social science, and public policy.* Port Washington, NY: Kennikat Press.

Lyles, K.L. (1996). Presidential expectations and judicial performance revisited: Law and politics in the federal district courts, 1960-1992. *Presidential Studies Quarterly*, 26(Spring), 447-472.

MacDonald, J.F. (1983). *Blacks and white TV: Afro-Americans in television since 1948.* Chicago, IL: Nelson-Hall Publishers.

MacPherson, C.B. (1962). *The political theory of possessive individualism: Hobbes to Locke.* New York: Oxford University Press.

Marcuse, H. (1964). *One dimensional man.* Boston, MA: Beacon Press.

Montgomery, D.E., Fine, M.A., and Myers, L.J. (1990). The development and validation of an instrument to assess an optimal Afrocentric world view. *Journal of Black Psychology*, 17(1), 37-54.

Morris, A.D. (1984). *The origins of the civil rights movement: Black communities organizing for change.* New York: The Free Press.

Mosse, G.L. (1978). *Toward the final solution: A history of European racism.* New York: Howard Fertig.

Myers, L.J. (1988). *Understanding an Afrocentric world view: Introduction to an optimal psychology.* Dubuque, IA: Kendall/Hunt Publishing Company.

Penna, S. and O'Brien, M. (1996). Postmodernism and social policy: A small step forwards? *Journal of Social Policy*, 25(1), 39-61.

Piven, F.F. and Cloward, R.A. (1971). *Regulating the poor: The functions of public welfare.* New York: Random House.

Piven, F.F. and Cloward, R. (1982). *The new class war.* New York: Pantheon.

Prigmore, C.S. and Atherton, C.R. (1986). *Social welfare policy: Analysis and formulation* (Second edition). Lexington, MA: D.C. Heath and Company.

Quadagno, J. (1994). *The color of welfare: How racism undermined the war on poverty.* New York: Oxford University Press.

Richan, W.C. (1988). *Beyond altruism: Social welfare policy in American society.* Binghamton, New York: The Haworth Press, Inc.

Rose, N. (1989). The political economy of welfare. *Journal of Sociology and Social Welfare*, 16(2), 87-108.

Schiele, J.H. (1997). The contour and meaning of Afrocentric social work. *Journal of Black Studies*, 27(6), 800-819.

Schiele, J.H. (1998). The personal responsibility act of 1996: The bitter and the sweet for African American families. *Families in Society*, 79(4), 424-432.

Seidman, S. (Ed.) (1994). *The postmodern turn: New perspectives on social theory*. New York: Cambridge University Press.

Semmes, C.E. (1993). Religion and the challenge of Afrocentric thought. *The Western Journal of Black Studies*, 17(3), 158-163.

Stefancic, J. and Delgado, R. (1996). *No mercy: How conservative think tanks and foundations changed America's social agenda*. Philadelphia, PA: Temple University Press.

Sullivan, P. (1994). Should spiritual principles guide social policy? No. In H.J. Karger and J. Midgley (Eds.), *Controversial issues in social policy* (pp. 69-74). Boston, MA: Allyn and Bacon.

Titterton, M. (1992). Managing threats to welfare: The search for a new paradigm. *Journal of Social Policy*, 21(1), 1-23.

Trattner, W.I. (1994). *From poor law to welfare state* (Fifth edition). New York: The Free Press.

U.S. Bureau of the Census (1998). *Statistical abstract of the United States, 1998*. Washington, DC: U.S. Government Printing Office.

Watson, D.L. (1990). *Lion in the lobby: The struggle of Clarence Mitchell, Jr., the 101st senator and the passage of civil rights laws*. New York: Morrow.

Weir, M., Orloff, A., and Skocpol, T. (Eds.) (1988). *The politics of social policy in the United States*. Princeton, NJ: Princeton University Press.

Wenocur, S. and Reisch, M. (1989). *From charity to enterprise: The development of American social work in a market economy*. Urbana, IL: University of Illinois Press.

Wice, P. (1992). *Judges and lawyers: The human side of justice*. New York: HarperCollins.

Willhelm, S. (1970). *Who needs the Negro?* Cambridge, MA: Schenkman Press.

Williams, C. (1993). *The rebirth of African civilization*. Chicago, IL: Third World Press.

Yang, C. (1996, December 16). Commentary: Let's stop beating up on legal immigrants. *Business Week*, 82.

Young, I.M. (1990). *Justice and the politics of difference*. Princeton, NJ: Princeton University Press.

Chapter 9

Akbar, N. (1976). Rhythmic patterns in African personality. In L. King, V. Dixon, and W. Nobles (Eds.), *African philosophy: Assumptions and paradigms for research on black people* (pp. 175-189). Los Angeles, CA: Fanon Center Publications.

Akbar, N. (1984). Afrocentric social sciences for human liberation. *Journal of Black Studies*, 14(4), 395-414.

Ani, M. (1994). *Yurugu: An African-centered critique of European cultural thought and behavior*. Trenton, NJ: Africa World Press.

Arvey, R.D. and Faley, R.H. (1988). *Fairness in selecting employees* (Second edition). New York: Addison-Wesley.

Asante, M.K. (1980). International/intercultural relations. In M.K. Asante and A. Vandi (Eds.), *Contemporary black thought* (pp. 43-58). Beverly Hills, CA: Sage.

Asante, M.K. (1988). *Afrocentricity*. Trenton, NJ: Africa World Press.

Asante, M.K. (1990). *Kemet, Afrocentricity, and knowledge*. Trenton, NJ: Africa World Press.

Billingsley, A. and Caldwell, C.H. (1994). The social relevance of the contemporary black church. *National Journal of Sociology*, 8(1/2), 1-23.

Blauner, R. (1972). *Racial oppression in America*. New York: Harper & Row.

Bloom, M., Fischer, J., and Orme, J. (1995). *Evaluating practice: Guidelines for the accountable professional* (Second edition). Boston, MA: Allyn and Bacon.

Brisbane, F.L. and Womble, M. (1991). *Working with African Americans: The professional's handbook*. Chicago, IL: HRDI International Press.

Chazan, N. (1993). Between liberalism and statism: African political cultures and democracy. In L. Diamond (Ed.), *Political culture and democracy in developing countries*, (pp. 67-105). Boulder, CO: Lynne Rienner.

Cook, N. and Kono, S. (1977). Black psychology: The third great tradition. *Journal of Black Psychology*, 3(2), 18-20.

Daly, A. (1982). *The impact of decentralization on organizational effectiveness in an urban county department of social services*. Unpublished doctoral dissertation. Ann Arbor, MI: University of Michigan.

Daly, A. (1994). African American and white managers: A comparison in one agency. *Journal of Community Practice*, 1(1), 57-79.

Eisenberger, R., Fasolo, P., and Davis-LaMastro, V. (1990). Perceived organizational support and employee diligence, commitment, and innovation. *Journal of Applied Psychology*, 75(1), 51-59.

Gyekye, K. (1992). Traditional political ideas: Their relevance to development in contemporary Africa. In K. Wiredu and K. Gyekye (Eds.), *Person and community: Ghanaian philosophical studies, I* (pp. 241-255). Washington, DC: The Council for Research in Values and Philosophy.

Hasenfeld, Y. (1983). *Human service organizations*. Englewood Cliffs, NJ: Prentice-Hall.

Hasenfeld, Y. (Ed.) (1992). *Human service organizations as complex organizations*. Thousand Oaks, CA: Sage.

Hasenfeld, Y. and English, R. (1974). *Human service organizations*. Ann Arbor, MI: University of Michigan Press.

Hunt, D. (1974). The black perspective on public management. *Public Administration Review*, 34(6), 520-525.

Kambon, K. (1992). *The African personality in America: An African-centered framework.* Tallahassee, FL: Nubian Nation Publication.

Kaplan, H. and Tausky, C. (1977). Humanism in organizations: A critical appraisal. *Public Administration Review*, 37(5), 171-180.

Karenga, M. (1993). *Introduction to black studies* (Second edition). Los Angeles, CA: University of Sankore Press.

Kershaw, T. (1992). Afrocentrism and the Afrocentric method. *The Western Journal of Black Studies*, 16(3), 160-168.

Lawrence, P.R. and Lorsch, J.W. (1967). *Organization and environment: Managing differentiation and integration.* Cambridge, MA: Harvard Graduate School of Business Administration.

Lieberson, S. (1980). *A piece of the pie: Blacks and white immigrants since 1880.* Berkeley, CA: University of California Press.

Lincoln, C.E. and Mamiya, L.H. (1990). *The black church in the African American experience.* Durham, NC: Duke University Press.

Lipsky, M. (1980). *Street-level bureaucracy.* New York: Russell Sage Foundation.

Litwak, E. (1978). Organizational constructs and mega bureaucracy. In R.S. Sarri and Y. Hansenfeld (Eds.), *The management of human services* (pp. 123-162). New York: Columbia University Press.

Longres, J.F. (1995). *Human behavior in the social environment* (Second edition). Itasca, IL: F.E. Peacock.

Martin, J.M. and Martin, E.P. (1995). *Social work and the black experience.* Washington, DC: National Association of Social Workers.

Nichols, E. (1987, September). *Counseling perspectives for a multi-ethnic and pluralistic work force.* Paper presented at the National Association of Social Workers Annual Conference, New Orleans, LA.

Nobles, W.W. (1980). African philosophy: Foundations for black psychology. In R. Jones (Ed.) *Black psychology* (Third edition) (pp. 23-35). New York: Harper & Row.

Perrow, C. (1978). Demystifying organizations. In R.S. Sarri and Y. Hasenfeld (Eds.), *The management of human services* (pp. 105-120). New York: Columbia University Press.

Schiele, J.H. (1997). An Afrocentric perspective on social welfare philosophy and policy. *Journal of Sociology and Social Welfare*, 24(2), 21-39.

Scott, R. (1967). The factory as a social service organization: Goal displacement in workshops for the blind. *Social Problems*, 15(2), 160-175.

Selznick, P. (1948). Foundation for the theory of organization. *American Sociological Review*, 13(1), 25-35.

Takaki, R. (1993). *A different mirror: A history of multicultural America.* Boston, MA: Little Brown and Company.

Warfield-Coppock, N. (1995). Toward a theory of Afrocentric organizations. *Journal of Black Psychology*, 21(1), 30-48.

Weber, M. (1946). *From Max Weber: Essays in sociology.* New York: Oxford University Press.

Williams, C. (1987). *The destruction of black civilization: Great issues of a race from 4500 B.C. to 2000 A.D.* Chicago, IL: Third World Press.

Witt, L.A. (1994). *Perceptions of organizational support and affectivity as predictors of job satisfaction.* Washington, DC: Office of Aviation Medicine, Federal Aviation Administration.

Chapter 10

Adorno, T. (1969). Sociology and empirical research. In T. Adorno, H. Albert, R. Dahrendorf, J. Habermas, H. Pilot, and K. Popper (Eds.), *The positivist dispute in German sociology* (G. Adey and D. Frisby, Trans.) (pp. 68-86). New York: HarperTorchbooks.

Akbar, N. (1979). African roots of black personality. In W.D. Smith, H. Kathleen, M.H. Burlew, and W.M. Whitney (Eds.), *Reflections on black psychology,* (pp. 79-87). Washington, DC: University Press of America.

Akbar, N. (1984). Afrocentric social sciences for human liberation. *Journal of Black Studies*, 14(4), 395-414.

Akbar, N. (1991). *Visions for black men.* Nashville, TN: Winston-Derek Publishers, Inc.

Akbar, N. (1994). *Light from ancient Africa.* Tallahassee, FL: Mind Productions and Associates.

Ani, M. (1994). *Yurugu: An African-centered critique of European cultural thought and behavior.* Trenton, NJ: Africa World Press.

Asante, M.K. (1987). *The Afrocentric idea.* Philadelphia, PA: Temple University Press.

Asante, M.K. (1988). *Afrocentricity.* Trenton, NJ: Africa World Press.

Asante, M.K. (1990). *Kemet, Afrocentricity, and knowledge.* Trenton, NJ: Africa World Press.

Astin, H.S. (1984). Academic scholarship and its rewards. In M. Steinkamp and M. Maehr (Eds.). *Advances in motivation and achievement* (Volume 2) (pp. 259-279). Greenwich: Jai Press.

Astin, H.S. and Davis, D.E. (1985). Research productivity across the life and career cycles: Facilitators and barriers for women. In M.F. Fox (Ed.), *Scholarly writing and publishing: Issues, problems, and solutions* (pp. 147-160). Boulder, CO: Westview Press.

Babbie, E. (1986). *Observing ourselves: Essays in social research.* Belmont, CA: Wadsworth Publishing Company.

Baldwin, J. (1981). Notes on an Afrocentric theory of black personality. *The Western Journal of Black Studies,* 5(3), 172-179.

Baldwin, J. (1985). Psychological aspects of European cosmology in American society. *The Western Journal of Black Studies*, 9(4), 216-223.

Baldwin, J. and Hopkins, R. (1990). African-American and European-American cultural differences as assessed by the worldviews paradigm: An empirical analysis. *The Western Journal of Black Studies*, 14(1), 38-52.

Bauman, Z. (1992). *Intimations of postmodernity.* New York: Routledge.

290 HUMAN SERVICES AND THE AFROCENTRIC PARADIGM

Bell, Y.R. (1994). A culturally sensitive analysis of black learning style. *Journal of Black Psychology*, 20(1), 47-61.

Blauner, R. and Wellman, D. (1973). Toward the decolonization of social research. In J. Ladner (Ed.), *The death of white sociology* (pp. 310-330). New York: Vintage Books.

Burgest, D.R. (1981). Theory on white supremacy and black oppression. *Black Books Bulletin*, 7(2), 26-30.

Burgest, D.R. (1982). Worldviews: Implications for social theory and third world people. In D.R. Burgest (Ed.), *Social work practice with minorities* (pp. 45-56). Metuchen, NJ: The Scarecrow Press.

Clarke, J.H. (1991). *Africans at the crossroads: Notes for an African world revolution*. Trenton, NJ: Africa World Press.

Davis, L. (1986). A feminist approach to social work research. *Affilia*, Spring, 2(1) 32-47.

Diop, C.A. (1991). *Civilization or barbarism: An authentic anthropology*. New York: Lawrence Hill Books.

Dixon, V. (1976). World views and research methodology. In L. King, V. Dixon, and W. Nobles (Eds.), *African philosophy: Assumptions and paradigms for research on black persons* (pp. 51-93). Los Angeles, CA: Fanon Center Publications.

Ezeabasili, N. (1977). *African science: Myth or reality?* New York: Vantage Press.

Feyerabend, P. (1981). *Problems of empiricism*. Cambridge, UK: Cambridge University Press.

Foucault, M. (1977). *Power/knowledge*. New York: Pantheon.

Fraser, M.W. (1993, January). *Scholarship in social work: Imperfect methods, approximate truths, and emerging challenges*. Paper presented at the 6th National Symposium on Doctoral Research and Social Work Practice, Ohio State University, College of Social Work, Columbus, OH.

Gadamer, H. (1989). *Truth and method* (Second edition) (J. Weinsheimer and D. Marshall, Trans.). New York: Crossroad.

Geertz, C. (1979). From the native's point of view: On the nature of anthropological understanding. In P. Rabinow and W. Sullivan (Eds.), *Interpretive social science* (pp. 225-242). Berkeley, CA: University of California Press.

Gilgun, J.F. (1994). Hand into glove: The grounded theory approach and social work practice research. In E. Sherman and W. Reid (Eds.), *Qualitative research in social work* (pp. 115-125). New York: Columbia University Press.

Gyekye, K. (1995). An essay on African philosophical thought—The Akan conceptual scheme. In A.G. Mosely (Ed.), *African philosophy: Selected readings* (pp. 339-349). Englewood Cliffs, NJ: Prentice-Hall.

Habermas, J. (1971). *Knowledge and human interests*. Boston, MA: Beacon Press.

Harding, S. (1991). *Whose science? Whose knowledge? Thinking from women's lives*. Ithaca, NY: Cornell University Press.

Harris, N. (1992). A philosophical basis for an Afrocentric orientation. *The Western Journal of Black Studies*, 16(3), 154-159.

Harrison, W.D.(1994). The inevitability of integrated methods. In E. Sherman and W. Reid (Eds.), *Qualitative research in social work* (pp. 409-422). New York: Columbia University Press.

Heineman-Pieper, M. (1981). The obsolete scientific imperative in social work research. *Social Service Review*, 55(3), 371-397.

Heineman-Pieper, M. (1989). The heuristic paradigm: A unifying and comprehensive approach to research. *Smith College Studies in Social Work*, 60(1), 8-34.

Herskovits, M.J. (1941). *The myth of the Negro past.* New York: Harper & Row.

Hill, R.B. (1980). Impediments and opportunities for black research organizations. In L.S. Yearwood (Ed.), *Black organizations: Issues on survival techniques* (pp. 193-196). Lanham, MD: University Press of America.

Holmes, G.E. (1992). Social work research and the empowerment paradigm. In D. Saleebey (Ed.), *The strengths perspective in social work practice* (pp. 158-168). New York: Longman.

Horkheimer, M. and Adorno, M. (1994). *Dialectic of enlightenment* (J. Cumming, Trans.). Originally published in 1944. Reprint, New York: Continuum.

Horton, R. (1993). *Patterns of thought in Africa and the west: Essays on magic, religion and science.* New York: Cambridge University Press.

James, G.G. (1954). *Stolen legacy.* New York: Philosophical Library.

Kambon, K. (1992). *The African personality in America: An African-centered framework.* Tallahassee, FL: Nubian Nation Publication.

Karenga, M. (1989). *Selections from the Husia: Sacred wisdom of ancient Egypt.* Los Angeles, CA: University of Sankore Press.

Kerlinger, F. (1979). *Behavioral research.* New York: Holt, Rinehart and Winston.

Kershaw, T. (1992). Afrocentrism and the Afrocentric method. *The Western Journal of Black Studies*, 16(3), 160-168.

Keto, C.T. (1989). *The African centered perspective of history.* Blackwood, NJ: K.A. Publications.

Long, J.S. and Fox, M.F. (1995). Scientific careers: Universalism and particularism. *Annual Review of Sociology*, 21, 45-71.

Lyotard, J. (1984). *The postmodern condition.* Minneapolis, MN: University of Minnesota Press.

Mannheim, K. (1936). *Ideology and utopia.* (L. Wirth, Trans.) New York: Harvest Books.

Marcuse, H. (1964). *One dimensional man.* Boston, MA: Beacon Press.

Mark, R. (1996). *Research made simple: A handbook for social workers.* Thousand Oaks, CA: Sage.

Martin, J.M. and Martin, E.P. (1985). *The helping tradition in the black family and community.* Silver Spring, MD: National Association of Social Workers.

Mbiti, J. (1970). *African religions and philosophy.* Garden City, NY: Anchor Books.

Mosse, G.L. (1978). *Toward the final solution: A history of European racism.* New York: Howard Fertig.

Myers, L.J. (1988). *Understanding an Afrocentric world view: Introduction to an optimal psychology.* Dubuque, IA: Kendall/Hunt Publishing Company.

Nichols, E. (1987, September). *Counseling perspectives for a multi-ethnic and pluralistic workforce.* Paper presented at the National Association of Social Workers Annual Conference, New Orleans, LA.

Nobles, W.W. (1980). African philosophy: Foundations for black psychology. In R. Jones (Ed.), *Black psychology* (Second edition) (pp. 23-35). New York: Harper & Row.

Popper, K. (1969). The logic of the social sciences. In T. Adorno, H. Albert, R. Dahrendorf, J. Habermas, H. Pilot, and K. Popper (Eds.), *The positivist dispute in German sociology* (G. Adey and D. Frisby, Trans.) (pp. 87-104). New York: HarperTorchbooks.

Popper, K. (1972). *Objective knowledge.* Oxford: Clarendon Press.

Reinharz, S. (1992). *Feminist methods in social research.* New York: Oxford University Press.

Schiele, J.H. (1991). An epistemological perspective on intelligence assessment among African-American children. *Journal of Black Psychology*, 17(2), 23-36.

Schiele, J.H. (1994). Afrocentricity as an alternative world view for equality. *Journal of Progressive Human Services*, 5(1), 5-25.

Schiele, J.H. (1996). Afrocentricity: An emerging paradigm in social work practice. *Social Work*, 41(3), 284-294.

Schiele, J.H. and Francis, E.A. (1996). The status of former CSWE ethnic minority doctoral fellows in social work academia. *Journal of Social Work Education*, 32(1), 31-44.

Seidman, S. (1994). The end of sociological theory. In S. Seidman (Ed.), *The postmodern turn: New perspectives on social theory* (pp. 119-139). New York: Cambridge University Press.

Semmes, C.E. (1981). Foundations of an Afrocentric social science: Implications for curriculum-building, theory, and research in black studies. *Journal of Black Studies*, 12(1), 3-17.

Smith, J.K. (1993). *After the demise of empiricism.* Norwood, NJ: Ablex Publishing Company.

Solomon, B. (1976). *Black empowerment: Social work in oppressed communities.* New York: Columbia University Press.

Sudarkasa, N. (1988). Interpreting the African heritage in Afro-American family organization. In H.P. McAdoo (Ed.), *Black families* (Second edition) (pp. 27-43). Beverly Hills, CA: Sage.

Tucker, R.C. (1978). *The Marx-Engels reader.* New York: W.W. Norton and Company.

Tyson, K. (1995). *New foundations for scientific social and behavioral research: The heuristic paradigm.* Boston, MA: Allyn and Bacon.

Van Sertima, I. (Ed.) (1989). *Nile Valley civilizations.* Atlanta, GA: Morehouse College.

Werner, O. (1994, December). *Four fundamental problems of ethnography and their implication for public policy.* Paper presented at the Ethnographic Research and Urban Policy Problems Conference, Washington, DC.

Williams, C. (1987). *The destruction of black civilization.* Chicago, IL: Third World Press.

Young, I.M. (1990). *Justice and the politics of difference.* Princeton, NJ: Princeton University Press.

Zahan, D. (1979). *The religion, spirituality, and thought of traditional Africa.* Chicago, IL: University of Chicago Press.

Chapter 11

Asante, M.K. (1990). *Kemet, Afrocentricity, and knowledge.* Trenton, NJ: Africa World Press.

Baker, D.R. and Wilson, M.K. (1992). An evaluation of scholarly productivity of doctoral graduates. *Journal of Social Work Education,* 28(2), 204-213.

Bauman, Z. (1992). *Intimations of postmodernity.* New York: Routledge.

Bloom, M., Fischer, J., and Orme, J. (1995). *Evaluating practice: Guidelines for the accountable professional* (Second edition). Boston, MA: Allyn and Bacon.

Burgest, D.R. (1981). Publish or perish: Some major considerations for black educators. *Black Caucus Journal,* 12(1), 13-17.

Cabral, A. (1973). *Return to the source.* New York: Monthly Review Press.

Dove, N. (1995). An African-centered critique of Marx's logic. *Western Journal of Black Studies,* 19(4), 260-271.

Fanon, F. (1961). *Black skin, white masks.* New York: Grove Press.

Finnegan, R. (1970). *Oral literature in Africa.* New York: Oxford University Press.

Foucault, M. (1977). *Power/knowledge.* New York: Pantheon.

Freire, P. (1970). *Pedagogy of the oppressed.* New York: Seabury Press.

Green, R.G., Hutchison, E.D., and Sar, B.K. (1990). *The research productivity of social work doctoral graduates: 1960-1988.* Unpublished manuscript.

Green, R.G., Hutchison, E.D., and Sar, B.K. (1992). Evaluating scholarly performance: The productivity of graduates of social work doctoral programs. *Social Service Review,* 66(3), 441-466.

Gyekye, K. (1987). *An essay on African philosophical thought: The Akan conceptual scheme.* New York: Cambridge University Press.

Harris, L. (1993). Postmodernism and utopia, an unholy alliance. In M. Cross and M. Keith (Eds.), *Racism, the city, and the state* (pp. 31-44). New York: Routledge.

Herbert, J.I. (1998). African American entrepreneurship and work force diversity. In A. Daly (Ed.), *Workplace diversity, issues, and perspectives* (pp. 331-340). Washington, DC: National Association of Social Workers.

Horton, R. (1993). *Patterns of thought in Africa and the west: Essays on magic, religion and science.* New York: Cambridge University Press.

Jansson, B.S. (1997). *The reluctant welfare state: A history of American social welfare policies* (Third edition). Pacific Grove, CA: Brooks/Cole.

Johnson, H.W. and Hull, G.H. (1995). Publication productivity of BSW faculty. *Journal of Social Work Education,* 31(3), 358-368.

Judd, C.M., Smith, E.R., and Kidder, L.H. (1991). *Research methods in social relations* (Sixth edition). Fort Worth, TX: Holt, Rinehart and Winston.

Kambon, K. (1992). *The African personality in America: An African-centered framework*. Tallahassee, FL: Nubian Nation Publication.

Karger, H.J. (1994). Is privatization a positive trend in social services? No. In H.J. Karger and J. Midgley (Eds.), *Controversial issues in social policy* (pp. 110-116). Boston, MA: Allyn and Bacon.

Karger, H.J. and Stoesz, D. (1998). *American social welfare policy: A pluralist approach* (Third edition). New York: Longman.

Kerlinger, F. (1979). *Behavioral research*. New York: Holt, Rinehart and Winston.

Kohl, L.F. (1989). *The politics of individualism: Parties and the American character in the Jacksonian era*. New York: Oxford University Press.

Marcuse, H. (1964). *One dimensional man*. Boston, MA: Beacon Press.

Mbiti, J. (1970). *African religions and philosophy*. Garden City, NY: Anchor Books.

Okpewho, I. (1992). *African oral literature: Backgrounds, character, and continuity*. Bloomington, IN: Indiana University Press.

Quadagno, J. (1994). *The color of welfare: How racism undermined the war on poverty*. New York: Oxford University Press.

Rothenberg, P. (1990). The construction, deconstruction, and reconstruction of difference. *Hypatia*, 5(1), 42-57.

Schiele, J.H. (1991). Publication productivity of African-American social work faculty. *Journal of Social Work Education*, 27(2), 125-134.

Schiele, J.H. (in press). Mutations of Eurocentric domination and their implications for African American families. In J. Young and L. Fenwick (Eds.), *Our children, youth, and families: What we must do*. Thousand Oaks, CA: Sage.

Schiele, J.H. and Francis, E.A. (1996). The status of former CSWE ethnic minority doctoral fellows in social work academia. *Journal of Social Work Education*, 32(1), 31-44.

Seidman, S. (1994). The end of sociological theory. In S. Seidman (Ed.), *The postmodern turn: New perspectives on social theory* (pp. 119-139). New York: Cambridge University Press.

Smith, J.K. (1993). *After the demise of empiricism*. Norwood, NJ: Ablex Publishing Company.

Stoesz, D. (1994). Is privatization a positive trend in social services? Yes. In H.J. Karger and J. Midgley (Ed.), *Controversial issues in social policy* (pp. 108-110). Boston, MA: Allyn and Bacon.

Tyson, K. (1995). *New foundations for scientific social and behavioral research: The heuristic paradigm*. Boston, MA: Allyn and Bacon.

U.S. Bureau of the Census (1998). *Statistical abstract of the United States, 1998*. Washington, DC: U.S. Government Printing Office.

Walker, W.T. (1995). *Somebody's calling my name*. New York: Judson Press.

Williams, C. (1987). *The destruction of black civilization*. Chicago, IL: Third World Press.

Wilson, A.N. (1993). *The falsification of Afrikan consciousness: Eurocentric history, psychiatry and the politics of white supremacy*. New York: Afrikan World Infosystems.

Index

9780789005663